Clinical Manual of
Alzheimer Disease and
Other Dementias

Clinical Manual of
Alzheimer Disease and
Other Dementias

Edited by

Myron F. Weiner, M.D.

Clinical Professor of Psychiatry and
Neurology and Neurotherapeutics
Aradine S. Ard Chair in Brain Science
Dorothy L. and John P. Harbin Chair in Alzheimer's Disease Research
University of Texas Southwestern Medical Center at Dallas, Texas

Anne M. Lipton, M.D., Ph.D.

Diplomate in Neurology
American Board of Psychiatry and Neurology

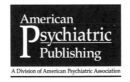

American
Psychiatric
Publishing
A Division of American Psychiatric Association

Washington, DC
London, England

If you would like to buy between 25 and 99 copies of this or any other American Psychiatric Publishing title, you are eligible for a 20% discount; please contact Customer Service at appi@psych.org or 800-368-5777. If you wish to buy 100 or more copies of the same title, please e-mail us at bulksales@psych.org for a price quote.

Copyright © 2012 American Psychiatric Association
ALL RIGHTS RESERVED

Manufactured in the United States of America on acid-free paper
15 14 13 12 11   5 4 3 2 1
First Edition

Typeset in Adobe's AGaramond and Formata.

American Psychiatric Publishing
1000 Wilson Boulevard
Arlington, VA 22209-3901
www.appi.org

Library of Congress Cataloging-in-Publication Data
Clinical manual of Alzheimer disease and other dementias / edited by Myron F. Weiner, Anne M. Lipton. — 1st ed.
    p. ; cm.
    Includes bibliographical references and index.
    ISBN 978-1-58562-422-5 (pbk. : alk. paper)
    I. Weiner, Myron F., 1934– II. Lipton, Anne M., 1966– III. American Psychiatric Association.
    [DNLM: 1. Alzheimer Disease. 2. Dementia. WT 155]
    616.8'31–dc23   2011042750

British Library Cataloguing in Publication Data
A CIP record is available from the British Library.

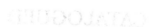

To Doris Svetlik
for her selfless devotion to the clinical care
of patients with dementia

and

Marsha Ard and John Harbin
for their support of Dr. Weiner's research on the treatment
and management of Alzheimer disease and related illnesses

Contents

7 Vascular Cognitive Disorder. 171

Cassandra E. I. Szoeke, Ph.D., F.R.A.C.P., M.B.B.S.,
B.Sc. (Hons.)
Stephen Campbell, F.R.A.C.P., M.Ch.B.S., B.Sc.
Edmond Chiu, A.M., M.B.B.S., D.P.M., F.R.A.N.Z.C.P.
David Ames, B.A., M.D., F.R.C.Psych., F.R.A.N.Z.C.P.

8 Dementia With Lewy Bodies and Other Synucleinopathies 193

Rawan Tarawneh, M.D.
James E. Galvin, M.D., M.Sc.

List of Tables

List of Figures

Contributors

David Ames, B.A., M.D., F.R.C.Psych., F.R.A.N.Z.C.P.
University of Melbourne Professor of Ageing and Health; Director, National Ageing Research Institute, Royal Melbourne Hospital, Melbourne, Victoria, Australia

Erin D. Bigler, Ph.D.
Professor, Department of Psychology and Neuroscience Center, Brigham Young University, Provo, Utah

Malaz Boustani, M.D., M.P.H.
Assistant Professor, Department of Medicine, Indiana University School of Medicine, Indianapolis, Indiana

Adam Boxer, M.D., Ph.D.
Vera and George Graziadio Chair in Alzheimer's Disease Research; Director, Alzheimer's Disease and Frontotemporal Dementia Clinical Trials Program; and Assistant Professor, Department of Neurology, University of California, San Francisco, San Francisco, California

Mary F. Bret, M.D.
Associate Professor, Department of Psychiatry, University of Texas Southwestern Medical Center, Dallas, Texas

Stephen Campbell, F.R.A.C.P., M.Ch.B.S., B.Sc.
Geriatrician, Department of Aged Care, Austin and Repatriation Hospital, Melbourne, Victoria, Australia

Edmond Chiu, A.M., M.B.B.S., D.P.M., F.R.A.N.Z.C.P.
Professorial Fellow, Academic Unit for Psychiatry of Old Age, University of Melbourne, Melbourne; Department of Psychiatry, Normanby House, St George's Hospital, Kew, Victoria, Australia

C. Munro Cullum, Ph.D., A.B.P.P.
Professor, Departments of Psychiatry and Neurology, University of Texas Southwestern Medical Center, Dallas, Texas

Martin R. Farlow, M.D.
Professor, Department of Neurology, Indiana University School of Medicine, Indianapolis, Indiana

Norman L. Foster, M.D.
Professor, Department of Neurology; Director, Center for Alzheimer's Care, Imaging and Research; Senior Investigator, The Brain Institute, University of Utah, Salt Lake City, Utah

James E. Galvin, M.D., M.Sc.
Clinical Professor of Neurology and Psychiatry and Clinical Director, Pearl Barlow Center for Memory Evaluation and Treatment, NYU Langone Medical Center, New York, New York

Robert Garrett, M.D.
Assistant Professor, Department of Psychiatry, University of Texas Southwestern Medical Center, Dallas, Texas

Yonas E. Geda, M.D, M.Sc.
Associate Professor of Neurology and Psychiatry, Department Vice Chair and Research Committee Chair, Psychiatry and Psychology; and Consultant, Division of Epidemiology, Department of Health Sciences Research, College of Medicine, Mayo Clinic, Rochester, Minnesota

David S. Geldmacher, M.D.
Charles and Patsy Collat Endowed Professor of Neurology and Director, Division of Memory Disorders and Behavioral Neurology, Department of Neurology, University of Alabama at Birmingham, Birmingham, Alabama

Laura H. Lacritz, Ph.D., A.B.P.P.
Associate Professor, Department of Psychiatry, University of Texas Southwestern Medical Center, Dallas, Texas

Anne M. Lipton, M.D., Ph.D.
Diplomate in Neurology, American Board of Psychiatry and Neurology

Constantine G. Lyketsos, M.D., M.H.S.
Professor, Department of Psychiatry, The Johns Hopkins Bayview Medical Center, Baltimore, Maryland

Kristin Martin-Cook, M.S., C.C.R.C.
Family Services Coordinator, Memory Research Unit, Department of Neurology, University of Texas Southwestern Medical Center, Dallas, Texas

Ronald C. Petersen, Ph.D., M.D.
Professor of Neurology, Cora Kanow Professor of Alzheimer's Disease Research, Department of Neurology, College of Medicine, Mayo Clinic, Rochester, Minnesota

Mary Quiceno, M.D.
Assistant Professor, Department of Neurology and Neurotherapeutics, University of Texas Southwestern Medical Center, Dallas, Texas

Danielle F. Richards
Banner Alzheimer's Institute, Tucson, Arizona

Craig D. Rubin, M.D.
Professor, Department of Medicine, University of Texas Southwestern Medical Center, Dallas, Texas

Martin Steinberg, M.D.
Assistant Professor, Department of Psychiatry, Johns Hopkins University School of Medicine, Baltimore, Maryland

Cassandra E.I. Szoeke, Ph.D., F.R.A.C.P., M.B.B.S., B.Sc. (Hons.)
Neurologist, Departments of Psychiatry and Neurology, University of Melbourne, Melbourne, Victoria, Australia

Rawan Tarawneh, M.D.
Department of Neurology, Washington University School of Medicine, St. Louis, Missouri

Pierre N. Tariot, M.D.
Research Professor of Psychiatry, University of Arizona College of Medicine; Director, Memory Disorders Center, Banner Alzheimer's Institute, Phoenix, Arizona

Myron F. Weiner, M.D.
Clinical Professor of Psychiatry and Neurology and Neurotherapeutics, Aradine S. Ard Chair in Brain Science, and Dorothy L. and John P. Harbin Chair in Alzheimer's Disease Research, University of Texas Southwestern Medical Center at Dallas, Dallas, Texas

Roy Yaari, M.D., M.A.S.
Associate Director, Memory Disorders Clinic, Banner Alzheimer's Institute, Phoenix, Arizona

Edward Y. Zamrini, M.D.
Professor of Neurology and Director of Clinical Trials, Center for Alzheimer's Care, Imaging and Research, University of Utah, Salt Lake City, Utah

Disclosure of Competing Interests

The following contributors to this book have indicated a financial interest in or other affiliation with a commercial supporter, a manufacturer of a commercial product, a provider of a commercial service, a nongovernmental organization, and/ or a government agency, as listed below:

Erin D. Bigler, Ph.D.—The author codirects the Neuropsychological Research and Assessment Clinic, which is part of the clinical psychology Ph.D. program. While most of this is training-oriented for a university-sponsored no-cost neuropsychology service to the community, some fee for service does occur, including dementia and competency evaluations. On occasion, this will require medicolegal expert testimony, especially for the individual with an acquired dementia. The author's research is supported by a National Institute of Mental Health grant (R01 MH1084795) and a National Institutes of Health grant (R01 HD048946-01 AZ).

Adam Boxer, M.D., Ph.D.—*Research funding:* Allon Therapeutics, Avid, Élan, Forest, Genentech, Janssen, Medivation, Pfizer; *Grants:* National Institutes of Health (R01 AG038791 [PI], R01 AG031278 [PI]), Alzheimer's Drug Discovery Foundation, CurePSP, Hellman Family Foundation, Tau Research Consortium; *Consultant:* Bristol-Myers Squibb, Genentech, Phloronol, Registrat-Mapi, and TauRx

Edmond Chiu, A.M., M.B.B.S., D.P.M., F.R.A.N.Z.C.P.—*Speaker honoraria:* Eisai, Pfizer, Servier

Martin R. Farlow, M.D.—*Research funding:* Bristol-Myers Squibb, Danone Research, Élan Pharmaceuticals, Eli Lilly, Genentech, Novartis Pharmaceuticals, OctaPharma, Pfizer, Sanofi-Aventis, Sonexa Therapeutics; *Consultant:* Accera, Astellas Pharma U.S., Baxter Healthcare, Bayer Pharmaceuticals, Bristol-Myers Squibb, DDB Remedy, Eisai Medical Research, GE Healthcare, Helicon, Medavante, Medivation, Merck, Novartis Pharmaceuticals, Pfizer, Prana Biotechnology, QR Pharma, Sanofi-Aventis Group, Toyama Chemical; *Speaker:* Eisai Medical Research, Forest, Pfizer, Novartis Pharmaceuticals; *Ownership:* Partial ownership of Chemigen, Inc.

Norman L. Foster, M.D.—*Consultant:* GE Healthcare; *Other:* serves on a Diagnostic Adjudication Committee for Bristol-Myers Squibb, and is an investigator in clinicaltrials currently funded by Pfizer, Inc. In the past 36 months, the author has served on scientific advisory boards for Wyeth/Élan Pharmaceuticals and Janssen Alzheimer Immunotherapy, and has been an investigator in clinical trials funded by Janssen Alzheimer Immunotherapy, Eli Lilly, Baxter Bioscience, Merck, Myriad Genetics, and Eisai.

David S. Geldmacher, M.D.—*Research support (contracted through the University of Virginia):* Eisai, Élan, Janssen Alzheimer Immunotherapy, Medivation, Novartis, Pfizer; *Consultant:* GlaxoSmithKline

Anne M. Lipton, M.D., Ph.D.—*Research grant:* Novartis Pharmaceuticals; *Consultant:* Axona; *Speaker's bureau honoraria:* Forest Pharmaceuticals

Constantine G. Lyketsos, M.D., M.H.S.—*Grant support (research or CME):* Associated Jewish Federation of Baltimore, AstraZeneca, Bristol-Myers, Eisai, Élan, Eli Lilly, Forest, GlaxoSmithKline, National Football League (NFL), National Institute on Aging; National Institute of Mental Health, Novartis, Ortho-McNeil, Pfizer, Weinberg Foundation; *Consultant/advisor:* Adlyfe, AstraZeneca, Eisai, Élan, Eli Lilly, Forest, Genentech, GlaxoSmithKline, Lundbeck, Merz, NFL Players Association, NFL Benefits Office; Novartis, Pfizer, Supernus, Takeda, Wyeth; *Honorarium or travel support:* Forest, GlaxoSmithKline, Health Monitor, Pfizer

Mary Quiceno, M.D.—*Advisory panel payment:* Accera

Cassandra E. I. Szoeke, Ph.D., F.R.A.C.P., M.B.B.S., B.Sc. (Hons.)—The author may accrue revenue on pending patent (filed 2003): diagnostic assay for seizure prediction. She has held consultancy and speaker roles for Pfizer, Sanofi-Aventis, Mayne Pharma, Merck, and Lundbeck. She is a clinical consultant to the Australian Commonwealth Science Research and Industry Organisation.

Pierre N. Tariot, M.D.—*Research support:* Abbott Laboratories, AstraZeneca, Avid, Baxter Healthcare, Bristol-Myers Squibb, Élan, Eli Lilly, GE, Genentech, GlaxoSmithKline, Medivation, Merck, Pfizer, Toyama, Wyeth Laboratories; *Other research support:* Alzheimer's Association, Arizona Department of Health Services, Institute for Mental Health Research, National Institute on Aging, National Institute of Mental Health; *Consultant:* Abbott Laboratories, Acadia, AC Immune, Allergan, AstraZeneca, Avid, Baxter Healthcare, Bristol-Myers Squibb, Eisai, Élan, Eli Lilly, Epix Pharmaceuticals, Forest Laboratories, Genentech, GlaxoSmithKline, Medavante, Medivation, Merck, Novartis, Pfizer, Sanofi-Aventis, Schering-Plough, Toyama, Worldwide Clinical Trials; Wyeth Laboratories; *Investments (stock options):* Adamas, Medavante; *Patents:* author is listed as contributor to a patent, "Biomarkers of Alzheimer's Disease"

Myron F. Weiner, M.D.—Bristol-Myers Squibb, Novartis

Roy Yaari, M.D., M.A.S.—*Research support:* Abbott Laboratories, AstraZeneca, Avid, Baxter Healthcare, Bristol-Myers Squibb, Élan, Eli Lilly, GlaxoSmithKline, Medivation, Merck, Pfizer, Toyama, Wyeth Laboratories

The following contributors to this book indicated that they have no competing interests or affiliations to declare:

David Ames, B.A., M.D., F.R.C.Psych., F.R.A.N.Z.C.P.
Malaz Boustani, M.D., M.P.H.
C. Munro Cullum, Ph.D., A.B.P.P.
James E. Galvin, M.D., M.Sc.
Robert Garrett, M.D.
Yonas E. Geda, M.D, M.Sc.
Laura H. Lacritz, Ph.D., A.B.P.P.
Kristin Martin-Cook, M.S., C.C.R.C.
Ronald C. Petersen, Ph.D., M.D.
Danielle F. Richards
Craig D. Rubin, M.D.
Martin Steinberg, M.D.
Rawan Tarawneh, M.D.
Edward Y. Zamrini, M.D.

Introduction

Dementia is a threshold diagnosis based on level of function; however, the clinical presentation of dementia may point to the underlying disease or pathophysiological process. We speak of persons as suffering from dementia when, as a result of impaired cognition, they have significant impairment of social or occupational functioning that is a decline from a previous level of function. It is clear, in the case of neurodegenerative diseases, that the underlying processes may not initially be functionally symptomatic and that there may be symptoms and biological factors that increase the certainty of evolution to a dementia syndrome. Since the preparation of this volume, new criteria have been proposed for Alzheimer disease, including criteria for preclinical Alzheimer disease (Sperling et al. 2011), mild cognitive impairment due to Alzheimer disease (Albert et al. 2011), and dementia due to Alzheimer disease (McKhann et al. 2011). Although these criteria will not have immediate impact on clinical practice, they will aid in early detection and diagnostic certainty, and will facilitate clinical and basic science research.

Although subsumed under the DSM-IV-TR category of cognitive disorders (American Psychiatric Association 2000), the conditions leading to dementia clearly have broader effects than on cognition alone, including on psychosis, mood disorder, and various disturbed and disturbing behaviors. We hope that we may eventually become able to arrest dementia-producing disorders before they reach the level of dementia. This means that clinicians need to increase their sensitivity to those persons at high risk or in the early stage of potentially dementing illnesses, as has happened, for example, with syphilis. The widespread use of antibiotics in developed countries has almost eliminated neurosyphilis, one of the major causes of long-term institutionalization in years past. A disease such as syphilis differs in important ways from a disease like Alzheimer disease. Syphilis may be thought of as a single genotype or agent with many phenotypes or clinical manifestations as the disease progresses (e.g., chancre, generalized skin rash, meningoencephalitis, gumma), and one type of treatment is effective in arresting all stages of the disease. By contrast, a disease such as Alzheimer disease is a single pathological phenotype (neuritic plaques, neurofibrillary tangles, loss of synapses), but it is likely to have many genotypes. As with atherosclerosis, there may be many contributing factors to a final common pathway, and multiple factors may need to be addressed to treat or arrest the disease. There may not be a silver bullet for Alzheimer disease.

This manual is a bare-bones distillation and update of the material contained in *The American Psychiatric Publishing Textbook of Alzheimer Disease and Other Dementias* (Weiner and Lipton 2009). It is meant to serve busy clinicians as a practical tool. For these reasons, 11 of the original 26 chapters have been deleted and others condensed or combined to address the immediate needs of clinicians. For example, the former chapter on biomarkers has been subsumed into the chapter on medical evaluation. On the other hand, the neuropsychiatric examination is still presented separately from the medical evaluation to emphasize the tools most readily available to the psychiatrist, which are eliciting the history and performing a mental status examination. Psychiatrists should be comfortable ordering appropriate laboratory and imaging studies but may sometimes have to turn to their internal medicine or neurological colleagues for additional evaluation or interpretation. Psychiatrists' special skills are in managing emotional and behavioral symptoms, assisting patients and their families, and, finally, contributing to the management of dementia patients in long-term-care facilities. Psychiatrists can play a vital part in helping family members adapt to their roles as caregivers, maintaining patients in the family setting, and bridging the gap between home care and long-term institutional care.

Part I of this book is devoted to assessment and diagnosis. Drug treatment is addressed in the first three chapters of Part II. The first two address behavioral issues. One chapter reviews treatment of psychiatric syndromes in dementia patients, and the second covers symptom-related treatments and general psychopharmacology. The third in the series deals with medications to improve or maintain cognitive and other functions in Alzheimer disease and supporting family caregivers.

Those readers interested in a broader view of the dementia syndrome, including its history, epidemiology, and future treatment, can find this material in *The American Psychiatric Publishing Textbook of Alzheimer Disease and Other Dementias* (Weiner and Lipton 2009). That text also includes discussions of legal and ethical issues.

Acknowledgments

Thanks to Dr. Bob Hales and Mr. John McDuffie of American Psychiatric Publishing for extending the invitation to create this manual and to Ms. Bessie Jones for helping to keep us in touch. Dr. Matthew Warren went over the manuscript word by word, making valuable suggestions for clarifying the text. Mr. Jed Falkowski assumed the responsibility for checking the reference section of each chapter against the text and physically assembling the final manuscript and digital files for submission. Ms. Barbara Davis updated the Resources section.

We thank the chapter authors for once more working with us to produce this clinical manual. On the home front, we thank Jeanette Weiner for her tolerance and Lee Lipton for his support in the course of a move to Ireland.

Myron F. Weiner, M.D.

Anne M. Lipton, M.D., Ph.D.

References

Albert MS, DeKosky ST, Dickson D, et al: The diagnosis of mild cognitive impairment due to Alzheimer's disease: recommendations from the National Institute on Aging–Alzheimer's Association workgroups on diagnostic guidelines for Alzheimer's disease. Alzheimers Dement 7:270–279, 2011 [Epub 2011 Apr 21]

American Psychiatric Association: Diagnostic and Statistical Manual of Mental Disorders, 4th Edition, Text Revision. Washington, DC, American Psychiatric Association, 2000

McKhann GM, Knopman DS, Chertkow H, et al: The diagnosis of dementia due to Alzheimer's disease: recommendations from the National Institute on Aging–Alzheimer's Association workgroups on diagnostic guidelines for Alzheimer's disease. Alzheimers Dement 7:263–269, 2011 [Epub 2011 Apr 21]

Sperling RA, Aisen PS, Beckett LA, et al: Toward defining the preclinical stages of Alzheimer's disease: recommendations from the National Institute on Aging–Alzheimer's Association workgroups on diagnostic guidelines for Alzheimer's disease. Alzheimer's Dement 7:280–292, 2011 [Epub 2011 Apr 21]

Weiner MF, Lipton AM: The American Psychiatric Publishing Textbook of Alzheimer's Disease and Other Dementias. Washington, DC, American Psychiatric Publishing, 2009

PART I

Assessment and Diagnosis

1

Neuropsychiatric Assessment and Diagnosis

Myron F. Weiner, M.D.

Robert Garrett, M.D.

Mary E. Bret, M.D.

Cognitive dysfunction manifests in many ways, including memory slips, inappropriate social behavior, suspiciousness, perceptual distortions, poor hygiene, and hoarding. Mild levels of cognitive inefficiency are part of the average aging process, but more severe impairment in cognitive spheres such as memory, language, and judgment often herald the onset of a dementing disorder.

In this chapter, we review the DSM-IV-TR cognitive disorders (American Psychiatric Association 2000), other cognitive syndromes, and other psychiatric disorders that may confound the diagnosis of cognitive disorders. This material anticipates Chapter 2, which involves detecting the illnesses or conditions underlying DSM-IV-TR syndromes, and also Chapter 12, which deals with psychiatric disorders in persons with dementia.

DSM-IV-TR Cognitive Disorders

DSM-IV-TR diagnoses are symptom clusters that meet a threshold of "clinically significant distress or impairment in social, occupational, or other important areas of functioning" (American Psychiatric Association 2000, p. 8). Thus, many persons with early dementing diseases do not meet the criteria for dementia. Increasingly, the goal for diagnosis of cognitive disorders has become early detection. For this reason, clinicians are now more likely to diagnose Alzheimer disease before patients meet full DSM-IV-TR criteria for dementia of the Alzheimer's type. In addition, many disorders that lead to dementia do not meet the DSM impaired memory criterion. For example, persons with frontotemporal dementias may present first with deficits in language, executive function, or judgment. Furthermore, despite the definition of dementia as a cognitive disorder, behavioral and emotional symptoms are intrinsic to the diseases underlying the cognitive disorders.

DSM-IV (American Psychiatric Association 1994) replaced the earlier DSM diagnostic category of organic mental disorders with that of cognitive disorders (this classification was retained in DSM-IV-TR; see Table 1–1).

The cognitive disorders are overlapping symptom complexes that often manifest in the course of the same underlying disease. For example, an evolving Pick disease might be diagnosed first as a personality change due to a general medical condition. As executive function and information processing become more impaired, the disorder would become diagnosable as a dementia. Often, several disorders affecting mental function coexist. Persons with cognitive impairment often become delirious, and major depression may coexist with dementia. Persons with Down syndrome often develop Alzheimer disease. Also, a dementing illness may complicate schizophrenia or bipolar disorder.

Normal Cognitive Aging

Differentiating normal aging from pathological cognitive decline is an issue for many persons and is of paramount significance for early intervention. Research in normal aging is complicated by the paucity of longitudinal studies. The most common studies compare different age groups, but they are confounded by cohort effects. Another confound in comparative studies is the influence of diseases such as hypertension and diabetes on cognition. Controlled

Table 1–1. DSM-IV-TR classification of delirium, dementia, and amnestic and other cognitive disorders; and mental disorders due to a general medical condition not elsewhere classified

Delirium, Dementia, and Amnestic and Other Cognitive Disorders

DELIRIUM
293.0   Delirium Due to . . . *[Indicate the General Medical Condition]*
——.   Substance Intoxication Delirium *(refer to Substance-Related Disorders for substance-specific codes)*
——.–   Substance Withdrawal Delirium *(refer to Substance-Related Disorders for substance-specific codes)*
——.–   Delirium Due to Multiple Etiologies *(code each of the specific etiologies)*
780.09 Delirium NOS

DEMENTIA
294.xx Dementia of the Alzheimer's Type, With Early Onset *(also code 331.0 Alzheimer's disease on Axis III)*
   .10   Without Behavioral Disturbance
   .11   With Behavioral Disturbance
294.xx Dementia of the Alzheimer's Type, With Late Onset *(also code 331.0 Alzheimer's disease on Axis III)*
   .10   Without Behavioral Disturbance
   .11   With Behavioral Disturbance
290.xx Vascular Dementia
   .40   Uncomplicated
   .41   With Delirium
   .42   With Delusions
   .43   With Depressed Mood
         Specify if: With Behavioral Disturbance
Code presence or absence of a behavioral disturbance in the fifth digit for Dementia Due to a General Medical Condition:
   0 = Without Behavioral Disturbance
   1 = With Behavioral Disturbance
294.1x Dementia Due to HIV Disease *(also code 042 HIV on Axis III)*
294.1x Dementia Due to Head Trauma *(also code 854.00 head injury on Axis III)*
294.1x Dementia Due to Parkinson's Disease *(also code 331.82 Dementia with Lewy bodies on Axis III)*
294.1x Dementia Due to Huntington's Disease *(also code 333.4 Huntington's disease on Axis III)*

Table 1–1.   DSM-IV-TR classification of delirium, dementia, and amnestic and other cognitive disorders; and mental disorders due to a general medical condition not elsewhere classified *(continued)*

DEMENTIA *(continued)*
294.1x Dementia Due to Pick's Disease *(also code 331.11 Pick's disease on Axis III)*
294.1x Dementia Due to Creutzfeldt-Jakob Disease *(also code 046.1 Creutzfeldt-Jakob disease on Axis III)*
294.1x Dementia Due to . . . *[Indicate the General Medical Condition not listed above] (also code the general medical condition on Axis III)*
——.— Substance-Induced Persisting Dementia *(refer to Substance-Related Disorders for substance-specific codes)*
——.— Dementia Due to Multiple Etiologies *(code each of the specific etiologies)*
294.8 Dementia NOS

AMNESTIC DISORDERS
294.0 Amnestic Disorder Due to . . . *[Indicate the General Medical Condition]*
       Specify if: Transient/Chronic
——.– Substance-Induced Persisting Amnestic Disorder
       (refer to Substance-Related Disorders for substance-specific codes)
294.8 Amnestic Disorder NOS

OTHER COGNITIVE DISORDERS
294.9 Cognitive Disorder NOS

**Mental Disorders Due to a General Medical Condition
Not Elsewhere Classified**
293.89 Catatonic Disorder Due to . . . *[Indicate the General Medical Condition]*
293.9 Mental Disorder NOS Due to . . . *[Indicate the General Medical Condition]*
310.1 Personality Change Due to . . . *[Indicate the General Medical Condition]*
       Specify type: Labile Type/Disinhibited Type/
       Aggressive Type/Apathetic Type/Paranoid Type/
       Other Type/Combined Type/Unspecified Type

Source.   Reprinted from American Psychiatric Association: *Diagnostic and Statistical Manual of Mental Disorders,* 4th Edition, Text Revision. Washington, DC, American Psychiatric Association, 2000. Copyright 2000, American Psychiatric Association. Used with permission.

studies that exclude persons with such conditions find less difference between younger adults and elders. In one such study, healthy adults ranging in age from 50 to 82 years learned word lists as well as younger adults did (Gunstad et al. 2006). Nevertheless, although vocabulary and general knowledge remain stable with aging, speed of information processing and psychomotor performance decline.

Memory

Impaired memory becomes more prevalent with aging. In a survey of memory function performed among community-dwelling elderly persons in the United States, 4% of individuals between ages 65 and 69 years and 36% of persons age 85 years or older had moderate to severe memory problems (Federal Interagency Forum on Aging-Related Statistics 2000). Most elders report forgetting names frequently, losing objects such as keys, and forgetting telephone numbers. Older adults recall as well as younger adults the gist of material they have learned but recall details less well. Because they rely on their general knowledge to supplement their memory, older adults are also more prone to errors in recall.

The current conceptualization of memory includes conscious and unconscious memory (Figure 1–1). *Conscious (explicit, declarative) memory* includes recall of people, places, objects, facts, and events. It includes episodic memory, semantic memory, and working memory. *Episodic memory* deals with time-associated memories stored for minutes to years (e.g., what a person did yesterday). *Semantic memory* involves facts, such as the color of an orange, learned over periods of time ranging from minutes to years. *Working memory* is the ability to manipulate over seconds to minutes information that may not be stored, such as retaining a new telephone number before dialing. *Unconscious (implicit, procedural) memory* deals with sequences of events involving the motor system (e.g., skills such as riding a bicycle) that do not require conscious recall. It also includes classical conditioning, habits, habituation (desensitization), and priming (the increased ability to recognize stimuli based on recent experience with them).

Through rehearsal, conscious memory of the steps in performing complex tasks can become unconscious. The various memory functions appear to involve different mechanisms and different brain circuitry (reviewed in Budson and Price 2005). Short-term memory is achieved by neurotransmitter-

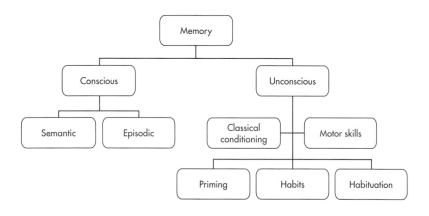

Figure 1–1.   Structure of memory.

Source.   Reprinted from Weiner MF, Garrett R, Bret ME: "Neuropsychiatric Assessment and Diagnosis," in *The American Psychiatric Publishing Textbook of Alzheimer Disease and Other Dementias.* Edited by Weiner MF, Lipton AM. Washington, DC, American Psychiatric Publishing, 2009, pp. 39–70. Copyright 2009, American Psychiatric Publishing. Used with permission.

induced long-term potentiation that strengthens synaptic connections. It can be disrupted by blocking the action of acetylcholine. The long-term storage of memories involves the outgrowth of new axon terminals and the development of new synapses. This process can be blocked by protein synthesis inhibitors.

The prefrontal cortex appears to be the site of working memory. The hippocampus transfers memory from short-term to long-term storage, and the portions of the cortex that originally processed the information are the sites of long-term storage of explicit memory (Squire 1992). The corpus striatum and cerebellum form part of the circuitry for procedural memory (Wenk 1999).

Little change occurs in working memory with age (Drachman and Leavitt 1972). Encoding and retrieval from episodic memory appear to decline, especially when the information cannot be placed in context, but vocabulary, general information, and recall of past historical or personal events remain relatively intact. Healthy elders' memory is generally preserved for relevant, well-learned material, but their ability to process novel information declines (Petersen et al. 1992). Slowing the presentation of new information helps normal elders, and cuing helps them retrieve more effectively from recent memory; however, memory aids are not very helpful when Alzheimer disease reaches the level of dementia.

Executive Function

Although the most common cognitive complaint of elders is impaired recall of names and recent events, the greatest age-associated cognitive decline is in executive function, possibly related primarily to loss of synapses in the prefrontal cortex and loss of dopaminergic input to the prefrontal cortex from the corpus striatum. Decline in executive function manifests as failure to suppress interfering information, the making of perseverative errors, and difficulty organizing working memory. Loss of dopaminergic function in the caudate nucleus and the putamen through reduction of dopamine D_2 and D_3 receptors and dopamine transporter accounts for almost all of the variance in recognition and working memory tasks (for review, see Hedden and Gabrieli 2005). In one study, older adults who were examined with functional magnetic resonance imaging (MRI) techniques during cognitive tasks showed bilateral prefrontal cortical activation, whereas younger persons showed only unilateral activation, suggesting that elders compensate by recruiting more neuronal circuits (Persson et al. 2004).

The Complaint of Cognitive Impairment

Of specific importance to the psychiatrist is that the complaint of cognitive impairment may be a means to deal with emotional issues or with an aspect of marital discord, as illustrated in the following case:

> A 60-year-old woman complained of impaired memory and concentration. Her medical history indicated that she had been evaluated medically for several physical complaints with no definite findings. Her husband reported that he had not observed difficulty with her cognitive functioning. A complete battery of blood tests and a urinalysis were performed and were negative or within normal limits. A complete neurological evaluation, including computed tomography of the head and an electroencephalogram, was negative.
>
> Neuropsychological testing showed no clinically meaningful impairment, but personality testing showed her to be highly anxious and highly preoccupied with physical symptoms. To the psychiatric examiner, she confided

that her greatest problem was her chronic marital conflict. This patient was assured that she did not have a brain disorder and was helped to draw her husband into brief marital counseling.

A clue that the investigation of a person for cognitive impairment stems from a marital problem is the complaint by a spouse of her partner's selective inattention. It is expressed as "He shuts me out" or "He can hear everyone else but me." For this reason, it is our practice to observe the interaction of the partners, bearing in mind that cognitive impairment can be the source of the strain in a relationship as well as its product.

Mild Cognitive Impairment

The term *mild cognitive impairment* (MCI; Petersen et al. 1997) does not appear in DSM-IV-TR. Individuals with MCI have complaints of poor memory, have normal activities of daily living and normal general cognitive function, have abnormal memory function for age, and do not meet the criteria for dementia but are at increased risk (see Chapter 6, "Mild Cognitive Impairment"). Many persons with MCI would be diagnosed by clinicians as having early Alzheimer disease. Indeed, a postmortem study of persons with MCI diagnosed by the Petersen criteria showed that all of these individuals had pathological findings involving medial temporal lobe structures suggestive of evolving Alzheimer disease (Petersen et al. 2006). Those at greatest risk for conversion to Alzheimer disease have severe memory impairment plus impairment in one or more other cognitive domains (Tabert et al. 2006).

In our experience, the most sensitive clinical tests for incipient Alzheimer disease include tests of concentration, recent memory (recall of three or four words after a brief distraction), and remote memory. Assessment of remote memory is confounded by education when general knowledge questions, such as names of past presidents of the United States or historical events, are used. Remote memory is more effectively tested by gathering information from knowledgeable informants that is relevant to the person being examined, such as family events or the number, names, and ages of grandchildren. Another sensitive indicator is loss of the abstract attitude—detected by the similarities and proverbs part of the mental status examination. Proverb interpretation, however, is highly culture bound and may yield false-positive results in persons from other cultures. Performance on the similarities subtest, although not culture bound, is related strongly to education and intelligence. Early in the course of the illness, patients with Alzheimer disease may also demonstrate impaired verbal fluency (e.g., difficulty naming all the animals they can think of in the next minute), dysnomia (difficulty with object naming), constructional dyspraxia (difficulty drawing simple geometrical figures such as intersecting pentagons), and executive dysfunction (difficulty drawing the face of a clock and setting the time). There are no clinical criteria for diagnosis of prodromal non-Alzheimer cognitive disorders.

Dementia

Dementia is an impairment of multiple cognitive abilities, including memory, that is sufficient to interfere with self-maintenance, work, or social relationships. The diagnosis is based on a patient's history (usually supplied by informants other than the patient) and clinical examination.

The diagnosis of dementia is complicated by the enormous variation across individuals. Many persons who have declined cognitively may still function at a level comparable to that of an average person their own age. Therefore, clinicians must compare a patient's present abilities with his or her own past abilities, usually by retrospective accounts furnished by patients or their families. However, family members' accounts are subject to bias. Family members often minimize deficits by stating that a loved one who appears impaired on clinical examination was never good with numbers or interested in reading or current events. Individual family members' biases are minimized through the use of multiple informants and simple scales assessing activities of daily living.

The DSM-IV-TR criteria for dementia (see Table 1–2) include the clinical means to elicit the diagnostic signs and symptoms. Table 1–3 indicates the criteria for diagnosing specific dementias. *A DSM-IV-TR diagnosis of dementia does not imply either continued progression or irreversibility.*

Minor degrees of cognitive impairment, especially cognitive impairment due to medications or metabolic disorders, are frequently reversible, but a full-blown dementia syndrome is rarely reversible. In 1992, *treatable* causes of dementia accounted for about 10.5% of cases and included neurosyphilis, fungal

Table 1–2. General diagnostic criteria for dementia based on DSM-IV-TR criteria

A. The development of multiple cognitive deficits manifested by both

(1) memory impairment (impaired ability to learn new information and to recall previously learned information)

(a) Working memory can be assessed by digit span forward and in reverse, with a discrepancy of three digits or more suggesting impairment. Short-term memory can be tested by asking the examinee to recall three words presented by the examiner after an interval of 5 minutes. Short-term memory can also be tested by presenting three objects without naming them, covering them up, and asking the examinee to name them 5 minutes later. Another test of short-term memory is to read a short paragraph aloud to the examinee and then ask the examinee to tell what he or she recalls.

(b) Long-term memory is tested by asking the examinee for personal information that can be validated by the accompanying person (date of birth, graduation from high school, marriage, etc.) and by asking for facts of common knowledge compatible with the examinee's education and cultural background, including questions such as the name of the president of the United States, names of the immediate past presidents, the state capital, or the location of the U.S. Capitol.

(2) one (or more) of the following cognitive disturbances:

(a) aphasia (language disturbance), including, in addition to the classic aphasias, difficulty with word finding and confrontational naming. Word finding difficulty is evidenced in advanced dementia by empty speech devoid of nouns and verbs, with relative preservation of socially overlearned speech, such as "How are you?" Earlier, it can be demonstrated by asking the subject to name as many animals as possible in 1 minute. Patients with Alzheimer disease will typically name fewer than 10 animals and will often repeat names. They also have difficulty naming the parts of a watch (watchband, stem, back, crystal), making paraphasic errors (e.g., *strap* for band or *lens* for crystal) or describing functions (e.g., "It's how you set it" for watch stem) instead.

(b) apraxia (inability to carry out motor activities despite intact motor function, e.g., strength and coordination). This difficulty is demonstrated when the examinee is asked, for example, to demonstrate how to turn a key in a lock.

(c) agnosia (failure to recognize or identify objects despite intact sensory function).

Table 1–2. General diagnostic criteria for dementia based on DSM-IV-TR criteria *(continued)*

A.   The development of multiple cognitive deficits manifested by both *(continued)*

(2)   one (or more) of the following cognitive disturbances *(continued):*

(d)   disturbance in executive functioning (i.e., planning, organizing, sequencing, abstracting).

1.   Impaired planning, organizing, and sequencing are indicated by an examinee's inability to deal with interpersonal, family, and employment-related issues and to describe logically how they might be dealt with. Changes in long-standing habits and personal hygiene may reflect executive dysfunction. The best source of information about executive functioning may be the examinee's history, but executive functioning may also be evaluated by asking the examinee how to deal with problems that individuals might encounter in daily life, such as an overdrawn bank account or a medical emergency. Executive functioning can also be assessed by asking examinees to perform serial tasks, such as going through the steps of mailing a letter (i.e., folding the paper, inserting it into an envelope, addressing the envelope, placing a stamp on it, and sealing it).

2.   Impaired abstracting ability is evidenced by the examinee's inability to abstractly categorize the similarity between objects such as a chair and a table, or a knife and a fork, or for highly educated persons, between a poem and a statue, or praise and punishment. Impaired abstracting ability is also evidenced by the examinee's inability to abstractly interpret common proverbs.

B.   The cognitive deficits in Criteria A1 and A2 each cause significant impairment in social or occupational functioning and represent a significant decline from a previous level of functioning.

C.   The deficits do not occur exclusively during the course of delirium.

Table 1–3.   DSM-IV-TR diagnostic criteria for specific dementia syndromes

Diagnostic criteria for dementia of the Alzheimer's type

A.   The development of multiple cognitive deficits manifested by both

   (1)   memory impairment (impaired ability to learn new information or to recall previously learned information)

   (2)   one (or more) of the following cognitive disturbances:

      (a)   aphasia (language disturbance)

      (b)   apraxia (impaired ability to carry out motor activities despite intact motor function)

      (c)   agnosia (failure to recognize or identify objects despite intact sensory function)

      (d)   disturbance in executive functioning (i.e., planning, organizing, sequencing, abstracting)

B.   The cognitive deficits in Criteria A1 and A2 each cause significant impairment in social or occupational functioning and represent a significant decline from a previous level of functioning.

C.   The course is characterized by gradual onset and continuing cognitive decline.

D.   The cognitive deficits in Criteria A1 and A2 are not due to any of the following:

   (1)   other central nervous system conditions that cause progressive deficits in memory and cognition (e.g., cerebrovascular disease, Parkinson's disease, Huntington's disease, subdural hematoma, normal-pressure hydrocephalus, brain tumor)

   (2)   systemic conditions that are known to cause dementia (e.g., hypothyroidism, vitamin B_{12} or folic acid deficiency, niacin deficiency, hypercalcemia, neurosyphilis, HIV infection)

   (3)   substance-induced conditions

E.   The deficits do not occur exclusively during the course of a delirium.

F.   The disturbance is not better accounted for by another Axis I disorder (e.g., major depressive disorder, schizophrenia).

Table 1–3. DSM-IV-TR diagnostic criteria for specific dementia syndromes *(continued)*

Diagnostic criteria for vascular dementia

A. The development of multiple cognitive deficits manifested by both

    (1) memory impairment (impaired ability to learn new information or to recall previously learned information)

    (2) one (or more) of the following cognitive disturbances:

        (a) aphasia (language disturbance)

        (b) apraxia (impaired ability to carry out motor activities despite intact motor function)

        (c) agnosia (failure to recognize or identify objects despite intact sensory function)

        (d) disturbance in executive functioning (i.e., planning, organizing, sequencing, abstracting)

B. The cognitive deficits in Criteria A1 and A2 each cause significant impairment in social or occupational functioning and represent a significant decline from a previous level of functioning.

C. Focal neurological signs and symptoms (e.g., exaggeration of deep tendon reflexes, extensor plantar response, pseudobulbar palsy, gait abnormalities, weakness of an extremity) or laboratory evidence indicative of cerebrovascular disease (e.g., multiple infarctions involving cortex and underlying white matter) that is judged to be etiologically related to the disturbance.

D. The deficits do not occur exclusively during the course of a delirium.

Diagnostic criteria for dementia due to other general medical conditions

A. The development of multiple cognitive deficits manifested by both

    (1) memory impairment (impaired ability to learn new information or to recall previously learned information)

    (2) one (or more) of the following cognitive disturbances:

        (a) aphasia (language disturbance)

        (b) apraxia (impaired ability to carry out motor activities despite intact motor function)

        (c) agnosia (failure to recognize or identify objects despite intact sensory function)

        (d) disturbance in executive functioning (i.e., planning, organizing, sequencing, abstracting)

Table 1–3.   DSM-IV-TR diagnostic criteria for specific dementia syndromes *(continued)*

Diagnostic criteria for dementia due to other general medical conditions *(continued)*

B.   The cognitive deficits in Criteria A1 and A2 each cause significant impairment in social or occupational functioning and represent a significant decline from a previous level of functioning.

C.   There is evidence from the history, physical examination, or laboratory findings that the disturbance is the direct physiological consequence of a general medical condition other than Alzheimer's disease or cerebrovascular disease (e.g., HIV infection, traumatic brain injury, Parkinson's disease, Huntington's disease, Pick's disease, Creutzfeldt-Jakob disease, normal-pressure hydrocephalus, hypothyroidism, brain tumor, or vitamin B_{12} deficiency).

D.   The deficits do not occur exclusively during the course of a delirium.

Diagnostic criteria for substance-induced persisting dementia

A.   The development of multiple cognitive deficits manifested by both

(1)   memory impairment (impaired ability to learn new information or to recall previously learned information)

(2)   one (or more) of the following cognitive disturbances:

(a)   aphasia (language disturbance)

(b)   apraxia (impaired ability to carry out motor activities despite intact motor function)

(c)   agnosia (failure to recognize or identify objects despite intact sensory function)

(d)   disturbance in executive functioning (i.e., planning, organizing, sequencing, abstracting)

B.   The cognitive deficits in Criteria A1 and A2 each cause significant impairment in social or occupational functioning and represent a significant decline from a previous level of functioning.

C.   The deficits do not occur exclusively during the course of a delirium and persist beyond the usual duration of substance intoxication or withdrawal.

D.   There is evidence from the history, physical examination, or laboratory findings that the deficits are etiologically related to the persisting effects of substance use (e.g., a drug of abuse, a medication).

Table 1–3.   DSM-IV-TR diagnostic criteria for specific dementia syndromes *(continued)*

Diagnostic criteria for dementia due to multiple etiologies

A.   The development of multiple cognitive deficits manifested by both

   (1)   memory impairment (impaired ability to learn new information or to recall previously learned information)

   (2)   one (or more) of the following cognitive disturbances:

      (a)   aphasia (language disturbance)

      (b)   apraxia (impaired ability to carry out motor activities despite intact motor function)

      (c)   agnosia (failure to recognize or identify objects despite intact sensory function)

      (d)   disturbance in executive functioning (i.e., planning, organizing, sequencing, abstracting)

B.   The cognitive deficits in Criteria A1 and A2 each cause significant impairment in social or occupational functioning and represent a significant decline from a previous level of functioning.

C.   There is evidence from the history, physical examination, or laboratory findings that the disturbance has more than one etiology (e.g., head trauma plus chronic alcohol use, dementia of the Alzheimer's type with the subsequent development of vascular dementia).

D.   The deficits do not occur exclusively during the course of a delirium.

Source.   Reprinted from American Psychiatric Association: *Diagnostic and Statistical Manual of Mental Disorders,* 4th Edition, Text Revision. T, American Psychiatric Association, 2000. Copyright 2000, American Psychiatric Association. Used with permission.

infections, tumor, alcohol abuse, subdural hematoma, normal-pressure hydrocephalus, and epilepsy (Katzman 1992). Our present-day ability to treat Alzheimer disease and vascular dementia brings the percentage of treatable conditions to more than 70%. *Reversible* dementias, including those related to drug toxicity, metabolic disorders, vitamin B_{12} deficiency, and hypothyroidism, still account for less than 5% of cases.

Delirium

Delirium is a state of altered consciousness and cognition, usually of acute onset (hours or days) and of brief duration (days or weeks). The hallmark of delirium is impaired attention. Many persons may remain oriented to person, place, and time, but tests of sustained attention, such as digit span and months of the year in reverse, will reveal impairment. Sleep-wake disturbances are common, as are reduced or increased psychomotor activity. Hallucinations are also frequent. In one series of patients with delirium, 27% experienced visual hallucinations, 12.4% auditory hallucinations, and 2.7% tactile hallucinations (Webster and Holroyd 2000). The DSM-IV-TR criteria for delirium due to a general medical condition are presented in Table 1–4.

Delirium is very common in general hospital patients. In a prospective study of nonconfused individuals 65 years or older who were undergoing repair of hip fracture or elective hip replacement surgery, delirium was diagnosed in 20% (Duppils and Wikblad 2000). The onset of delirium was postoperative in 96% of patients and generally resolved within 48 hours. Predisposing factors were older age, cognitive impairment, and preexisting brain disease. There is also evidence that carrying the apolipoprotein E4 allele increases susceptibility to delirium (van Munster et al. 2009).

In many individuals, the first sign of a cognitive disorder may be postoperative delirium. In our experience, episodes of delirium frequently herald dementia with Lewy bodies. Delirium includes a greater degree of personality disorganization and clouding of consciousness than does dementia. Fluctuating cognitive ability occurs in dementia but not to the extent or with the rapidity (minutes or hours) that it occurs in delirium. Dementia patients usually give their best cognitive performance early in the day when they are not fatigued, under circumstances in which they do not feel challenged or anxious. Toward the end of the day, many persons with cognitive impairment become transiently delirious, a phenomenon often referred to as *sundowning*. The diagnosis of dementia cannot be made in the presence of delirium.

The following case of delirium (courtesy of Kip Queenan, M.D.) involves a patient seen in a general hospital.

A 73-year-old man was brought by police to a psychiatric emergency facility after emergency personnel received a 911 call from his wife, whom he had held down by force and threatened with a shotgun, believing her to be a bur-

Table 1–4. DSM-IV-TR diagnostic criteria for delirium due to a general medical condition

A. Disturbance of consciousness (i.e., reduced clarity of awareness of the environment) with reduced ability to focus, sustain, or shift attention.

B. A change in cognition (such as memory deficit, disorientation, language disturbance) or the development of a perceptual disturbance that is not better accounted for by a preexisting, established, or evolving dementia.

C. The disturbance develops over a short period of time (usually hours to days) and tends to fluctuate during the course of the day.

D. There is evidence from the history, physical examination, or laboratory findings that the disturbance is caused by the direct physiological consequences of a general medical condition.

Source. Reprinted from American Psychiatric Association: *Diagnostic and Statistical Manual of Mental Disorders,* 4th Edition, Text Revision. Washington, DC, American Psychiatric Association, 2000. Copyright 2000, American Psychiatric Association. Used with permission.

glar. The patient had developed a seizure disorder 10 years previously following surgical evacuation of a brain abscess, but he had been seizure free for many years while taking diphenylhydantoin. His wife dated his change in mental status to a month earlier, when he was hospitalized following a seizure. After his discharge from the hospital, the patient began having periods of confusion and irritability. These symptoms worsened after he was prescribed and started taking quetiapine and levetiracetam.

The patient's family reported a history of memory problems since his brain surgery. The patient had been a truck driver prior to his brain abscess; he had been retired since then. He had been independent in activities of daily living until his recent seizure, but his wife had been helping him with their finances ever since his surgery. In the previous 6 months, his cognition had declined. He needed his wife to help navigate while driving, and he was no longer keeping up with current events or hobbies.

Aside from hypertension and a craniotomy for evacuation of a brain abscess, the patient had no significant medical history. He did not use drugs or alcohol.

Laboratory studies were unremarkable aside from MRI evidence of encephalomalacia over the right parieto-occipital lobe, a left caudate infarct, and a left posterior cerebral artery watershed infarction.

On examination, the patient had problems with naming, comprehension, and repetition. His initial score on the Mini-Mental State Examination (MMSE) was 8; he was unable to draw a clock. He was very confused when admitted to the hospital, had visual hallucinations, and made numerous attempts to pull out his intravenous lines. He improved significantly within 24–48 hours after discontinuation of levetiracetam. He was thought to have had a mild dementia due to his brain injury and several nonobvious strokes with a superimposed delirium due to levetiracetam. At discharge, he was alert, oriented to person and place, and no longer hallucinating.

Amnestic Disorder

The primary manifestation of amnestic disorder is memory impairment. The DSM-IV-TR diagnostic criteria for this uncommon disorder are presented in Table 1–5. When part of a dementia syndrome, amnestic disorder is not diagnosed separately. The most common cause of persisting amnestic disorder (Korsakoff syndrome) is thiamine deficiency, which is typically associated with malnutrition accompanying long-term alcohol abuse and often preceded by the delirium, ophthalmoplegia, and ataxia of Wernicke encephalopathy. Persistent amnesia may result from many types of brain injury, the best known being bilateral hippocampal lesions, which impair recent memory and prevent additional storage, while not impairing memories that were stored before the injury (Zola-Morgan et al. 1986).

Amnestic episodes occur with the short-acting benzodiazepines. These episodes are usually transient but may confound diagnosis of dementia or amnestic disorder. It is important to consider amnestic disorders in the differential diagnosis, since they are reversible when due to drugs and partly reversible in Wernicke encephalopathy.

Other Cognitive Disorders

The category *cognitive disorder not otherwise specified* (NOS) indicates cognitive dysfunction presumed to be due to a general medical condition that does not meet criteria for delirium, dementia, or amnestic disorder. A common example is postconcussion disorder, with impaired memory or attention following head trauma. Another common example is postoperative cognitive dysfunction (POCD). In a prospective study, deficits were present at 1 week but largely gone 3 months after surgery; however, after 6 months, 29% continued to complain of cognitive deficits (Dijkstra et al. 1999). A prospective study of POCD in persons age 60 or older who had undergone major noncardiac surgery under general anesthesia showed cognitive dysfunction in 26% at 1 week after surgery and

Table 1–5.   DSM-IV-TR diagnostic criteria for amnestic disorder due to a general medical condition

A. The development of memory impairment as manifested by impairment in the ability to learn new information or the inability to recall previously learned information.

B. The memory disturbance causes significant impairment in social or occupational functioning and represents a significant decline from a previous level of functioning.

C. The memory disturbance does not occur exclusively during the course of a delirium or a dementia.

D. There is evidence from the history, physical examination, or laboratory findings that the disturbance is the direct physiological consequence of a general medical condition (including physical trauma).

Source.   Reprinted from American Psychiatric Association: *Diagnostic and Statistical Manual of Mental Disorders,* 4th Edition, Text Revision. Washington, DC, American Psychiatric Association, 2000. Copyright 2000, American Psychiatric Association. Used with permission.

in 10% at 3 months, compared with control rates of 3.4% and 2.8%, respectively (Biedler et al. 1999). Risk factors for early POCD were increasing age and duration of anesthesia, little education, a second operation, postoperative infection, and respiratory complications. However, a more recent meta-analysis of controlled surgical studies found no difference in POCD in the immediate postoperative period between general and regional anesthesia (Bryson and Wyand 2006).

Psychiatric Disorders

Major Depressive Disorder

Among the group of psychiatric disorders that should be considered in the assessment of a person with cognitive complaints or symptoms, the most common is major depression. Depression must be considered in the evaluation of a person with a cognitive complaint, as a primary diagnosis or a complication of an underlying disease. Many depressed persons experience cognitive impairment, although the severity of their impairment does not correspond with the severity of their depressive symptoms. Although Sternberg and Jarvik (1976) reported that short-term memory deficits are correctable by successful treatment with antidepressants, and Greenwald et al. (1989) found that MMSE scores improved after successful treatment, more recent studies suggest that following remission of depressive symptoms (Nebes et al. 2003), deficits persist in cognitive functions, including working memory, speed of information processing, episodic memory, and attention.

The response of both depressive and cognitive symptoms to antidepressant treatment does not firmly establish a sole diagnosis of depression in elderly patients. Of 23 elderly patients who had amelioration of cognitive symptoms with treatment of their depression, nearly half later developed a dementing illness (Alexopoulos et al. 1993).

The level of depressive comorbidity in Alzheimer disease is highly controversial (see Chapter 12, "Treatment of Psychiatric Disorders in People With Dementia"), in part due to the substantial overlap of depressive symptoms with the symptoms of Alzheimer disease. In our experience, depressive syndromes are a common cause of cognitive complaints in persons without demonstrable brain pathology. There is an approximately 20% prevalence of major depression in the first 2 years after stroke (Robinson 2003), and depression is also frequent in patients with Parkinson disease (McDonald et al. 2003).

The DSM-IV-TR criteria for a major depressive episode are presented in Table 1–6. Differentiation between the cognitive impairment of depression and that due to degenerative or metabolic brain disorder is based on the following:

1. Onset of depressive symptoms preceding cognitive impairment
2. Sudden, fairly recent (weeks or months), and often identifiable onset of cognitive impairment, in terms of both time and emotionally important life events (loss of job or spouse)
3. Patients' emphasizing inability to think, concentrate, and remember
4. Signs and symptoms of depression
5. Objective cognitive testing showing patients' deficits to be less severe than their complaints, with performance improved by encouragement, cuing, and structure
6. Depressed patients' more commonly giving "I don't know" answers in contrast to making near misses, confabulating, or repeating (perseverating) answers
7. Normal electroencephalogram
8. Absence of any condition known to affect brain function

Table 1–6.   DSM-IV-TR criteria for major depressive episode

A.   Five (or more) of the following symptoms have been present during the same 2-week period and represent a change from previous functioning; at least one of the symptoms is either (1) depressed mood or (2) loss of interest or pleasure.

Note: Do not include symptoms that are clearly due to a general medical condition, or mood-incongruent delusions or hallucinations.

(1)   depressed mood most of the day, nearly every day, as indicated by either subjective report (e.g., feels sad or empty) or observation made by others (e.g., appears tearful)

(2)   markedly diminished interest or pleasure in all, or almost all, activities most of the day, nearly every day (as indicated by either subjective account or observation made by others)

(3)   significant weight loss when not dieting or weight gain (e.g., a change of more than 5% of body weight in a month), or decrease or increase in appetite nearly every day

(4)   insomnia or hypersomnia nearly every day

(5)   psychomotor agitation or retardation nearly every day (observable by others, not merely subjective feelings of restlessness or being slowed down)

(6)   fatigue or loss of energy nearly every day

(7)   feelings of worthlessness or excessive or inappropriate guilt (which may be delusional) nearly every day (not merely self-reproach or guilt about being sick)

(8)   diminished ability to think or concentrate, or indecisiveness, nearly every day (either by subjective account or as observed by others)

(9)   recurrent thoughts of death (not just fear of dying), recurrent suicidal ideation without a specific plan, or a suicide attempt or a specific plan for committing suicide

B.   The symptoms do not meet criteria for a mixed episode.

C.   The symptoms cause clinically significant distress or impairment in social, occupational, or other important areas of functioning.

D.   The symptoms are not due to the direct physiological effects of a substance (e.g., a drug of abuse, a medication) or a general medical condition (e.g., hypothyroidism).

E.   The symptoms are not better accounted for by bereavement, i.e., after the loss of a loved one; the symptoms persist for longer than 2 months or are characterized by marked functional impairment, morbid preoccupation with worthlessness, suicidal ideation, psychotic symptoms, or psychomotor retardation.

Source.   Reprinted from American Psychiatric Association 2000. Copyright 2000, American Psychiatric Association. Used with permission.

Brain imaging is not useful in differentiating depression from a dementing illness. On the other hand, neuropsychological testing can help.

Bipolar Disorder

The depressive phase of bipolar disorder should be clinically evaluated as described above for major depressive disorder. The manic phase is not usually confused with cognitive disorders, but persons with frontotemporal dementias are often confused with manic patients because of their impulsivity, disinhibition, and poor judgment.

Mood Disorder Due to a General Medical Condition

Mood disorder due to a general medical condition and substance-induced mood disorder can be confused with dementia because of the many overlapping signs of both dementia and depression. The essential feature of mood disorder due to a general medical condition is prominent and persistent mood alteration associated with a general medical condition, including carcinoma of the pancreas (Carney et al. 2003) and hepatitis C (Angelino and Treisman 2006). Hyper- or hypothyroidism and hyper- or hypoadrenocorticism can cause depression or mania. DSM-IV-TR criteria for mood disorder due to a general medical condition are listed in Table 1–7.

Substance-Induced Mood Disorder

Substance-induced mood disorder (see Table 1–8) is characterized by prominent and persistent mood alteration associated with substance use. Depressive symptoms may be caused by drugs, including reserpine, methyldopa, β-blockers, interferon, and some hallucinogens. Exogenous steroids can cause depression or mania.

Anxiety Disorder Due to a General Medical Condition

Generalized anxiety or recurrent panic attacks are the chief characteristics of anxiety disorders due to a general medical condition. Endocrine disorders such as hyperthyroidism and hypothyroidism, pheochromocytoma, hypercortisolism, and fasting hypoglycemia are potential causative factors, along with a host of others. DSM-IV-TR criteria for anxiety disorder due to a general medical condition are listed in Table 1–9.

Table 1–7.   DSM-IV-TR diagnostic criteria for mood disorder due to a general medical condition

A.   A prominent and persistent disturbance in mood predominates in the clinical picture and is characterized by either (or both) of the following:

(1)   depressed mood or markedly diminished interest or pleasure in all, or almost all, activities

(2)   elevated, expansive, or irritable mood

B.   There is evidence from the history, physical examination, or laboratory findings that the disturbance is the direct physiological consequence of a general medical condition.

C.   The disturbance is not better accounted for by another mental disorder (e.g., adjustment disorder with depressed mood in response to the stress of having a general medical condition).

D.   The disturbance does not occur exclusively during the course of a delirium.

E.   The symptoms cause clinically significant distress or impairment in social, occupational, or other important areas of functioning.

Source.   Reprinted from American Psychiatric Association: *Diagnostic and Statistical Manual of Mental Disorders,* 4th Edition, Text Revision. Washington, DC, American Psychiatric Association, 2000. Copyright 2000, American Psychiatric Association. Used with permission.

Schizophrenia

Schizophrenia may be a direct cause of impaired cognition (Keefe and Eesley 2006) or may coexist with a cognitive disorder. Psychotic symptoms that occur in persons with cognitive disorders tend to differ from those of schizophrenia. Persons with cognitive disorders rarely develop organized delusional systems with bizarre content. They often accuse others of stealing or attempting to break in to their homes, but are unable to offer explanations. The hallucinations of persons with cognitive disorders such as dementia with Lewy bodies, Parkinson disease with dementia, or Alzheimer disease tend to be visual, whereas those of schizophrenia are more commonly auditory and accusatory. Schizophrenia usually begins early in life and remains present through the life span. Hallucinations and delusions are generally prominent in the early and middle course of the illness but frequently lessen later on. Few individuals with schizophrenia are able to maintain employment or normal social relationships in the early and middle years of their lives. Thus, an adequate history from family members or caregivers documenting normal adulthood is

Table 1–8.   DSM-IV-TR diagnostic criteria for substance-induced mood disorder

A. A prominent and persistent disturbance in mood predominates in the clinical picture and is characterized by either (or both) of the following:

   (1) depressed mood or markedly diminished interest or pleasure in all, or almost all, activities

   (2) elevated, expansive, or irritable mood

B. There is evidence from the history, physical examination, or laboratory findings of either (1) or (2):

   (1) the symptoms in Criterion A developed during, or within a month of, substance intoxication or withdrawal

   (2) medication use is etiologically related to the disturbance

C. The disturbance is not better accounted for by a mood disorder that is not substance induced. Evidence that the symptoms are better accounted for by a mood disorder that is not substance induced might include the following: the symptoms precede the onset of the substance use (or medication use); the symptoms persist for a substantial period of time (e.g., about a month) after the cessation of acute withdrawal or severe intoxication or are substantially in excess of what would be expected given the type or amount of the substance used or the duration of use; or there is other evidence that suggests the existence of an independent non-substance-induced mood disorder (e.g., a history of recurrent major depressive episodes).

D. The disturbance does not occur exclusively during the course of a delirium.

E. The symptoms cause clinically significant distress or impairment in social, occupational, or other important areas of functioning.

Source.   Reprinted from American Psychiatric Association: *Diagnostic and Statistical Manual of Mental Disorders,* 4th Edition, Text Revision. Washington, DC, American Psychiatric Association, 2000. Copyright 2000, American Psychiatric Association. Used with permission.

usually sufficient to distinguish schizophrenia from a cognitive disorder with psychosis. In rare cases, a high-functioning individual with schizophrenia may not have his or her illness diagnosed until later adulthood. In addition, schizophrenia can emerge in the fourth to sixth decades of life. Considerable evidence suggests that the cognitive deficits of schizophrenia precede the psychotic symptoms and are relatively stable over the course of illness despite the presence or absence of active psychosis (Green 2006).

Table 1–9. DSM-IV-TR diagnostic criteria for anxiety disorder due to a general medical condition

A. Prominent anxiety, panic attacks, or obsessions or compulsions predominate in the clinical picture.

B. There is evidence from the history, physical examination, or laboratory findings that the disturbance is the direct physiological consequence of a general medical condition.

C. The disturbance is not better accounted for by another mental disorder (e.g., adjustment disorder with anxiety in which the stressor is a serious general medical condition).

D. The disturbance does not occur exclusively during the course of a delirium.

E. The disturbance causes clinically significant distress or impairment in social, occupational, or other important areas of functioning.

Source. Reprinted from American Psychiatric Association: *Diagnostic and Statistical Manual of Mental Disorders,* 4th Edition, Text Revision. Washington, DC, American Psychiatric Association, 2000. Copyright 2000, American Psychiatric Association. Used with permission.

Delusional Disorder

Delusional disorders need to be distinguished from cognitive disorders accompanied by delusions because of differences in their management and outcome. The delusions that characterize delusional disorders are commonly erotomanic, grandiose, jealous, persecutory, or somatic. They are expressed with certainty, and attempts to question patients about them are met with anger and increasing mistrust. Delusions of persons with progressive neurodegenerative disorders are less firmly held, transient, and rarely systematized. Among these delusions is that of the phantom boarder—an unseen person who the cognitively impaired person believes is in the house. More commonly, delusions in cognitive disorders are readily seen in terms of wishful thinking, such as an elderly woman's belief that her children still live with her and are going to school.

Psychotic Disorder Due to a General Medical Condition

DSM-IV-TR diagnostic criteria for psychotic disorder due to a general medical condition are presented in Table 1–10. The criteria specifically exclude psychosis during delirium. Hallucinations and delusions are the most common symptoms of this disorder. Etiologies vary widely but may include inflammatory

Table 1–10.   DSM-IV-TR diagnostic criteria for psychotic disorder due to a general medical condition

A.   Prominent hallucinations or delusions.

B.   There is evidence from the history, physical examination, or laboratory findings that the disturbance is the direct physiological consequence of a general medical condition.

C.   The disturbance is not better accounted for by another mental disorder.

D.   The disturbance does not occur exclusively during the course of a delirium.

Source.   Reprinted from American Psychiatric Association: *Diagnostic and Statistical Manual of Mental Disorders,* 4th Edition, Text Revision. Washington, DC, American Psychiatric Association, 2000. Copyright 2000, American Psychiatric Association. Used with permission.

disorders of the brain (e.g., paraneoplastic syndrome) and meninges, brain tumors, and seizure disorders.

Personality Change Due to a General Medical Condition

General medical conditions may exaggerate preexisting personality traits or cause a change in personality. There are many patterns, but emotional instability, recurrent outbursts of aggression or rage, impaired social judgment, apathy, suspiciousness, and paranoid ideation are frequent. Encephalitis, brain tumors, head trauma, multiple sclerosis, frontotemporal degenerative diseases, and strokes are common causes of personality changes. These symptoms may also occur as interictal phenomena in temporal lobe epilepsy. The DSM-IV-TR criteria for personality change due to a general medical condition are presented in Table 1–11. Although many such cases do not meet criteria for dementia, their functional deficits may be just as severe.

Down Syndrome

Family members and health care professionals who provide care for persons with mental retardation face the issue of cognitive decline in aging patients with Down syndrome. Patients with Down syndrome who live past age 35 years demonstrate the microscopic pathology of Alzheimer disease, but not all develop dementia (Oliver et al. 1998). It is important in this population, as in all others, to seek remediable causes of functional decline.

Table 1–11.   DSM-IV-TR diagnostic criteria for personality change due to a general medical condition

A.   A persistent personality disturbance that represents a change from the individual's previous characteristic personality pattern. (In children, the disturbance involves a marked deviation from normal development or a significant change in the child's usual behavior patterns lasting at least 1 year.)

B.   There is evidence from the history, physical examination, or laboratory findings that the disturbance is the direct physiological consequence of a general medical condition.

C.   The disturbance is not better accounted for by another mental disorder (including other mental disorders due to a general medical condition).

D.   The disturbance does not occur exclusively during the course of a delirium.

E.   The disturbance causes clinically significant distress or impairment in social, occupational, or other important areas of functioning.

Source.   Reprinted from American Psychiatric Association: *Diagnostic and Statistical Manual of Mental Disorders,* 4th Edition, Text Revision. Washington, DC, American Psychiatric Association, 2000. Copyright 2000, American Psychiatric Association. Used with permission.

Other Psychiatric Disorders

Ganser Syndrome

Ganser syndrome is subsumed in DSM-IV-TR under the heading of dissociative disorder NOS. The psychological mechanism is that of conversion disorder, and in fact the syndrome has been termed *conversion pseudodementia* (Hepple 2004). Ganser syndrome differs from malingering in that the mechanism appears to be unconscious. In this syndrome, ludicrous approximate answers (vorbeireden) or responses are made to simple questions or commands, indicating that the patient clearly understands the questions and unconsciously gives incorrect responses (Goldin and MacDonald 1955). When asked to add 2 + 2, the patient may answer 5. The patient may point down when asked to point up, and then point up when asked to point down. Ganser syndrome is frequently accompanied by complaints of auditory and visual hallucinations, circumscribed amnesia, and disorientation. Neuropsychological testing yields highly inconsistent performance (Heron et al. 1991), as is also seen in malingering. These symptoms develop rapidly and usually occur in response to a severe environmental stress, such as facing trial or imprisonment. They are usually short-lived and require no active treatment.

Malingering

Impaired cognition may be pretended for various types of gain. The effects of trivial head injuries may be magnified to escape hard labor or to gain monetary compensation. Mental status examination and neuropsychological testing of the individual who is feigning impaired cognition show inconsistent deficits, with better performance on many items that call for high-level integration than on some items calling for lesser levels of cognitive function. For example, simple similarities will not be understood, whereas more complicated similarities will call forth an abstract response; or digit span, a simple test of attention, will be limited to three digits, whereas the patient can follow complicated directions to the restroom.

Senile Squalor

The phenomenon of senile squalor is well known to those who work with adult protective services. Reviewed by Snowdon et al. (2007), senile squalor consists of self-neglect or neglect of one's surroundings, accompanied by hoarding and social isolation to which the individual is completely oblivious. The place of residence is disorganized, dirty, and filled with useless objects or materials. The exterior of the residence is usually dilapidated as well. At times, numerous animals described as "pets" are also in the dwelling and are also not well cared for. Attempts have been made to understand this phenomenon in terms of psychiatric disorders such as obsessive-compulsive personality disorder or obsessive-compulsive disorder, but most individuals with this set of behaviors functioned well earlier in life. It seems likely that these individuals suffer significant deficits in frontal brain circuits that are variable in origin. Studies such as functional neuroimaging have not been performed on these individuals because of their general unwillingness to participate in medical investigations. Longitudinal observations of these individuals have also not been possible, because they generally refuse follow-up by social agencies.

Speech and Language

Speech and language are affected in many cognitive disorders. Speech tends to be slow in diseases of the basal ganglia, Parkinson disease, and vascular dementia; explosive or slurred in progressive supranuclear palsy; and poorly articulated in multiple sclerosis or following stroke. Disorders of language (aphasias) often result from regional brain damage and are often confused with dementia. The history of aphasia patients will usually reveal a brain insult, most often stroke or head trauma. There are usually neurological deficits such as hemiparesis (especially in the Broca type), unilateral hyperreflexia, and visual field deficits. In general, anomia that progresses to aphasia suggests neurodegenerative disease; aphasia that resolves over time to anomia generally results from acute brain injury.

The categorization of aphasias is based on the language functions (e.g., fluency, comprehension, repetition) they impair. Global aphasia impairs all language functions and occurs in large left-hemisphere strokes. Anomic aphasia, by contrast, primarily affects word finding, may be related to lesions of the left angular or left posterior middle temporal gyrus, and is common in Alzheimer disease. Broca (anterior, nonfluent) aphasia impairs verbal fluency, repetition, and naming and results from lesions of the posterior inferior portion of the left (or dominant) frontal lobe. In Broca aphasia, speech requires great effort and is agrammatical, with the patient omitting word modifiers such as articles, prepositions, and conjunctions. For example, a person who wants to go to the bathroom might say, "Want...go...bath...room," with great effort and great relief after having expressed himself or herself. These patients generally understand what is said to them and can obey commands but have difficulty with repetition, reading aloud, and writing. Although they have difficulty with naming, they are helped by prompts.

Patients with Wernicke (posterior, fluent) aphasia have fluent, paraphasic, neologistic speech with poor comprehension, repetition, and naming. The naming difficulty is not usually aided by prompting. Reading and writing are also impaired. Speech tends to have little informational content and relies on indefinite words and phrases. The sentence "I want to go to the bathroom" might be rendered by a fluent aphasic patient as "I wish to go to the you-know bath place now soon," with no awareness of the peculiarity of his or her speech. Word approximations (paraphasias) may be based on similar sounds or phonemes (phonemic paraphasia), such as "meek" for "meat," or similar meanings (semantic paraphasia), such as "writer" for "pencil." The tissue damage in this syndrome is to the posterior superior portion of the first temporal gyrus of the dominant hemisphere.

Among the frontotemporal dementias are progressive aphasias without history of brain insult or localizing neurological signs. These include primary progressive aphasia and semantic dementia. For more detailed discussions of primary progressive aphasia and semantic dementia, see Chapter 3, "Neuropsychological Assessment," and Chapter 9, "Frontotemporal Dementia and Other Tauopathies."

Mild difficulty with retrieval of nouns (dysnomia) occurs early in the course of Alzheimer disease. More pronounced language disturbance occurs later in the disease, including fluent aphasia, perseveration, and palilalia (echoing one's own speech), and may culminate in mutism. In response to a request to write a sentence, the following material was produced by a man with Alzheimer disease who had prominent language dysfunction.

> Sou you can right so he can write this is zold This is so some belt so the right food can you can right so can rin so you can right the right So you can right so that you can right.

Figure 1–2 presents an algorithm for the differential diagnosis of aphasia based on language function.

Clinical Techniques and Tools for Diagnosing Cognitive Dysfunction

Clinical evaluation begins with history taking and direct examination of patients. History taking involves the patient, a knowledgeable informant, and all pertinent medical information. Direct access to medical records is important because lay informants often do not accurately recall medical events or the outcomes of various laboratory tests.

In addition to eliciting information concerning patients' cognitive abilities, the clinician seeks evidence of emotional or interpersonal contributions to the presenting symptoms. Patients' emotional responses to their mental difficulties are evaluated, and an attempt is made to determine family strengths and weaknesses. Patients' personality patterns are also considered. This information helps shape the plan of management.

History Taking

Ideally, medical records are reviewed in advance of examining the patient. When possible, we obtain a history from a family informant before examining the patient. We also ask what medications are being taken. When possible, we inter-

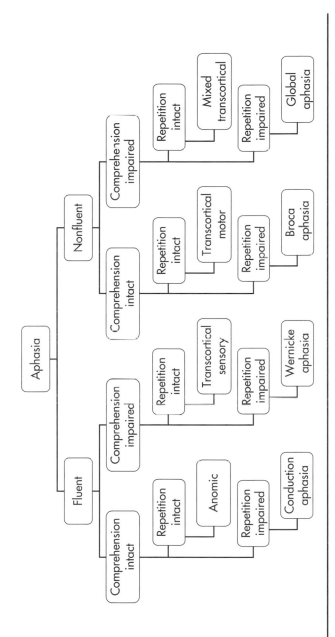

Figure 1–2. Language algorithm for the differential diagnosis of aphasia.

Source. Reprinted from Weiner MF, Garrett R, Bret ME: "Neuropsychiatric Assessment and Diagnosis," in *The American Psychiatric Publishing Textbook of Alzheimer Disease and Other Dementias.* Edited by Weiner MF, Lipton AM. Washington, DC, American Psychiatric Publishing, 2009, pp. 39–70. Copyright 2009, American Psychiatric Publishing. Used with permission.

view a patient in the presence of a family member to ensure the accuracy of factual information and to ascertain how the patient's performance during the examination compares with his or her daily performance. A patient is interviewed alone if unaccompanied or if he or she objects to having others in the examination room. When possible, time is allowed to interview the accompanying person alone; family members often withhold information in a patient's presence out of concern that they may humiliate or anger the patient. Typical information withheld concerns patients' paranoid thinking, hallucinations, or incontinence. Having a friend or relative present is a comfort to most persons with cognitive impairment. Thus, history taking tends to be a three-way conversation rather than a formal interview. In the flow of the conversation, many clues emerge concerning the relationship between patients and significant others, the impact of patients on their families, and the impact of others on the patients. Husbands often resent their wives' diminished ability to maintain their household. Dependent spouses may resent having to be responsible for their formerly dominant spouses. In many cases, tension exists between spouses because one does not believe that the other truly cannot learn, remember, or understand. For example, a man who knew his wife had Alzheimer disease chided her for reading romance novels instead of reading more substantial works, as she had done earlier in her life. Examining one spouse in the presence of the other can be helpful in dealing with the intact spouse's denial and in demonstrating how to deal with defects in the other's ability to remember, plan, and cooperate.

Mental Status Examination

The mental status examination is performed with consideration for patients' frustration tolerance and is tailored to their level of cognitive performance. For example, when it becomes obvious that the patient is not oriented to year and month, we do not usually inquire about orientation to day and date. When the patient is irritable or easily frustrated, we abbreviate each category of inquiry. We treat all responses as equally valid, whether correct or not, and we praise the patient for effort by saying "good" or "that's fine" after a series of responses. Exceptions to this general approach are when formal testing of cognition is done for scientific studies, when completeness is important, or when we suspect that the patient is not making an effort to perform the task, and we may withhold praise until the patient has made adequate effort or urge the patient to focus attention on the task at hand.

Attention is tested by both forward and reverse digit span. Working memory is tested by asking patients to recall three words following 5 minutes of distraction. This test can be performed with objects presented verbally or objects shown to the patient without naming them. Response to cuing is also important, because it helps to distinguish retrieval deficits from failure to encode. Testing remote memory is more difficult. Patients with little formal education can be asked about current events that fall within their range of interest; this is done most effectively when an outside informant is asked about recent events in the patient's life (e.g., family birthdays and other family events).

Routine examination of language function includes assessment of articulation, fluency, comprehension, repetition, naming, reading, and the ability to write sentences (see the following section for a more detailed language examination). Language fluency encompasses delays in word finding, paraphasias, and neologisms. Word fluency (the ability to generate a list of words), a very sensitive indicator of cognitive impairment, can be tested by asking patients to name all the animals they can think of in 1 minute. The average score for high school graduates is 18 (±6) (Goodglass and Kaplan 1972).

Comprehension tests begin with graded tasks, such as asking patients to point to one, two, and three objects in the room, and then proceed to asking simple logic questions such as "Is my cousin's mother a man or a woman?"

Naming tests should include the parts of objects, such as the parts of a watch (stem, watchband, back or case, face, crystal or glass) or the parts of a shirt. Reading ability should be considered in the context of patients' education. Writing ability is assessed by asking patients to write a dictated sentence and by then asking them to compose a sentence of their own. We test calculating ability with a simple problem in multiplication.

Praxis is evaluated by asking patients to imitate an action performed by the examiner, to perform simple motor acts in response to the examiner's request, and to copy a set of simple geometric figures (we use a Greek/open cross and a triangle within a triangle). Drawing a cube is used to detect constructional dyspraxia in mildly impaired, well-educated persons. In our experience, cognitively intact persons 80 years and older do not draw the cube well.

Fund of information is assessed by using a standard set of questions ranging from simple to difficult and by evaluating the responses in relation to patients' level of education and job achievement.

Ability to think abstractly is assessed by using similarities and proverbs, but this evaluation requires consideration of patients' education, cultural background, and native language. Impairment of abstract reasoning can be inferred from part-object substitution in tests of ideomotor praxis, such as using one's fingers as the teeth of a comb while pretending to comb one's hair, and from inability in clock drawing to set the time at 8:20 because no 20 is on the clock (see description of Clock Drawing Test in section "Quantifying Aspects of Dementing Illness" later in this chapter). Judgment may be estimated by asking patients questions on how they would manage certain life situations, such as "What would you do if the electric company called and told you that the last check you wrote them was returned because of insufficient funds?" However, judgment is better assessed from history by an informant than by direct evaluation of the patient.

Elements of the mental status examination that detect executive dysfunction include assessments of ideomotor and constructional praxis, abstract reasoning, and judgment. Likewise, portions of the neurological examination, including the Luria hand sequence (Weiner et al. 2011), go–no-go tasks, and reciprocal motor tasks, detect executive dysfunction. Clock drawing is a useful test of executive function. Executive dysfunction is also detectable in the course of the history taking—for example, as mistakes in social judgment such as inappropriate sexual advances—and in the course of the mental status examination—for example, with inappropriate handling of objects (utilization behavior), such as grasping the examiner's tie, or inappropriate laughter or flirtation.

Examination of Language

A basic language evaluation samples spontaneous speech, comprehension abilities, repetition and prosody, naming, and category generation. Spontaneous speech is usually elicited in history taking but can also be elicited by asking patients to describe a drawing or photograph. Language expression and comprehension can be assessed in a graded fashion; naming of pictures can be assessed by starting with a common object (e.g., an automobile) and later showing an uncommon object (e.g., a hammock). Naming ability can progress from pointing to one object to pointing to a series of objects. Repetition ability is tested in an increasingly more complicated way, beginning with single words and extending to phrases, sentences, and several-sentence utterances. Word lists are generated to test ability to generate categories (e.g., "Name all the animals you can think of in 1 minute"), a type of semantic task. Reading and writing sentences is useful as well.

Disruptions in the motor cortex and the language cortex of the brain result in misarticulation. The difficulty is apparent in patients who use the wrong sound for letters in words, such as a "b" sound for a "v" sound. Articulation problems are rare in cortical dementias and suggest other problems, such as stroke, that may affect motor cortex or motor tracts. A phonemic paraphasia is the substitution of one sound in a word for another, as in /pot/ for /cot/. Verbal apraxias manifest as searching to find the correct placement of sounds, such as /pot, lot, rot, cot/; this problem represents an inability to place the tongue properly to form sounds accurately.

Deficits in fluency include halting speech, long pauses, interjections while searching for words, stuttering, and monotonous tone of voice. Many words are completely eliminated in dysfluent speech, giving it the character of "telegram speech." Articles, function words, conjunctions, and prepositions all may be lost, leaving the listener with a bare set of content words. For example, dysfluent speech will have decreased verbal output, decreased phrase length, effortful speech, and loss of prosody (e.g., "I go store").

Repetition requires intact hearing, an intact articulatory inventory, and fluent speech (if the stimulus is longer than a word). Agrammatic speech may result in mismatches between subjects and verbs, or misuse of person, number, and gender markers (e.g., "Me go store").

Semantics is a set of acceptable interpretations to each entity that is accepted as a word or a sentence, to include words that fit the intent of the speaker and convey the message most easily to the listener. For example, the word *can* is the verb meaning "to be able to" or the noun meaning "a receptacle made out of tin." Ambiguous sentences use this multiplicity of meanings to generate several interpretations for a sentence's meaning. Ambiguous sentences can be interpreted in several ways. For example, the sentence "Children hate annoying parents" could mean "children hate to annoy their parents" or "children hate parents who annoy them." Generating interpretations of ambiguous sentences is one way of testing for semantic abilities, as are naming objects in pictures and generating names in a given category.

Persons with early Alzheimer disease have generally intact language. The ability to articulate, to form grammatical sentences, and to repeat is not affected until late in the disorder. The first sign of language disturbance will probably occur at the semantic level, with the inability to retrieve words, although their meaning is retained.

Speech in frontotemporal dementias may become markedly less fluent and slower, while demonstrating obvious grammatical struggles. Speech gradually deteriorates further, as does language function in all the cortical dementias in the middle and late stages.

In primary progressive aphasia (Kertesz and Munoz 2003), phonological errors in speech are evident early (e.g., /efelant/ for /elephant/). Anomia is initially mild. Comprehension is relatively good. Suggested diagnostic criteria include the gradual loss of word finding, object naming, syntax, or word comprehension in the absence of stroke or tumor, with loss of day-to-day function attributable to loss of language abilities. Loss of syntax and word naming abilities cause speech to be slow and deliberate.

In the semantic dementia presentation of frontotemporal dementia, patients have relatively intact syntax and phonology/pronunciation skills, but a marked inability to generate words in a semantic category (e.g., animal naming). Category fluency is reduced. Semantic relationships between pictures are poor. In testing with pictures cut out from magazines, patients are asked about the connection between groups within a similar category (e.g., camels and pyramids).

Repetition is typically intact in patients with Alzheimer disease and semantic dementia. Testing involves, for example, having a person repeat three words, then three phrases, and then three simple sentences. Repetition is very poor in primary progressive aphasia.

Characterizing Dementing Illnesses

Dementing illnesses can be characterized as cortical or subcortical (see also Chapter 3, "Neuropsychological Assessment"). *Cortical dementias* usually present as one of two overlapping groups: *frontotemporal* or *temporoparietal.* A frontal dementia presentation can be due to Pick disease or anterior cerebral artery stroke. A common presentation is progressive personality change and breakdown in social conduct. Other features are defective judgment, difficulty in focusing attention, apathy, disinhibition, silliness, echoing words, mirroring others' behavior, unawareness of deficit, difficulty in following instructions (often manifested as motor dyspraxia), and often a slightly prancing gait. Personality changes often antedate cognitive symptoms in fronto-temporal dementias. In primary progressive aphasia, initial symptoms include difficulty with verbal expression. Normal-pressure hydrocephalus often includes frontal signs, such as complete indifference to urinary incontinence. Temporoparietal dementia, the most common presentation of Alzheimer disease, is accompanied by naming difficulties and constructional dyspraxia, with relative preservation of personality. Persons with cortical dementias may or may not be aware of their deficits. Figure 1–3 presents a language algorithm for the diagnosis of cortical dementias.

Subcortical dementias, with primary pathology in the thalami, basal ganglia, rostral brain stem, and their frontal projections, overlap in symptoms with frontal dementias but also usually involve speech and motor abnormalities. The most prominent symptoms include overall slowing of movement and cognitive processing, deficits in social judgment, and mood change. Causes of subcortical dementia include cerebrovascular disease, Parkinson disease, Huntington disease, Wilson disease, and progressive supranuclear palsy.

Quantifying Cognitive Impairment

Commonly used measures of cognitive/executive function are also presented in Chapter 3 ("Neuropsychological Assessment"). The Mini-Mental State Examination (Folstein et al. 1975) is the most widely used brief cognitive assessment tool. It requires 10–15 minutes to administer. A perfect score is 30 points. The MMSE is confounded by premorbid intelligence and education. The originators indicate that a score ≤23 by a person with a high school education is suggestive of dementia. A cutoff score of 18 is suggested for those with an eighth-grade education or less. Crum et al. (1993) published a table with suggested normal values in relation to age and education. The MMSE is not sensitive, does not examine executive function, and will frequently not detect impairment in highly educated persons, but its brevity and the minimal training required make it useful in conjunction with the Clock Drawing Test (see below) as a screening test for cognitive impairment and for following the progression of cognitive disorders. The MMSE is protected by copyright and must be ordered from Psychological Assessment Resources, P.O. Box 998, Odessa, FL 33556 (1-800-331-8378).

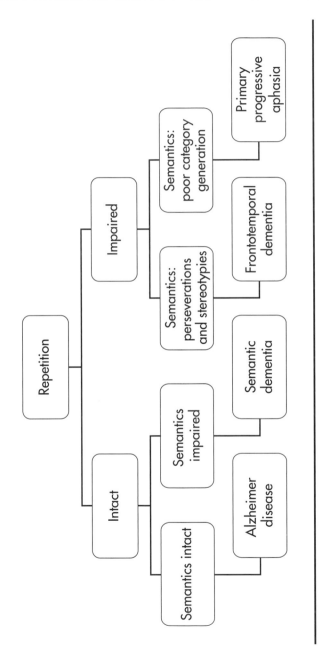

Figure 1–3.   Language algorithm for the diagnosis of cortical dementias. *Source.*   Reprinted from Weiner MF, Garrett R, Bret ME: "Neuropsychiatric Assessment and Diagnosis," in *The American Psychiatric Publishing Textbook of Alzheimer Disease and Other Dementias.* Edited by Weiner MF, Lipton AM. Washington, DC, American Psychiatric Publishing, 2009, pp. 39–70. Copyright 2009, American Psychiatric Publishing. Used with permission.

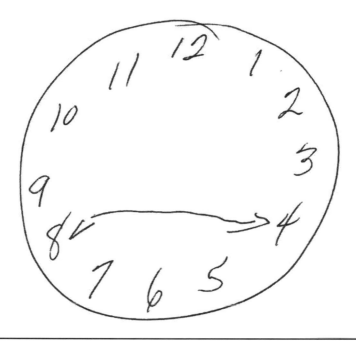

Figure 1–4. Clock drawn by early Alzheimer disease patient, Mini-Mental State Examination score=27.
Source. Reprinted from Weiner MF, Garrett R, Bret ME: "Neuropsychiatric Assessment and Diagnosis," in *The American Psychiatric Publishing Textbook of Alzheimer Disease and Other Dementias.* Edited by Weiner MF, Lipton AM. Washington, DC, American Psychiatric Publishing, 2009, pp. 39–70. Copyright 2009, American Psychiatric Publishing. Used with permission.

Because it involves planning, sequencing, and abstract reasoning, the Clock Drawing Test is a simple means to detect executive dysfunction (Nolan and Mohs 1994). The subject is presented with a blank page and asked to draw the face of a clock and to place the numbers in the correct positions. After drawing a circle and placing the numbers, the subject is asked to draw in the hands indicating the time as 20 minutes after 8. Scoring is as follows: 1 point for drawing a closed circle, 1 point for placing numbers correctly, 1 point for including all correct numbers, and 1 point for placing the hands in the correct positions. There is no cutoff score, but any score <4 raises the suspicion of executive impairment. Distortions due to tremor are disregarded. Figures 1–4 and 1–5 show

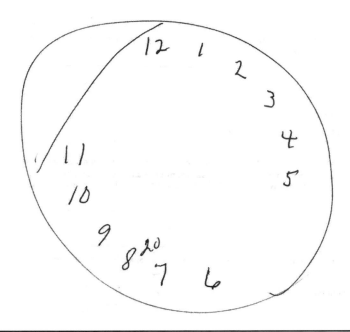

Figure 1–5.   Clock drawn by early Alzheimer disease patient, Mini-Mental State Examination score = 28.

Source.   Reprinted from Weiner MF, Garrett R, Bret ME: "Neuropsychiatric Assessment and Diagnosis," in *The American Psychiatric Publishing Textbook of Alzheimer Disease and Other Dementias.* Edited by Weiner MF, Lipton AM. Washington, DC, American Psychiatric Publishing, 2009, pp. 39–70. Copyright 2009, American Psychiatric Publishing. Used with permission.

deficits in persons diagnosed clinically with Alzheimer disease whose MMSE scores were within the normal range for their age. Figure 1–4 shows early impairment of clock drawing in a person with early Alzheimer disease who scored 27 points on the MMSE. Figure 1–5 shows the clock drawn by a person with early Alzheimer disease who scored 28 on the MMSE.

The Montreal Cognitive Assessment (MoCA; Nasreddine et al. 2005) is a more sensitive instrument than the MMSE. It requires about 15 minutes to administer. The MoCA samples executive function in addition to other cognitive domains and was specifically designed to detect MCI. The score range is 0–30 (with a suggested cutoff of <27 points for detection of MCI). The instrument may be downloaded free from www.mocatest.org.

Readers interested in other scales for quantifying noncognitive aspects of dementia are referred to the book by Burns et al. (1999).

Key Clinical Points

- Cognitive impairment is detected from history and mental status examination, not from laboratory tests.

- Neuropsychiatric symptoms—for example, behavioral, emotional, vegetative, ideational, and perceptual disturbances—are regular components of cognitive disorders.

- Assessment of language can help greatly in the differential diagnosis of cognitive disorders.

- Instruments, such as the Mini-Mental State Examination, Clock Drawing Test, and Montreal Cognitive Assessment, are available to quantify cognitive impairment.

References

Alexopoulos GS, Meyers BS, Young RC: The course of geriatric depression with "reversible dementia": a controlled study. Am J Psychiatry 150:1693–1699, 1993

American Psychiatric Association: Diagnostic and Statistical Manual of Mental Disorders, 4th Edition. Washington, DC, American Psychiatric Association, 1994

American Psychiatric Association: Diagnostic and Statistical Manual of Mental Disorders, 4th Edition, Text Revision. Washington, DC, American Psychiatric Association, 2000

Angelino AF, Treisman GJ: Evidence-informed assessment and treatment of depression in HCV and interferon-treated patients. Int Rev Psychiatry 17:471–476, 2006

Biedler A, Juckenhöfel S, Larsen R, et al: Postoperative cognition disorders in elderly patients: results of the "International Study of Postoperative Cognitive Dysfunction (ISPOCD 1)" [in German]. Anaesthesist 48:884–895, 1999

Bryson GL, Wyand A: Evidence-based clinical update: general anesthesia and the risk of delirium and postoperative cognitive dysfunction. Can J Anaesth 53:669–677, 2006

Budson AE, Price BH: Memory dysfunction. N Engl J Med 352:692–699, 2005

Burns A, Lawlor B, Craig S: Assessment Scales in Old Age Psychiatry. London, Martin Dunitz, 1999

Carney CP, Jones L, Woolson RF, et al: Relationship between depression and pancreatic cancer in the general population. Psychosom Med 65:884–888, 2003

Crum RM, Anthony JC, Bassett SS, et al: Population-based norms for the Mini-Mental State Examination by age and educational level. JAMA 269:2386–2391, 1993

Dijkstra JB, Houx PJ, Jolles J: Cognition after major surgery in the elderly: test performance and complaints. Br J Anaesth 82:867–874, 1999

Drachman DA, Leavitt J: Memory impairment in the aged: storage versus retrieval deficit. J Exp Psychol 93:302–308, 1972

Duppils GS, Wikblad K: Acute confusional states in patients undergoing hip surgery: a prospective observation study. Gerontology 46:36–43, 2000

Federal Interagency Forum on Aging-Related Statistics: Older Americans 2000: Key Indicators of Well-Being. Washington, DC, Government Printing Office, 2000

Folstein MF, Folstein SE, McHugh PR: "Mini-mental state": a practical method for grading the cognitive state of patients for the clinician. J Psychiatr Res 12:189–198, 1975

Goldin S, MacDonald JE: The Ganser state. J Ment Sci 101:267–280, 1955

Goodglass H, Kaplan E: The Assessment of Aphasia and Related Disorders. Philadelphia, PA, Lea & Febiger, 1972

Green MJ: Cognitive impairment and functional outcome in schizophrenia and bipolar disorder. J Clin Psychiatry 67 (suppl 9):3–8, 2006

Greenwald BS, Kramer-Ginsberg E, Marin DB, et al: Dementia with coexistent major depression. Am J Psychiatry 146:1472–1478, 1989

Gunstad J, Paul RH, Brickman AM, et al: Patterns of cognitive performance in middle-aged and older adults. J Geriatr Psychiatry Neurol 19:59–64, 2006

Hedden T, Gabrieli JD: Healthy and pathological processes in adult development: new evidence from neuroimaging of the aging brain. Curr Opin Neurol 18:740–747, 2005

Hepple J: Conversion pseudodementia in older people: a descriptive case series. Int J Geriat Psychiatry 19:961–967, 2004

Heron EA, Kritchevsky M, Delis DC: Neuropsychological presentation of Ganser symptoms. J Clin Exp Neuropsychol 13:656–666, 1991

Katzman R: Diagnosis and management of dementia, in Principles of Geriatric Neurology. Edited by Katzman R, Rowe JW. Philadelphia, PA, FA Davis, 1992, pp 167–206

Keefe RSE, Eesley CE: Neurocognitive impairments, in The American Psychiatric Publishing Textbook of Schizophrenia. Edited by Lieberman JA, Stroup TS, Perkins DO. Washington, DC, American Psychiatric Publishing, 2006, pp 245–260

Kertesz A, Munoz D: Primary progressive aphasia and Pick's complex, J Neurol Sci 206:97–107, 2003

McDonald WM, Richard IH, DeLong MR: Prevalence, etiology, and treatment of depression in Parkinson's disease. Biol Psychiatry 54:363–375, 2003

Nasreddine ZS, Phillips NA, Bédirian V, et al: The Montreal Cognitive Assessment, MoCA: a brief screening tool for mild cognitive impairment. J Am Geriatr Soc 53:695–699, 2005

Nebes RD, Pollock BG, Houck PR, et al: Persistence of cognitive impairment in geriatric patients following antidepressant treatment: a randomized, double-blind clinical trial with nortriptyline and paroxetine. J Psychiatr Res 37:99–108, 2003

Nolan KA, Mohs RC: Screening for dementia in family practice, in Alzheimer's Disease: A Guide to Practical Management, Part II. Edited by Richter RW, Blass JP. St Louis, MO, Mosby–Year Book, 1994, pp 81–95

Oliver C, Crayton L, Holland A, et al: A four-year prospective study of age-related cognitive change in adults with Down's syndrome. Psychol Med 28:1365–1377, 1998

Persson J, Sylvester CY, Nelson JK, et al: Selection requirements during verb generation: differential recruitment in older and younger adults. Neuroimage 23:1382–1390, 2004

Petersen RC, Smith G, Kokmen E, et al: Memory function in normal aging. Neurology 42:396–401, 1992

Petersen RC, Smith GE, Waring SC, et al: Aging, memory, and mild cognitive impairment. Int Psychogeriatr 9 (suppl 1):65–69, 1997

Petersen RC, Parisi JE, Dickson DW, et al: Neuropathologic features of amnestic mild cognitive impairment. Arch Neurol 63:665–672, 2006

Robinson RG: Poststroke depression: prevalence, diagnosis, treatment, and disease progression. Biol Psychiatry 54:376–387, 2003

Snowdon J, Shah A, Halliday G: Severe domestic squalor: a review. Int Psychogeriatr 19:37–51, 2007

Squire LR: Declarative and nondeclarative memory: multiple brain systems supporting learning and memory. J Cogn Neurosci 4:231–243, 1992

Sternberg DE, Jarvik ME: Memory functions in depression: improvement with antidepressant medication. Arch Gen Psychiatry 33:219–224, 1976

Tabert MH, Manley JJ, Liu X, et al: Neuropsychological prediction of conversion to Alzheimer disease in patients with mild cognitive impairment. Arch Gen Psychiatry 63:916–924, 2006

van Munster BC, Korevaar J, Zwinderman AH, et al: The association between delirium and the apolipoprotein E epsilon 4 allele: new study results and a meta-analysis. Am J Geriatr Psychiatry 17:856–862, 2009

Webster R, Holroyd S: Prevalence of psychotic symptoms in delirium. Psychosomatics 41:519–522, 2000

Weiner MF, Hynan LS, Rossetti H, et al: Luria's three-step test: what is it and what does it tell us? Int Psychogeriatr May 4, 2011 (Epub ahead of print)

Wenk GL: Functional neuroanatomy of learning and memory, in Neurobiology of Mental Illness. Edited by Charney DS, Nestler EJ, Bunney BS. New York, Oxford University Press, 1999

Zola-Morgan S, Squire LR, Amaral DG: Human amnesia and the medial temporal region: enduring memory impairment following a bilateral lesion limited to field CA1 of the hippocampus. J Neurosci 6:2950–2967, 1986

Further Reading

Blazer DG, Steffens DC: The American Psychiatric Publishing Textbook of Geriatric Psychiatry. Washington, DC, American Psychiatric Publishing, 2009

Cummings JL, Mega M: Neuropsychiatry and Behavioral Neuroscience. New York, Oxford University Press, 2003

Miller BL, Cummings JL: The Human Frontal Lobes: Functions and Disorders, 2nd Edition. New York, Guilford, 2006

2

Medical and Neurological Evaluation and Diagnosis

Anne M. Lipton, M.D., Ph.D.

Craig D. Rubin, M.D.

The development of subjective or objective cognitive impairment or the sudden worsening of cognitive impairment or behavior in a person with known dementia is an indication for medical evaluation. Important elements of such an evaluation are summarized in Table 2–1. Additional studies used for selected patients are listed in Table 2–2. For each patient, the physician uses clinical judgment to tailor the assessment, especially to identify reversible or partially reversible causes of cognitive dysfunction, including depression, medications, and hypothyroidism.

47

Table 2–1. Medical evaluation of cognitive dysfunction

History and physical examination

Neurological examination

Mental status examination

    Attention and concentration, recent and remote memory, language, executive functioning, and visuospatial skills

    Mini-Mental State Examination or comparable objective screening measure

    Assessment of mood

Blood tests

    Blood chemistries: electrolytes, blood urea nitrogen, creatinine, glucose, and liver function tests

    Complete blood count and differential

    Folate

    Homocysteine

    Lipid profile

    Thyroid-stimulating hormone

    Vitamin B_{12} level

    Serological tests for syphilis (rapid plasma reagin and treponemal tests), if indicated

Computed tomography (CT) or magnetic resonance imaging (MRI) of the brain

Setting

The medical and neurological evaluation of persons with cognitive impairment is generally performed in an outpatient setting. Hospitalization is required only when behavioral symptoms make outpatient evaluation impossible or when it is suspected that an emergency medical or surgical procedure might be needed. Otherwise, hospitalization may actually have transient deleterious effects, because some individuals become more confused in a hospital environment. In fact, cognitive impairment is an independent risk factor for developing in-hospital delirium.

History

The diagnostic process begins with history taking, including obtaining information from a person with close knowledge of the patient, an accurate accounting of all medications and supplements, and a review of medical records.

Table 2–2.   Medical evaluation of cognitive dysfunction: additional measures

Neuropsychological testing

Blood tests

Antinuclear antibodies

Calcium

Ceruloplasmin

DNA studies: presenilin 1, CAG repeats, ataxia profile

Erythrocyte sedimentation rate

HIV tests

Liver function tests

Magnesium

Methylmalonic acid

Paraneoplastic antibodies (anti-Hu, anti-MaTa, anti-Ri, anti-Yo)

Porphyrins

Vasculitis workup: protein C and S activity, activated protein C resistance, antithrombin III, factor V Leiden, lupus anticoagulant, prothrombin 20201A

Lumbar puncture

Routine studies

Cell count and differential

Total protein

Glucose

VDRL (Venereal Disease Research Laboratory) test

Gram stain

Bacterial culture

Additional studies

Amyloid-beta peptide 42 ($A\beta_{42}$) and tau protein concentrations

Acid-fast bacillus stain and culture

Cryptococcal antigen

Cytology

Fungal culture

Table 2–2.   Medical evaluation of cognitive dysfunction: additional measures *(continued)*

Lumbar puncture *(continued)*

Additional studies *(continued)*

Immunoglobulin G index/synthesis rate

Lyme titer or polymerase chain reaction (PCR)

Oligoclonal bands

Viral tests: titers and PCR (cytomegalovirus, herpes simplex, varicella zoster)

14-3-3 protein

Whipple antibody by PCR

Urine tests

Urinalysis

24-hour urine copper

24-hour urine heavy metals

24-hour urine porphyrins

Toxicology screen

Electroencephalogram

Cisternogram

Arteriography (invasive or noninvasive)

Single-photon emission computed tomography (SPECT)

Positron emission tomography (PET)

The history of the present illness should be gathered with regard to the patient's and family's chief current concern, the first cognitive and/or behavioral problem(s) noted, the onset and course of the problem(s), and other problems that may have developed. The patient's age, level of education, current or prior occupation, and baseline functioning are important.

The onset of symptoms guides evaluation and diagnosis. An acute onset (minutes or hours) suggests delirium and a large differential diagnosis that includes infectious, toxic/metabolic, medication side-effect, vascular, traumatic, psychiatric, and multifactorial causes. Subacute onset (over days to weeks) suggests infectious, toxic/metabolic, or neoplastic origin. A gradual progressive decline over months to years is more typical of degenerative disorders.

Dating the onset of cognitive or behavioral difficulties is often difficult. The "unmasking" of chronic cognitive impairment may be perceived as an acute decline in cognition and function when a spouse who has been compensating for a patient dies or leaves the home for other reasons. A family may also be unaware of any significant changes until a loved one is hospitalized for a medical illness or a surgical procedure. The combination of an unfamiliar environment and a medical illness or a surgical procedure often unmasks preexisting dementia and may also precipitate delirium in a person with cognitive impairment. Therefore, it is important to reevaluate the person for cognitive impairment once a delirium has resolved.

Symptomatic improvement is associated with trauma, acute vascular disorders, and acute toxic and metabolic disorders. Fluctuations in cognitive dysfunction may occur more commonly in certain dementing illnesses, such as dementia with Lewy bodies. In most dementing illnesses, cognitive impairment fluctuates, depending on the complexity of the environment, emotional strain, fatigue, general physical health, and time of day. Symptoms are frequently worse in the evenings.

Frequently, the first symptoms noted in a dementing illness are loss of initiative and loss of interest in activities that were formerly pleasurable. Individuals with impaired frontal lobe function may show apathy and/or disinhibition. Suspiciousness and irritability may accompany early dementing illness, as may depression or elation and grandiosity. Vivid hallucinations are frequent in dementia with Lewy bodies. Tactile hallucinations and illusions are common in delirium. Auditory hallucinations in individuals with dementia tend to be of familiar others speaking or music playing, whereas accusatory or threatening voices that speak through the radio or television are more characteristic of schizophrenia. Sleepwalking and rapid eye movement (REM) sleep behavior disorder may precede the onset of synucleinopathies such as Parkinson disease and dementia with Lewy bodies (see Chapter 8, "Dementia With Lewy Bodies and Other Synucleinopathies").

Neurological symptoms often suggest specific dementia diagnoses. Such symptoms may include loss of consciousness, seizures, loss of coordination, gait and balance problems, movement disorders, weakness (generalized or localized), impairment of vision or hearing, and other cranial nerve dysfunction. Seizures should always be considered in the differential diagnosis of cognitive dysfunction. Partial complex seizures can cause intermittent behavioral disruption, which is often, but not always, accompanied by motor stereotypy and postictal sleepiness. Seizures may point to a primary seizure disorder or to other conditions, such as neoplasm, in which seizures are secondary. Gait apraxia and early urinary incontinence are associated with normal-pressure hydrocephalus. The combination of dysarthria and paralysis of gaze suggests progressive supranuclear palsy. Unilateral limb apraxia suggests corticobasal ganglionic degeneration or frontotemporal dementia. Bradykinesia may indicate depression, early Parkinson disease, or another subcortical process. Lack of coordination and sensory and cranial nerve symptoms may indicate multiple sclerosis or progressive supranuclear palsy. Choreiform movements accompany Wilson disease and Huntington disease, whereas myoclonic jerks accompany Creutzfeldt-Jakob disease (CJD) and mid- to late-stage Alzheimer disease. Lateralized abnormalities of strength, tone, reflexes, or sensation suggest a possible vascular origin. Visual field deficits point to possible vascular or neoplastic disease, whereas unilateral hearing loss raises a concern for possible neoplasm.

A personal or family history of a disease or disorder may be associated with cognitive decline. Diabetes, hypertension, strokes, hypercholesterolemia, heart disease, and signs of generalized atherosclerosis are risk factors for vascular dementia. Severe renal or hepatic disease may produce metabolic encephalopathy. HIV seropositivity raises the possibility of direct effects of the virus on the brain or an opportunistic brain infection. Huntington and Wilson diseases exemplify familial diseases associated with dementia. Alzheimer disease rarely occurs as an autosomal dominant familial disease. Nearly half of frontotemporal dementias may be hereditary (Chow et al. 1999).

Many medications can impair cognitive function, including anticholinergic agents (including some medications for bladder incontinence), diphenhydramine (a frequent ingredient in over-the-counter sleep aids), benzodiazepine hypnotics and tranquilizers, barbiturates, anticonvulsants, propranolol, and cardiac glycosides. Episodes of confusion in persons with porphyria may be induced by various medications, including barbiturates and benzodiazepines.

History of alcohol abuse may point to the origin of an amnestic disorder or dementia, especially in patients who have had repeated episodes of delirium tremens. Other substance abuse may also cause cognitive impairment.

Environmental toxins, such as arsenic, mercury, lead, organic solvents, and organophosphate insecticides, can produce encephalopathies, usually accompanied by severe systemic symptoms.

Physical Examination

Funduscopic examination may reveal optic atrophy in the case of multiple sclerosis or papilledema in the case of increased intracranial pressure such as that caused by a tumor. Cardiovascular examination may demonstrate an irregular rhythm consistent with atrial fibrillation and increased risk for stroke. Carotid bruits may be an indicator of stenosis. Abdominal examination may reveal hepatomegaly. Examination of the skin and extremities may reveal signs of vasculitis such as petechiae.

Neurological Examination

Cranial Nerves

Cranial nerve examination may include assessment of olfaction, but the relationship of olfactory deficits to dementing illness remains controversial. Although the wide consensus is that olfactory deficits occur in Alzheimer disease and Parkinson disease (Mesholam et al. 1998), such deficits also occur in elders without dementing illness. Anosmia of sudden onset may point to a significant head injury.

Visual and auditory acuity are important to test, because sensory impairment may influence mental status testing. Pupillary abnormalities occur with neurosyphilis but may also result from cataract surgery. The typical Argyll Robertson pupil seen with neurosyphilis is small, irregular, and reactive to accommodation but not to light. Retinal examination may reveal damage from long-standing hypertension or diabetes. Impairment of gaze in progressive supranuclear palsy usually affects downward gaze first, then upward gaze, and finally horizontal gaze.

Asymmetry of the facial muscles in the lower part of the face occurs with an upper motor neuron lesion such as a stroke or tumor. Weakness of muscles (e.g., tongue, sternocleidomastoid, trapezius) supplied by other cranial nerves and/or altered facial sensation may also suggest a stroke.

Motor System

Patients are assessed for muscle bulk, tone, and strength, as well as for any apraxia or abnormal involuntary movements, such as tremor, dyskinesia, or chorea. Increased resistance to passive movement (rigidity) is common as dementia progresses. The occurrence of rigidity early in the course of a dementing illness may indicate a parkinsonian syndrome, especially when accompanied by tremor or other parkinsonian symptoms. Clonus may be demonstrable in patients with upper motor neuron damage due to a stroke or spinal damage. Myoclonus—a lightning-like jerk of a limb, limbs, or the entire body—may be induced by testing reflexes (reflex myoclonus) or by suddenly startling the patient (startle reflex), such as by a loud noise. Myoclonus in the setting of rapidly progressive dementia should raise the possibility of CJD, but myoclonus may occur later in the course of other dementias, such as Alzheimer disease and Lewy body disease.

Parkinsonism

Bradykinesia, resting tremor, rigidity, and postural instability are the cardinal signs of idiopathic Parkinson disease. The presence of two or three but not all of these signs suggests secondary parkinsonism, such as medication-induced parkinsonism, or Parkinson-plus syndromes such as Lewy body disease. Other parkinsonian features that may be seen in Parkinson disease and related syndromes include restriction of extraocular movements, masklike facies, hypophonia, dysarthria, dysphagia, collapsing movements, micrographia, stooped posture, slow gait, turning en bloc, festinating gait, and decreased arm swing with walking. Consideration should be given, especially in elderly patients, to other factors such as muscle deconditioning and medications that may cause or contribute to some of these symptoms.

Sensation

Vibration sense in the lower extremities is frequently reduced in the elderly, but position sense is not. Sensory neuropathies, which are characterized by loss of vibratory and pinprick sensation in the periphery and are greatest distally, occur in individuals with hypothyroidism, significant alcohol use, diabetes, syphilis, and vitamin B_{12} deficiency. In the case of the tabes dorsalis syndrome of neurosyphilis, both vibratory and position sense are frequently impaired due to involvement of the dorsal columns.

Reflexes

Deep tendon reflexes are generally reduced in sensory neuropathy. Increased deep tendon reflexes may accompany the sensory neuropathy of vitamin B_{12} deficiency. Asymmetric reflexes and the presence of a plantar extensor response (Babinski reflex) suggest upper motor neuron pathology. Frontal release signs, also called frontal reflexes or primitive reflexes (grasp, palmomental, rooting, snout, sucking), may be seen even in healthy elderly persons. These signs are therefore relatively nonspecific, except when seen in younger adult patients and in the context of other frontal abnormalities on neurological or mental status examination.

Gait and Posture

Gait tends to slow with aging, and tandem walking may be difficult for elders. The cautious or "senile" gait of older persons is characterized by a narrow or slightly wide base, short stride length, and en bloc turning. Gait apraxia or "magnetic" gait, in which a patient has difficulty initiating steps, raises the possibility of normal-pressure hydrocephalus.

Laboratory Studies

Blood

For the clinical evaluation of dementia, the Quality Standards Subcommittee of the American Academy of Neurology (Knopman et al. 2001) recommends routine blood tests, including serum electrolytes; glucose, blood urea nitrogen/creatinine, folate, and vitamin B_{12} concentrations; and thyroid-stimulating hormone. Syphilis testing is recommended only for clinical suspicion of neurosyphilis.

Low-normal levels of vitamin B_{12} (<400 pg/mL) have been associated with neuropsychiatric symptoms, so levels in this range may indicate a need for supplementation, especially in an individual presenting with cognitive deficits. Methylmalonic acid may be checked to help decide the question of supplementation and whether folate should also be added, as levels are elevated in vitamin B_{12} deficiency but not folate deficiency. Factors leading to low B_{12} levels also raise levels of methylmalonic acid and homocysteine. Because elevated homocysteine level (above 15 μmol/L) is associated with risk for vascular disease, low or low-normal B_{12} or methylmalonic acid level above 950 nmol/L can be treated with oral cobalamin supplements.

A lipid profile is advisable because hypercholesterolemia is an independent and treatable risk factor for cerebrovascular disease.

Serum ceruloplasmin and 24-hour urinary copper are determined in possible cases of Wilson disease, as in a young person (age <40 years) presenting with cognitive impairment. It is also necessary to measure 24-hour urine copper output because serum ceruloplasmin may be low or normal in a person with Wilson disease.

If there is a suspicion of covert or unreported drug use or of exposure to toxins such as lead or mercury, appropriate toxicological testing may be performed. When indicated, serum levels of medications that produce confusion (including digitalis, anticonvulsants, and lithium) may be useful.

Urine

A urinary tract infection may cause confusion and pychosis in elderly patients and patients with dementia. Special urine studies (see Table 2–2) may be indicated in individuals with suspected exposure to heavy metals, substance abuse, Wilson disease (see subsection "Blood" above), or porphyria.

Spinal Fluid

Routine use of lumbar puncture is not included in the recommendations of the American Academy of Neurology (Knopman et al. 2001) for evaluation of dementia. However, the procedure is indicated in patients with positive syphilis serology, known or suspected cases of rapidly progressive dementia, HIV/AIDS, or suspected central nervous system infection.

The 14-3-3 protein may be a useful cerebrospinal fluid marker for the diagnosis of CJD. Levels of this protein are high in 95% of patients with sporadic CJD (Zerr et al. 1998), but the sensitivity and specificity of the 14-3-3 protein test vary between the different subtypes of sporadic CJD. The sensitivity of the 14-3-3 test is higher in patients with molecular features of classic sporadic CJD than in patients with the nonclassic CJD subgroups (94% vs. 77%).

Special Diagnostic Procedures

Genetic Markers

Genetic markers are not recommended for routine diagnostic purposes (Knopman et al. 2001) or for asymptomatic persons concerned about the future development of dementing illness. Genetic testing may be appropriate for some asymptomatic persons in selected cases of hereditary dementing illnesses, such as Huntington disease, in which genetic testing can confirm a diagnosis or detect presymptomatic disease. It may also be warranted in some cases of familial early-onset Alzheimer disease with autosomal dominant penetrance. Inheritance of the cholesterol-transporting protein apolipoprotein E4 is associated with late-onset familial and sporadic Alzheimer disease, but this marker cannot be used alone as a diagnostic test or to predict the onset of Alzheimer disease. Therefore, the test is not recommended for asymptomatic persons. However, in persons who meet clinical criteria for Alzheimer disease, the presence of an E4 allele increases the specificity of the diagnosis from 55% to 84% (Mayeux et al. 1998). Multiple genetic loci and genes are associated with inherited frontotemporal lobar degeneration, but genetic testing is available only in research centers.

Neuroimaging

An extensive overview of neuroimaging is presented in Chapter 4. Performing structural neuroimaging, brain magnetic resonance imaging (MRI), or computed tomography (CT) of the head is a guideline recommendation by the American Academy of Neurology (Knopman et al. 2001). Brain MRI is the structural neuroimaging test of choice. It is not necessary to perform brain MRI with contrast medium, but gadolinium may be indicated if the history or examination raises concern about neoplasm or infection. In our experience, structural imaging rarely leads to the discovery of treatable causes for cognitive impairment in persons with slowly progressive cognitive impairment who have normal physical and neurological examinations. Functional neuroimaging, such as positron emission tomography (PET) or single-photon emission computed tomography, may be employed in diagnostic dilemmas. PET has been approved by Medicare as a diagnostic procedure for differentiating frontotemporal dementia from Alzheimer disease.

Radionuclide cisternography is used to differentiate between communicating and noncommunicating hydrocephalus and helps establish the diagnosis of normal-pressure hydrocephalus by demonstrating reflux into the ventricles and delayed pericerebral diffusion.

Other Diagnostic Procedures

Angiography

Intracerebral angiography should be performed for specific indications, such as diagnosis of aneurysms, vascular malformations, occluded arteries and veins, and mass lesions such as hemorrhages, abscesses, and neoplasms. Contrast medium injected percutaneously into a carotid, brachial, or femoral artery allows visualization of the entire circulation of the neck and brain. Risks of this procedure include embolization, as well as arterial spasm and occlusion.

Magnetic resonance and CT angiography, which produce computer-generated images of the major cervical and intracranial arteries, are much more benign and less expensive techniques, but they are somewhat less precise. These techniques involve the intravenous injection of a small amount of contrast material.

Carotid and Transcranial Sonography

Evidence of generalized arteriosclerosis, carotid bruits, transient ischemic attacks, or stroke warrants sonographic investigation of the carotid and intracranial vasculature. Patients with evidence of stroke on history, examination, or neuroimaging are referred for echocardiography to be evaluated for any cardiac source of emboli. Patients with evidence of large-vessel cerebrovascular disease are referred for cerebral angiography. Transcranial Doppler imaging may be performed to image the intracranial vasculature, including the circle of Willis.

Electroencephalography

The electroencephalogram (EEG) is of limited value in the evaluation of cognitive impairment. Electroencephalographic findings in Alzheimer disease include slowing of the posterior dominant rhythm, an increase in diffuse slow (theta or delta) activity, and generalized bursts of slow activity, but none of these findings is specific or sensitive for Alzheimer disease. Most persons with severe to moderate Alzheimer disease have such electroencephalographic abnormalities, reflecting the degree of impairment of cortical function. However, the EEG is often normal early in the illness (Markand 1990).

Most persons with frontotemporal dementia (Pick disease) have normal EEGs. Patients with Huntington disease typically have low voltage (Robinson et al. 1994), but this pattern is neither sensitive nor specific. The presence of triphasic waves frequently indicates a delirium due to toxic or metabolic disorders (Engel and Romano 1959).

Electroencephalography can be useful in the diagnosis of patients with rapidly progressive cognitive deterioration in whom CJD is considered in the differential.

In persons with CJD, the electroencephalographic pattern is distinctive. In the initial phase of the illness, electroencephalographic changes consist of a progressive disorganization of background rhythms and increased amounts of generalized slow (theta-delta) activity. As the disease progresses, the EEG is characterized by periodic, bilaterally synchronous, sharply contoured biphasic and triphasic waves, which appear at irregular intervals of one or two per second (Brenner 1999). Similar electroencephalographic findings have been reported in rare cases of lithium intoxication, baclofen-associated encephalopathy, myoencephalopathy ragged–red fiber disease, and HIV encephalopathy (Brenner 1999).

Electroencephalographic studies are most widely performed in the evaluation of cognitively impaired persons who appear to have epileptic seizures. Several studies indicate that epilepsy complicates Alzheimer disease. Amatniek et al. (2006) found an 8% cumulative incidence of seizures over 7 years. The diagnosis of Alzheimer disease or other dementia increases the risk of unprovoked seizures approximately sixfold (Hesdorffer et al. 1996). However, persons with dementing illness are also at high risk for other paroxysmal events that mimic epileptic seizures, including transient ischemic attacks, syncopal episodes, and acute behavioral disturbances. Electroencephalography is often the best way to establish the diagnosis, because the presence of paroxysmal generalized or focal spikes, sharp waves, or sharp and slow wave complexes (interictal epileptiform discharges) are highly predictive of epileptic seizures.

Quantitative electroencephalography and long-latency cortical evoked potentials such as the P300 do not seem to add to clinical diagnostic specificity in the dementing illnesses, although they remain as tools for clinical research. Neither technique is mentioned in published practice parameters for the diagnosis of dementia in the United States (Knopman et al. 2001) or Europe (Waldemar et al. 2007).

Brain Biopsy

Brain biopsy is reserved for situations in which a treatable illness is suspected. We reserve this procedure for suspected autoimmune cerebral vascular disease and infectious brain diseases not diagnosable by spinal fluid studies. Brain biopsy is of limited use in that only small amounts of tissue can be sampled, and the brain areas most affected by diseases such as Alzheimer disease are not readily accessible. Brain biopsy is generally not advisable simply to confirm suspected CJD because of the possibility of transmission to others and the untreatable nature of this illness.

How Much Evaluation Is Enough?

Opinions differ as to what constitutes an adequate laboratory workup for dementing illness. The Canadian guidelines (Mohr et al. 1995) suggest that blood urea nitrogen, vitamin B_{12}, folic acid, serologic test for syphilis, urinalysis, and erythrocyte sedimentation rate *not* be performed unless indicated by history or physical examination. They also suggest neuroimaging only if patients are younger than 60 years, or if there is use of anticoagulants or a history of bleeding disorder, recent head trauma, cancers that metastasize to brain, unexplained neurological symptoms, rapid progress of disease, dementia duration of less than 2 years, or urinary incontinence and gait disorder suggestive of normal-pressure hydrocephalus. As noted above, the American Academy of Neurology recommendations (Knopman et al. 2001) include routine blood tests such as serum electrolytes; glucose, blood urea nitrogen/creatinine, folate, and vitamin B_{12} concentrations; and thyroid function. Of these tests, blood urea nitrogen, creatinine, and vitamin B_{12} levels are not recommended on a routine basis by the European Federation of Neurological Societies guidelines (Waldemar et al. 2007). Syphilis serology is recommended only if there is clinical suspicion of neurosyphilis. Structural neuroimaging with CT or MRI is now a guideline recommendation of the American Academy of Neurology (Knopman et al. 2001).

A minimum medical workup for dementia includes a history (with careful scrutiny of medications), physical and neurological examination, mental status examination, brain MRI (preferably) or CT of the head, and some laboratory studies. Routine laboratory tests, such as complete blood count and differential, lipid profile, electrolytes, urea nitrogen, creatinine, and blood glucose, are helpful in identifying underlying medical conditions. Laboratory workup for dementia often includes thyroid-stimulating hormone, vitamin B_{12}, and folate. Erythrocyte sedimentation rate, calcium, magnesium, and liver function tests may be indicated in some cases. Lumbar puncture is indicated if an infectious, inflammatory, or autoimmune disorder is suspected. An EEG should be ordered if epilepsy or CJD is suspected. Functional neuroimaging is important for the differential diagnosis of atypical dementias.

How Often Are Evaluations Indicated?

Brief reevaluations should be done at least yearly, including an interim clinical history, a neurological examination, and mental status testing. Monitoring progression of the illness through history and examination and by noting the response to any treatment may help to confirm the original diagnosis or raise doubt if the typical clinical course and findings are not observed. An unusually fast progression may raise suspicion for an illness such as CJD. Marked improvement may suggest a reversible disease such as depression that may remit or respond to treatment. New focal signs may point to a vascular or neoplastic component. More comprehensive evaluations are indicated when such new findings arise, particularly when a reversible component of cognitive impairment is suspected.

Additional comprehensive evaluations are not indicated when an adequately diagnosed disease process is following its predicted course. A minimum evaluation in these cases includes a medication check and medical examination, including brief mental status testing.

Conclusion

Although differences exist as to the exact procedures used to determine the etiology of cognitive impairment or dementing illness, the medical evaluation of cognitive impairment requires accurate history taking, mental status examination, physical and neurological evaluation, a relatively small number of blood tests, and neuroimaging. Illnesses that progress rapidly or that have an atypical course warrant more comprehensive investigation at a tertiary care center, where investigators have experience with a variety of dementing illnesses. As techniques and treatments evolve, methods such as functional neuroimaging may be used more frequently as a means for early detection and monitoring the course of treatment.

Key Clinical Points

- Potential identification of a reversible dementia etiology is an important reason for clinical evaluation.
- An acute onset suggests delirium rather than dementia.

- Recommended tests for dementia are serum electrolytes; glucose, blood urea nitrogen/creatinine, folate, and vitamin B_{12} concentrations; and thyroid-stimulating hormone.
- Structural neuroimaging is recommended for evaluation of suspected dementing illness.
- Genetic testing is generally not necessary or indicated in clinical evaluation of dementia.

References

Amatniek JC, Hauser WA, DelCastillo-Castaneda C, et al: Incidence and predictors of seizures in patients with Alzheimer's disease. Epilepsia 47:867–872, 2006

Brenner RP: EEG and dementia, in Electroencephalography: Basic Principles, Clinical Applications, and Related Fields. Edited by Niedermeyer E, Lopes da Silva F. Philadelphia, PA, Lippincott Williams & Wilkins, 1999

Chow TW, Miller BL, Hayashi VN, et al: Inheritance of frontotemporal dementia. Arch Neurol 56:817–822, 1999

Engel GE, Romano J: Delirium, a syndrome of cerebral insufficiency. J Chronic Dis 9:260–277, 1959

Hesdorffer DC, Hauser WA, Annegers JF, et al: Dementia and adult-onset unprovoked seizures. Neurology 46:727–730, 1996

Knopman DS, DeKosky ST, Cummings JL, et al: Practice parameter: diagnosis of dementia (an evidence-based review). Report of the Quality Standards Subcommittee of the American Academy of Neurology. Neurology 56:1143–1153, 2001

Markand ON: Organic brain syndromes and dementias, in Current Practice of Clinical Electroencephalography. Edited by Daly DD, Pedley TA. New York, Raven, 1990, pp 401–423

Mayeux R, Saunders AM, Shea S, et al: Utility of the apolipoprotein E genotype in the diagnosis of Alzheimer's disease. N Engl J Med 338:506–511, 1998

Mesholam RI, Moberg PJ Mahr RN, et al: Olfaction in neurodegenerative disease: a meta-analysis of olfactory functioning in Alzheimer's and Parkinson's diseases. Arch Neurol 55:84–90, 1998

Mohr E, Feldman H, Gauthier S: Canadian guidelines for the development of antidementia therapies: a conceptual summary. Can J Neurol Sci 22:62–71, 1995

Robinson DJ, Merskey H, Blume WT, et al: Electroencephalography as an aid in the exclusion of Alzheimer's disease. Arch Neurol 51:280–284, 1994

Waldemar G, Dubois B, Emre M, et al: Recommendations for the diagnosis and management of Alzheimer's disease and other disorders associated with dementia: EFNS guidelines. Eur J Neurol 14:e1–e26, 2007

Zerr I, Bodemer M, Gefeller O, et al: Detection of 14-3-3 protein in the cerebrospinal fluid supports the diagnosis of Creutzfeldt-Jakob disease. Ann Neurol 43:32–40, 1998

Further Reading

Cummings JL: Alzheimer disease. N Engl J Med 351:56–67, 2004

Rubin CD: The primary care of Alzheimer disease. Am J Med Sci 332:314–333, 2006

Selkoe D: Alzheimer disease: mechanistic understanding predicts novel therapies. Ann Intern Med 140:627–638, 2004

Trojanowski QJ: Biological markers for therapeutic trials in Alzheimer's disease. Proceedings of the Biological Markers Working Group: NIA initiative on neuroimaging in Alzheimer's disease. Neurobiol Aging 24:521–536, 2003

3

Neuropsychological Assessment

C. Munro Cullum, Ph.D., A.B.P.P.

Laura H. Lacritz, Ph.D., A.B.P.P.

Neuropsychological evaluation is often an important component of a dementia workup. In addition to characterizing level of cognitive functioning, neuropsychological assessment provides quantitative and qualitative information regarding specific cognitive strengths and weaknesses and enables comparison of cognitive patterns across disorders to assist with differential diagnosis. Serial testing extends the utility of baseline/diagnostic cognitive assessment by tracking areas of cognitive change over time, charting rate of progression, and aiding in treatment planning and in the making of recommendations for behavioral and environmental adaptations.

Table 3–1. Cognitive declines associated with aging

Speed of mental processing

New learning/episodic memory

Recall of details

Executive functioning

Visuospatial functioning

Word finding ability

Effect of Aging on Cognitive Function

In cross-sectional studies, many cognitive functions show lower performances with advancing age (see Table 3–1). However, so-called crystallized verbal abilities, such as vocabulary skills, fund of knowledge, and sight-word reading, do not deteriorate much, if at all, with age, and thus are often used in helping to estimate long-standing or premorbid levels of function (Salthouse 2010).

Comprehensive Neuropsychological Evaluation for Dementia

The comprehensive neuropsychological evaluation assesses multiple cognitive domains and abilities that are interpreted within the framework of an individual's life context and in relation to norm-referenced standard scores.

The Referral Question

When assistance with differential diagnosis is the primary purpose, a different group of tests is needed than when the goal of the examination is to document level of cognitive impairment. For example, evaluation of a patient in whom the diagnosis of Alzheimer disease has already been made will often involve less extensive testing than that of a patient who is referred for occasional memory problems at work and in whom the etiology of the problems is unclear. Table 3–2 lists some of the situations in which neuropsychological testing can be most helpful as an adjunctive procedure, and Table 3–3 lists referral situations that are more difficult to address from a neuropsychological perspective.

Table 3–2.   Typical clinical issues addressed by neuropsychology

Detect subtle deficits (particularly in high-functioning individuals)

Aid in differential diagnosis of dementia

Characterize pattern of function: localization, lateralization, multifocal, diffuse

Characterize cognitive strengths and weaknesses (help identify and develop appropriate compensatory strategies)

Assist in designing intervention strategies to help optimize patient functioning

Quantify preintervention to postintervention changes (medication trial)

Identify and assess impact of psychiatric factors on functional abilities

Determine need for rehabilitation services

Determine ability to return to work

Assist with disability determination and/or need for placement

Aid in clinical decision making and recommendations to patients (e.g., issues regarding driving, safely living alone, making independent judgments, need for placement)

Length of the Neuropsychological Examination

Neuropsychological evaluations vary in length, depending on many factors, including the referral question, patient's background (i.e., age and education), and patient's level of functioning. Brief screening batteries may be used to detect or rule out severe cognitive impairment, but more detailed examinations are typically needed to thoroughly address differential diagnostic issues and assist with recommendations for everyday living. Some evaluations may take less than an hour, but most routine examinations of persons with suspected dementing illness require several hours of testing in addition to a clinical interview.

Table 3–3.   More-difficult-to-address referral situations

Medically unstable patient

Acute or severe psychosis

Profound cognitive compromise

Precise prediction of clinical course

Differential diagnosis with complicated neuromedical history

Significant comorbid substance abuse

Neuropsychological Testing of Elders

Although many neuropsychological tests are sensitive to dementia, some are more appropriate than others for use with elderly patients and in cases of known cognitive impairment. A variety of brief cognitive screening measures and test batteries have been developed specifically for dementia patients.

Neuropsychological Evaluation of Cognitive Domains

Global Cognitive Status

Global cognitive status is typically assessed by screening tools with several different types of cognitive tasks or items, the scores on which are summed to yield a global score indicating level of impairment. In patients with dementia, brief cognitive screening tests are commonly used in clinical and research settings to provide a quick index of level of overall dementia severity. Such tools are limited, particularly when used in isolation, because of their brevity and insensitivity to subtle cognitive impairments. Table 3–4 lists some of the more commonly used screening tests.

Scores in the normal range on cognitive screening tests do not necessarily rule out dementing illness or cognitive impairment. As with other neurocognitive measures, these tasks are influenced by factors such as age, education, and ethnicity. As a result, careful interpretation and use of appropriate norms are important in the interpretation of findings.

When bedside examination and/or cognitive screening yields suspect findings, or when detailed information regarding cognitive status is desired, formal neuropsychological evaluation is in order.

Cognitive Domains Typically Assessed by the Neuropsychological Evaluation

Table 3–5 presents the cognitive domains typically assessed in a comprehensive neuropsychological evaluation, in addition to commonly used measures for each domain. There are many neuropsychological tests for these various ability areas, including standard clinical measures and even more tests developed for research questions.

Table 3–4. Common dementia screening tests

Mini-Mental State Examination (MMSE; Folstein et al. 1975)

Copyrighted and published by Psychological Assessment Resources

Time: 7 minutes

Most widely used cognitive screening test, available in multiple languages

30 total points (orientation, language, word recall, visuoconstruction)

Age- and education-adjusted norms (Crum et al. 1993; test manual)

Total score <24 suggests impairment (<27 in higher-functioning populations)

Three-word recall plus orientation items most sensitive to dementia

Various modified versions available

Montreal Cognitive Assessment (MoCA; Nasreddine et al. 2005)

Forms available at www.mocatest.org

Time: 5 minutes

Norms available

Available in multiple languages

Items: Trails, cube copy, clock draw, naming, 5-item word list, digit span, repetition, verbal fluency, similarities, orientation

Scoring=30 points total; >25/30=normal

Mini-Cog (Borson et al. 2000)

Time: 3 minutes; useful in multiethnic groups

Items: Three-word recall *(apple, table, penny)*, clock drawing

Scoring=3 points for words, 2 for clock

"Positive screen"=score of 0, or score of 1 or 2 with an abnormal clock

"Negative screen"=score of 1 or 2 with normal clock, or score of 3

Memory Impairment Screen (MIS; Buschke et al. 1999)

Four-word learning with delayed free recall+category cues

Scoring=(2×free recall)+cued recall

Score ≤4 suggests dementia, depending on base rate in population

Normative tables and cut scores included in the article

Table 3–4.   Common dementia screening tests *(continued)*

Mattis Dementia Rating Scale (DRS [Mattis 1988], DRS-2 [Jurica et al. 2002])

Available from Psychological Assessment Resources

A more detailed screening instrument than those listed above

Time: 30–40 minutes

Total score (144 possible points) is summed from the following subscales: Attention, Initiation and Perseveration, Construction, Conceptualization, and Memory

Score: 135–144 = normal; 125–134 = mild; 115–124 = mild to moderate; 105–114 = moderate; 95–104 = moderate to severe; <95 = severe

Intellectual Level

An estimate of global cognitive or intellectual abilities can be used to determine the extent to which current intellectual results reflect a decline from presumed premorbid abilities. In addition, having an estimate of overall intellectual ability is useful in interpreting the results from other measures (e.g., whether memory test results are lower than expected given an individual's intellectual level). Because intellectual assessment tools generally include multiple subtests, the pattern of subtest scores can be used to infer cognitive decline in addition to providing information relevant to specific cognitive strengths and weaknesses. For example, the ability to define words tends to remain intact well into the course of dementia, whereas the ability to interpret proverbs or assemble three-dimensional blocks to replicate patterns may be impaired early on. The Wechsler Adult Intelligence Scale, now in its fourth edition (WAIS-IV; Wechsler 2008), is the most popular means to assess adult intellectual capacity. Verbal and nonverbal/visuoperceptual intellectual abilities are assessed. Even though the utility of IQ scores may be limited and such scores are becoming less frequently used, composite scores can be derived that provide general descriptors regarding overall and specific intellectual or cognitive capacity. Various means of estimating global intellectual status also exist, including the WAIS-IV and short forms of the WAIS-IV (Sattler and Ryan 2009).

Attention and Concentration

In humans, attention and concentration underlie all higher neuropsychological processes. Attention reflects a complex array of activities involving the reticular, thalamic, and frontal systems of the brain (Wilkins et al. 1987). As cognitive

Table 3–5. Cognitive domains typically assessed in neuropsychological evaluation and relevant neuropsychological tests

Global cognitive status
Dementia Rating Scale–2 (Jurica et al. 2002)
Mini-Mental State Examination (Folstein et al. 1975)
Montreal Cognitive Assessment (Nasreddine et al. 2005)

Intellectual ability
Selected subtests from the WAIS-IV[a]

Premorbid intellectual level
Wide Range Achievement Test–4 (Wilkinson and Robertson 2006)

Executive function
Wisconsin Card Sorting Test (Heaton 1981)
Trail Making Test–Part B (Army Individual Test Battery 1944)

Attention/processing speed
Digit Span (WAIS-IV, or Repeatable Battery for the Assessment of Neuropsychological Status; RBANS; Randolph 1998)
Trail Making Test–Part A (Army Individual Test Battery 1944)

Language
Boston Naming Test (Kaplan et al. 1982)
Verbal Fluency: letter (FAS or CFL) and category (animals, fruits) fluency (Spreen and Benton 1977)
Vocabulary subtest (WAIS-IV)

Visuospatial skills
Block Design subtest (WAIS-IV)
Clock Drawing Test (Freedman et al. 2004)
Rey-Osterrieth Complex Figure: copy (Corwin and Bylsma 1993)

Learning and memory
Verbal learning and memory
California Verbal Learning Test, 2nd Edition (Delis et al. 2000)
Hopkins Verbal Learning Test—Revised (Benedict et al. 1998)
Logical Memory subtest (WMS-IV)

Table 3–5.   Cognitive domains typically assessed in neuropsychological evaluation and relevant neuropsychological tests *(continued)*

Learning and memory *(continued)*

Nonverbal memory

　Visual Reproduction subtest (WMS-IV)

　Rey-Osterrieth Complex Figure Test (Visser 1985): immediate and delayed recall

Psychomotor abilities

Finger Tapping Test (Reitan 1969)

Hand dynamometer

Note.　WAIS-IV = Wechsler Adult Intelligence Scale, 4th Edition (Wechsler 2008); WMS-IV = Wechsler Memory Scale, 4th Edition (Wechsler 2009).
[a]Selected subtests are often used to provide an estimate of current intellectual status (e.g., Vocabulary or Information + Block Design or Matrix Reasoning).

processes become impaired, the balance between vigilance to all novel stimuli and the focus on those stimuli most relevant to survival is frequently disrupted. Thus, impaired selective attention in patients with dementia leads them to be either highly distractible or excessively focused. Accompanying problems in sustaining or dividing attention are also usually present.

　Simple attention can be assessed by tasks such as digit span forward, which does not require mental manipulation of information. Patients must have intact basic attention to get through any neuropsychological test. Sustained attention may be evaluated through requiring patients to be vigilant for recurrent target stimuli in a long auditory or visual sequence. Divided attention or sequencing tasks may require patients to alternate responding on a number-letter sequencing test, such as the Trail Making Test (Army Individual Test Battery 1944).

　Because attention is ordered hierarchically, persons with mild impairment may have little difficulty with simple or sustained attention even though they may have difficulty alternating their attentional focus. Those with more severe impairment will often have difficulty with all levels of attentional processing beyond the most basic of tasks. Thus, if impairment is seen at a lower level of attention (e.g., using digit span forward), deficits in higher-order attentional skills will be present and should be factored into the evaluation plan as well as into the interpretation of other test results. If a patient fails to attend adequately to memory test stimuli at the encoding stage, delayed recall of that material cannot be validly tested.

Executive Function

Loss of executive processing abilities, such as organizing, planning, and evaluating one's own problem-solving behavior, is common in dementing illnesses. Executive functions are thought to be mediated primarily by frontal brain systems. Because this set of abilities represents the highest level of cognitive control and planning, executive functions rely heavily on a variety of supportive cognitive skills. Difficulties with planning, reasoning, and inhibition may manifest in many ways, and accurate assessment of this complex set of skills has proven challenging. Most commonly, these abilities are measured by neuropsychological tasks that depend on novel problem-solving skills, such as the Wisconsin Card Sorting Test (Heaton 1981). Other tasks that rely on guided generation, such as letter fluency and the switching of mental sets, are also used in the evaluation of executive functions. Cognitive screening measures and bedside mental status examinations are poor at elucidating executive function impairments, and a history of clear executive function–related problem behaviors may be needed to make inferences in the absence of more detailed testing.

Memory

Memory difficulties are the most common problems reported by persons with dementing illnesses and healthy elders. Memory constitutes a higher-order collection of mental processes that includes the collection, storage, and retrieval of information; it represents the integration of multiple functional brain systems.

Memory involves a number of sequential processes. Information initially enters sensory memory, a short-term storage modality. From sensory memory, information is transmitted to short-term memory (also called primary memory, immediate memory, working memory, and attention span). Short-term memory is a limited-capacity system in which information is maintained by continued attention and rehearsal. Short-term memory can be thought of as lasting briefly (only 20–30 seconds), with stored information replaced by new material unless rehearsal or some other retention strategy is introduced. Transfer of new information into long-term memory begins within the first second of exposure to the stimulus, providing for a 20- to 30-second overlap between short-term and long-term memory. The consolidation of material in long-term memory takes much longer and involves a gradual strengthening of the memory trace over a period of several minutes to several hours. This trace is highly unstable and easily subject to loss, as illustrated by anterograde amnesia in a postconcussive syndrome. Once information has entered long-term memory (of virtually unlimited capacity), it is maintained by repetition or organization through meaning and association.

Memory retrieval is the process of locating and accessing information from long-term storage. Retrieval can direct verbatim access to memory storage traces or access to a general idea or gist of the original material, with final output representing a reconstruction of this idea (Russell 1981). Another important distinction is between recall and recognition. To use an education analogy, free recall is measured by essay tests, whereas recognition memory is evaluated in multiple-choice tests. Problems in recognition memory often relate to faulty storage, but testing in a recognition format may improve performance in patients who have a primary deficit in retrieval. This distinction between free recall and recognition memory performance can be very useful in differentiating the cognitive impairment of depression from that of brain injury or dementing illness. Patients with Alzheimer disease typically exhibit difficulties in both free recall and recognition memory (storage and retrieval problems), whereas depressed patients and normal elders more frequently show only difficulties in free recall (retrieval problems) (Kaszniak et al. 1986); similar distinctions have also been reported between patients with Alzheimer disease and those with subcortical dementias.

Two of the major forms of memory storage are episodic and semantic. *Episodic memory* refers to memories that have been given a temporal and spatial coding (i.e., when and where something occurs, such as the birth of one's first child). *Semantic memory* is a verbally mediated memory that lacks a spatial or temporal context, such as factual knowledge. Both episodic memory and semantic memory are subsumed under the term *declarative memory. Nondeclarative memory,* sometimes called *implicit* or *procedural memory,* involves memory for overlearned skills and automatic perceptual or semantic processes that are not factually oriented.

No single measure assesses all dimensions of memory, and most of the popular clinical memory tests (i.e., recollecting recently presented information) assess declarative memory. Nevertheless, formal memory tests, particularly those assessing verbal memory, better discriminate cognitively impaired persons from normal elders than do simple mental status examinations or language tests. Word lists have proven very useful in the identification and differential diagnosis of memory disorders, because word lists lend themselves to a variety of scores that can be used to characterize the pattern of memory dysfunction (e.g., encoding vs. retrieval deficits). Popular verbal list–learning measures include the California Verbal Learning Test, 2nd Edition (CVLT-II; Delis et al. 2000), the Rey Auditory Verbal Learning Test (RAVLT; Lezak 1983), and the briefer Hopkins Verbal Learning Test—Revised (HVLT-R; Benedict et al. 1998). Such instruments have the advantage of multiple learning trials (vs. one-time exposure to stimuli), adequate length to require secondary (long-term) memory, a delay condition, and a recognition trial. The CVLT-II is unique in that it allows for the assessment and quantification of *how* learning occurs and what types of errors are made during learning and recall. HVLT-R is shorter and has multiple alternate forms.

In contrast to the word list–learning tasks, the Wechsler Memory Scale, now in its fourth edition (WMS-IV; Wechsler 2009), includes a very popular subtest, Logical Memory, which assesses recall for paragraph-length information. Performance on contextual memory tasks such as Logical Memory, in contrast to list-learning tasks, allows for comparison of patients' ability to encode stimuli of different levels of complexity and organization.

Visual memory is often evaluated by presenting a standard figure or set of visual designs to a patient to copy and to later recall following a delay. The Visual Reproduction subtest of the WMS-IV and the Rey-Osterrieth Complex Figure Test (Visser 1985) are examples of commonly used nonverbal memory tests. Differences in visual memory performances have been found as many as 10 years prior to eventual diagnosis when examining longitudinal data from control subjects who ultimately developed dementing illnesses (Kawas et al. 2003). However, older adults show greater variability on nonverbal memory tasks than do their younger counterparts. Thus, although such tasks may be sensitive to abnormal memory function, specificity is sometimes lacking in healthy elderly samples.

Visuospatial Functioning

Visuospatial processes are complex and involve a variety of functional systems in the brain, particularly the right hemisphere. Visuoconstructional functioning is frequently evaluated through use of various standard figure copies and drawings (e.g., clock, cube, cross), with characteristic declines in quality seen as dementia progresses. Drawings by patients with Alzheimer disease often exhibit oversimplification, poor angulation, and impaired perspective. Furthermore, they often display poor planning in their layout and presentation, which may reflect a combination of deficits in visuospatial as well as executive function skills. For example, a combination of deficits may lead to various different errors during clock drawing attempts (see Chapter 1, Figures 1–4 and 1–5). One of the more common neuropsychological measures of visuoconstruction is the WAIS Block Design subtest, which requires patients to assemble three-dimensional cubes to form a pattern matching that of the examiner's model or a drawing. In addition to central brain mechanisms, primary visual impairments and motor deficits may complicate graphomotor constructions by the elderly.

Language

Receptive language involves the comprehension of oral and written communication (see Chapter 1, "Neuropsychiatric Assessment and Diagnosis"). Comprehension deficits may involve misunderstanding of individual words or sentences. Visual comprehension of written material is based on auditory mastery and is also often disturbed when an individual has auditory comprehension deficits. The appreciation of nonverbal components of language, such as prosody and social perception, may also be impaired as part of a dementia syndrome.

Expressive language disturbances can take numerous forms as well. These include disturbances of articulation and word finding; paraphasia; and the loss of grammar, syntax, repetition, verbal fluency, and writing. Speaking requires the ability to articulate individual vowels, consonants, and syllables and to combine them in the appropriate order. To speak a word, one must locate it among the large repository of words previously learned. A person with cognitive impairment may be able to describe the use of an object but not name it. This dysnomia may be assessed through the Boston Naming Test and its derivations (Goodglass and Kaplan 1972; Lansing et al. 1999). *Paraphasia* refers to the production of unintended syllables, sounds, or words, such as substituting *knife* for *night* or *mother* for *woman*. Loss of grammar and syntax can also occur and may manifest as the inability to string more than two or three words together in spontaneous sentences. Similarly, patients may be able to produce spontaneous, normal speech but be unable to repeat words or sentences spoken by others.

Verbal fluency, the ability to produce words and sentences in uninterrupted strings, is affected by numerous factors, including executive dysfunction and dysnomia associated with frontal and temporal lobe lesions. Common fluency tasks include the generation of as many words as possible within a minute that begin with a specified letter or that belong to a specific category such as animals. Patients with Alzheimer disease commonly show deficits in verbal fluency tasks, and a number of studies have suggested relatively greater difficulty in category versus letter fluency (Epker et al. 1999).

Motor Abilities

Motor abilities range from simple functions such as strength and speed to more complex skilled movements (*praxis*). Basic motor deficits occur commonly in vascular and subcortical dementias. Simple motor strength is often assessed through use of a hand dynamometer. Manual speed may be tested through procedures or instruments requiring finger tapping or fine motor dexterity. Losses in motor strength and speed beyond expectations for a person's age and gender deserve further investigation, particularly when lateralized.

Apraxia refers to a disruption of complex skilled movements that does not arise from basic motor difficulties. Patients may be unable to carry out a motor response to command that is easily performed spontaneously (*ideomotor apraxia*). Alternatively, they may be unable to sequence motor acts toward a specific goal (*ideational apraxia*). Although they are one of the features of more advanced dementia, apraxias are uncommon in early Alzheimer disease. Evaluation of praxis often involves instructing the patient to pantomime a series of common activities (e.g., brushing teeth, using a comb) both through verbal command and by imitation, and these activities are scored on sections of tests such as the Boston Diagnostic Aphasia Examination (Goodglass et al. 2001).

Sensory-Perceptual Abilities

Primary sensory impairments are often detected before neuropsychological testing is conducted. Thus, although sensory-perceptual assessment is less often undertaken as part of the neuropsychological evaluation of dementia, a number of standardized tests exist that may be indicated—for example, in cases of suspected cerebrovascular disease, wherein focal sensory and/or motor deficits may be present. Several standardized sensorimotor tasks include measures of basic sensory-perceptual skills (e.g., simple touch, response to double simultaneous stimulation, finger graphesthesia, tactile gnosis, stereognosis).

Personality and Emotion

Clinical interviewing of patients with known or suspected cognitive impairment is sometimes challenging because of their level of cognitive impairment, expressive language deficits, amnesia, lack of insight into internal mood states, apathy, and/or uncooperativeness. The use of standardized clinical psychological tests and specific symptom questionnaires may allow patients to respond through a written, less personal modality and may be highly informative. Instruments such as the Beck Depression Inventory, 2nd Edition (Beck et al. 1996), and the Quick Inventory to Diagnose Depression (Rush et al. 2003) can be used to assess depressive symptoms, and other measures such as the Geriatric Depression Scale (Yesavage et al. 1983) and Cornell Scale for Depression in Dementia (Alexopoulos et al. 1988) have been developed specifically for elders. A careful assessment of physical versus emotional symptoms of depression is important, particularly given some of the physical limitations that may accompany diseases of the elderly. Severe depression may present with cognitive symptoms that should be carefully and systematically evaluated and quantified. The neuropsychological evaluation may be particularly helpful in distinguishing qualitative features of depression from those of dementia (McClintock et al. 2010).

Everyday Functional Abilities

Although the assessment of everyday functional abilities is often beyond the scope of the traditional neuropsychological examination, several standardized measures of instrumental activities of daily living are available for assessment of patients with dementia. Several popular examples are the Instrumental Activities of Daily Living Scale (Lawton and Brody 1969), Independent Living Scales (Loeb 1996), and Daily Activities Questionnaire (Oakley et al. 1993). Such instruments typically rely on caregiver report or require patients to perform tasks analogous to various daily functions, such as dressing, making change, check writing, or dialing a telephone. Although many of these measures can be time-consuming or rely exclusively on caregiver ratings, the Texas Functional Living Scale (Cullum et al. 2001) is a brief, quantitative, performance-based measure of simple everyday skills relevant to the functioning of patients with dementia. It has shown sensitivity to dementia, correlates well with the Mini-Mental State Examination in patients with Alzheimer disease (Weiner et al. 2006), shows improvement in response to acetylcholinesterase inhibitor treatment (Saine et al. 2002), and differentiates dementia patients needing different levels of nursing care (Weiner et al. 2007). Use of such measures can also facilitate a more direct communication of neuropsychological concepts to caregivers in terms of everyday function because these measures employ more tasks with face validity and perhaps ecological validity.

Neuropsychological Screening Batteries for Dementia

Brief Test Batteries for Clinical Settings

Although the tests discussed in the previous section are commonly used in the comprehensive neuropsychological evaluation of persons with known or suspected dementia, a number of briefer test batteries have been developed for use in clinical settings. One such battery is the Repeatable Battery for the Assessment of Neuropsychological Status (Randolph 1998), a 30- to 45-minute screening battery. The Consortium to Establish a Registry for Alzheimer's Disease (CERAD) neuropsychological battery (Morris 1989), developed specifically for persons with dementia, can be completed in 25–30 minutes. The CERAD battery has been used in many studies of dementia, and normative data for older populations are available (Welsh et al.1994). Chandler et al. (2005) developed a total score for the CERAD battery that has shown utility in characterizing patients with dementia and in charting overall progression over time (Rossetti et al. 2010).

Telecognitive Assessment

The availability of traditional face-to-face neuropsychological evaluations may be limited in certain circumstances, such as in rural communities, and a growing body of literature supports the use of videoconferencing in psychiatry (Hilty et al. 2002). Only a handful of studies have explored the feasibility of videoconferencing-based neuropsychological testing, or *telecognitive assessment,* in dementia. Cullum et al. (2006) examined the validity of telecognitive assessment by comparing face-to-face evaluations with those conducted by teleconferencing using a brief battery of standard clinical measures in a sample of 19 subjects with Alzheimer disease and 14 patients with mild cognitive impairment. There were high correlations and little bias between the testing conditions, suggesting feasibility, validity, and reliability of this emerging testing approach.

Interpretation of Neuropsychological Results

Neuropsychological assessment begins with a systematic inquiry into a person's medical and developmental history; language acquisition; school grades, as well as learning problems; military record; occupational history; and acquired insults to the central nervous system. Past psychiatric history and treatment are also important to assess within the context of the onset and progression of current symptoms and presenting complaints. Current medications are also reviewed.

Examination of an individual's performance on a test in comparison with the performance of others in the general population who share demographic similarities provides important comparative reference data that aid interpretation. A great challenge is the development of cross-cultural norms, which is important because cultural and linguistic backgrounds may have a large effect on some tests.

Regardless of the norms used, standard scores (t scores, z scores, percentile ranks, scaled scores, etc.) that are commonly derived from the raw test scores should be used as interpretive guidelines. These are ideally derived from large groups of people free from neuropsychiatric disorders, and application to the individual case may require adjustment. Other factors that come into play when considering the interpretation of standard or raw test scores include obtaining adequate effort from the individual and ensuring that he or she adequately hears and understands the test instructions.

Neuropsychological Profiles in Dementia

Alzheimer Disease

Early-stage Alzheimer disease is typically characterized by progressive impairment of new learning and recent (episodic) memory, although the often subtle nature of its onset, characteristically slow progression, and heterogeneity in behavioral expression may complicate early detection. Delayed recall of verbal material (whether assessed via paragraph or word list recall) has consistently been shown to be particularly sensitive to the types of early memory deficits characteristic of Alzheimer disease (see Table 3–6).

In general, individuals with Alzheimer disease show reduced encoding, consolidation, and storage of new information, as well as rapid forgetting of newly learned material. Careful quantitative as well as qualitative analysis of verbal learning and memory performances often reveals a "prototypical" pattern of findings on measures such as the CVLT-II. As noted in Table 3–6, patients with Alzheimer disease tend to show limited learning, sometimes recalling only the last few items presented, and they make characteristic intrusion errors during learning and recall of words, wherein they often respond with semantically related words rather than target list items. Cuing is less often helpful to these patients and may stimulate additional intrusions. Delayed recognition testing is also impaired, with high numbers of false-positive errors, reflecting the patients' deficits in encoding as well as retrieval. Patterns derived from such results can be used to aid in differential diagnosis, because dementia syndromes may demonstrate different profiles (see Table 3–7).

Following the onset of deterioration of episodic memory, additional cognitive declines are subsequently seen in executive functioning and aspects of language—most notably, prominent word finding difficulties and reduced verbal fluency. Visuospatial impairments are also common, as evidenced by visuoconstructional deficits and loss of direction sense/confusion. Gross visuospatial deficits may be identified by simple cognitive tasks such as clock drawing (Freedman et al. 1994), in which evidence of executive dysfunction may also be observed (e.g., problems setting the hands of the clock to a specified time, stimulus-bound responses).

Vascular Dementia

Considerable overlap exists between the cognitive impairments of Alzheimer disease and vascular dementia (see also Chapter 7, "Vascular Cognitive Disorder"), and the two illnesses may coexist. Despite an overlap in cognitive symptoms, neuropsychological evaluation may nevertheless assist with the diagnosis of vascular dementia through identifying focal neurocognitive impair-

Table 3–6.   Characteristics of memory dysfunction in Alzheimer disease

Impaired encoding (limited learning, decreased organization)

Rapid forgetting

Recency recall (recalling information from the end of a list or paragraph)

Intrusion errors during recall

Impaired recognition

ments, "spotty" neuropsychological profiles (e.g., a mixture of "cortical" and "subcortical" signs), and test results reflecting asymmetries in sensory and/or motor performance. Furthermore, vascular profiles may lack some of the features of the amnestic syndrome of Alzheimer disease. Serial neuropsychological testing can also help to characterize the pattern and trajectory of decline in such patients over time.

Frontotemporal Dementias

Frontotemporal dementias include a variety of disorders, such as behavioral-variant frontotemporal dementia, Pick disease (with or without Pick bodies), corticobasal ganglionic degeneration, nonspecific frontal gliosis, and various tauopathies, in addition to language-variant frontotemporal dementias that include primary progressive aphasia and semantic dementia. Characteristic symptoms include deficits in abstraction, executive function, self-awareness, and social behavior. Neuropsychological evaluation of these patients typically reveals prominent deficits in executive function and cognitive flexibility, in addition to behavioral symptoms that typify frontal lobe syndromes. In language-variant frontotemporal dementias, expressive language deficits in the form of fluent or nonfluent aphasia with marked word finding difficulty or loss of semantic knowledge are typically the first symptoms reported, although executive function impairments may also be present early in the course of the disease. Importantly, the deficits in executive functioning and language are typically more prominent than deficits in memory in this class of disorders, a fact that may assist in differential diagnosis (Neary et al. 1998) (see Table 3–7).

Table 3–7. Verbal learning and memory features in dementia syndromes

	Impaired encoding	Deficient recall	Intrusion errors	Perseveration errors	Impaired recognition
Alzheimer	++	++	++	–	++
Frontotemporal	+	+	–	+	+/–
Vascular	++	+	–	+/–	–
Subcortical	+/–	–	–	–	–
Depression	+/–	+/–	–	–	–

Note. Presence (+) or absence (–) of qualitative memory features on standardized word list–learning tasks.

Subcortical Dementias

Subcortical dementias frequently involve slowing of general information processing and reduced attention, in addition to problems with executive and visuospatial functions. Marked language deficits are characteristically absent, with the exception of reduced verbal fluency, and due to subcortical-cortical disconnections, the pattern of deficits can mimic frontal lobe dysfunction. The memory impairment associated with subcortical dysfunction (at least in milder cases) tends to manifest more as impaired retrieval and memory search mechanisms, because delayed recall testing often reveals some degree of impairment, while performance on cued recall and particularly recognition testing tends to be much better. This pattern suggests that patients are better able to encode and store more information than to spontaneously recall material. Cued recall and recognition testing of episodic memory is therefore critical in differential diagnosis. In cases of severe cognitive impairment, patients with subcortical dementias may be indistinguishable from those with cortical dementia due to the magnitude of their deficits.

Depression

The terms *dementia syndrome of depression* and *pseudodementia* have been used to designate reversible cognitive deficits experienced by some patients with severe depression (Wells 1979). The fact that dementia patients may experience depressive symptoms can complicate attempts to distinguish the functional dementia of depression from structural brain diseases. Individuals with depression sometimes resemble patients with subcortical dysfunction in their slowed information processing and failure to spontaneously employ active learning and memory search strategies (King and Caine 1990). When poor cognitive performance on formal neuropsychological testing has been seen in these patients, several characteristic features or trends have been observed. Attention may be reduced and/or variable across tasks. Depressed patients often show intact memory storage even though retrieval problems may occur, in contrast to individuals with Alzheimer disease, who have both impaired storage and retrieval, as demonstrated by poor performance and errors during recognition memory testing. However, persistence of deficits following recovery from depression may signal a dementing illness, so serial evaluations may be very useful. Neuropsychological patterns of performance can often be used to differentiate Alzheimer disease from cognitive difficulties secondary to depression. For many patients with depression, despite cognitive complaints, performance on formal neuropsychological examination may be normal or only slightly abnormal in effortful tests (McClintock et al. 2010). In cases where some cognitive inefficiencies are apparent, the disorders may coexist, and differential diagnosis may be challenging in a small proportion of patients. Accordingly, serial neuropsychological evaluations may be useful to monitor cognitive and memory abilities over time, because the cognitive difficulties in patients with uncomplicated depression would not be expected to progress.

Conclusion

Neuropsychological evaluation is a standard part of the comprehensive neurodiagnostic evaluation of cognitive concerns. Careful test selection and interpretation yield valuable information regarding the presence or absence of abnormal cognitive decline, can assist with differential diagnosis, and can be used for quantitative tracking of cognitive changes over time. Identifying specific cognitive functions that may be maintained or enhanced by new medications and quantifying treatment response also provide important opportunities for neurocognitive assessment. Obtaining an assessment of an individual's cognitive strengths and weaknesses can assist in treatment planning and providing sound recommendations to patients and their families.

Key Clinical Points

- Neuropsychological testing is the most sensitive means of evaluating cognition.

- Brief bedside tests of memory and cognition are available, but may be unreliable or insensitive, especially for individuals with mild impairments.

- Normal scores on brief cognitive screening tasks may be obtained by patients with mild impairments.

- Normal aging is associated with changes in some but not all cognitive abilities.

- Reference to test norms is important in interpreting neuropsychological test results.

- Patterns of neuropsychological test results may assist in differential diagnosis.

References

Alexopoulos GS, Abrams RC, Young RC, et al: Cornell Scale for Depression in Dementia. Biol Psychiatry 23:271–284, 1988

Army Individual Test Battery: Manual of Directions and Scoring. Washington, DC, War Department, Adjutant General's Office, 1944

Beck AT, Steer RA, Ball R, et al: Comparison of Beck Depression Inventories IA and -II in psychiatric outpatients. J Pers Assess 67:588–597, 1996

Benedict RHB, Schretlen D, Groninger L, et al: Hopkins Verbal Learning Test—Revised: normative data and analysis of inter-form and test-retest reliability. Clin Neuropsychol 12:43–55, 1998

Borson S, Scanlan J, Brush M, et al: The Mini-Cog: a cognitive "vital signs" measure for dementia screening in multi-lingual elderly. Int J Geriatr Psychiatry 15:1021–1027, 2000

Buschke H, Kuslansky G, Katz M, et al: Screening for dementia with the Memory Impairment Screen. Neurology 52:231–238, 1999

Chandler MJ, Lacritz LH, Hynan LS, et al: A total score for the CERAD Neuropsychological battery. Neurology 12:102–106, 2005

Corwin L, Bylsma FW: "Psychological Examination of Traumatic Encephalopathy" by A. Rey and "The Complex Figure Copy Test" by P. A. Osterrieth. The Clinical Neuropsychologist 7:3–21, 1993

Crum RM, Anthony JC, Bassett SS, et al: Population-based norms for the Mini-Mental State Examination by age and education level. JAMA 269:2386–2391, 1993

Cullum CM, Saine K, Chan LD, et al: Performance-based instrument to assess functional capacity in dementia: the Texas Functional Living Scale. Neuropsychiatry Neuropsychol Behav Neurol 14:103–108, 2001

Cullum CM, Weiner MF, Gehrmann H, et al: Feasibility of telecognitive assessment in dementia. Assessment 13:385–390, 2006

Cullum CM, Saine K, Weiner MF: The Texas Functional Living Scale. San Antonio, TX, Psychological Corporation, 2008

Delis DC, Kramer JH, Kaplan E, et al: California Verbal Learning Test, 2nd Edition, Adult Version. San Antonio, TX, Psychological Corporation, 2000

Epker MO, Lacritz LH, Cullum CM: Comparative analysis of qualitative verbal fluency performance in normal elderly and demented populations. J Clin Exp Neuropsychol 21:425–434, 1999

Folstein MF, Folstein SE, McHugh PR: "Mini-mental state": a practical method for grading the cognitive state of patients for the clinician. J Psychiatr Res 12:189–198, 1975

Freedman M, Leach L, Kaplan E, et al: Clock Drawing: A Neuropsychological Analysis. New York, Oxford University Press, 1994

Goodglass H, Kaplan E: The Assessment of Aphasia and Related Disorders. Philadelphia, PA, Lea & Febiger, 1972

Goodglass H, Kaplan E, Barresi B: Boston Diagnostic Aphasia Examination, 3rd Edition. Philadelphia, PA, Lippincott Williams & Wilkins, 2001

Heaton RK: Wisconsin Card Sorting Test Manual. Odessa, FL, Psychological Assessment Resources, 1981

Hilty DM, Luo JS, Morache C, et al: Telepsychiatry: an overview for psychiatrists. CNS Drugs 16:527–548, 2002

Jurica PJ, Leitten CL, Mattis S: Dementia Rating Scale–2: Professional Manual. Lutz, FL, Psychological Assessment Resources, 2002

Kaplan E, Goodglass H, Weintraub S: The Boston Naming Test. Philadelphia, PA, Lea & Febiger, 1982

Kaszniak AW, Poon LW, Riege W: Assessing memory deficits: an information-processing approach, in Handbook for Clinical Memory Assessment of Older Adults. Edited by Poon LW. Washington, DC, American Psychological Association, 1986

Kawas CH, Corrada MM, Brookmeyer R, et al: Visual memory predicts Alzheimer's disease more than a decade before diagnosis. Neurology 60:1089–1093, 2003

King DA, Caine DA: Depression, in Subcortical Dementia. Edited by Cummings JL. New York, Oxford University Press, 1990

Lansing AE, Ivnik RJ, Cullum CM, et al: An empirically derived short form of the Boston Naming Test. Arch Clin Neuropsychol 14:481–487, 1999

Lawton MP, Brody EM: Assessment of older people: self-maintaining and instrumental activities of daily living. Gerontologist 9:179–186, 1969

Lezak MD: Neuropsychological Assessment, 2nd Edition. New York, Oxford University Press, 1983

Loeb PA: Independent Living Scales. San Antonio, TX, Psychological Corporation, 1996

Mattis S: Dementia Rating Scale. Odessa, FL, Psychological Assessment Resources, 1988

McClintock SM, Husain MM, Greer TL, et al: Association between depression severity and neurocognitive function in major depressive disorder: a review and synthesis. Neuropsychology 24:9–34, 2010

Morris JC, Heyman A, Mohs RC, et al: The Consortium to Establish a Registry for Alzheimer's Disease (CERAD), part I: clinical and neuropsychological assessment of Alzheimer's disease. Neurology 39:1159–1165, 1989

Nasreddine ZS, Phillips NA, Bédirian V, et al: The Montreal Cognitive Assessment, MoCA: a brief screening tool for mild cognitive impairment. J Am Geriatr Soc 53:695–699, 2005

Neary D, Snowden JS, Gustafson L, et al: Frontotemporal lobar degeneration: a consensus on clinical diagnostic criteria. Neurology 51:1546–1554, 1998

Oakley F, Sunderland T, Hill JL, et al: A validation study of the Daily Activities Questionnaire: an activities of daily living assessment for people with Alzheimer's disease. J Outcome Meas 3:297–307, 1993

Randolph C: Repeatable Battery for the Assessment of Neuropsychological Status. Lutz, FL, Psychological Assessment Resources, 1998

Reitan RM: Manual for Administration of Neuropsychological Test Batteries for Adults and Children. Indianapolis, IN, Author, 1969

Rossetti HC, Munro Cullum C, Hynan LS, et al: The CERAD neuropsychologic battery total score and the progression of Alzheimer disease. Alzheimer Dis Assoc Disord 24:138–142, 2010

Rush AJ, Trivedi MH, Ibrahim HM, et al: The 16-item Quick Inventory of Depressive Symptomatology (QIDS), Clinician Rating (QIDS-C), and Self-Report (QIDS-SR): a psychometric evaluation in patients with chronic major depression. Biol Psychiatry 54:573–583, 2003

Russell EW: The pathology and clinical examination of memory, in Handbook of Clinical Neuropsychology. Edited by Filskov S, Boll T. New York, Wiley, 1981

Saine K, Cullum CM, Martin-Cook K, et al: Comparison of functional and cognitive donepezil effects in Alzheimer's disease. Int Psychogeriatr 14:181–185, 2002

Salthouse TA: Selective review of cognitive aging. J Int Neuropsychol Soc 16:754–760, 2010

Sattler JM, Ryan JJ: Assessment of the WAIS-IV. San Diego, CA, Jerome M Sattler, 2009

Spreen O, Benton AL: Neurosensory Center Comprehensive Examination for Aphasia. Victoria, Australia, University of Victoria Neuropsychology Laboratory, 1977

Visser RSH: Manual of the Complex Figure Test. Amsterdam, Swets & Zeitlinger, 1985

Wechsler D: Wechsler Adult Intelligence Scale, 4th Edition. San Antonio, TX, Psychological Corporation, 2008

Wechsler D: Wechsler Memory Scale, 4th Edition. San Antonio, TX, Psychological Corporation, 2009

Weiner MF, Gehrmann HR, Hynan LS, et al: Comparison of the test of everyday functional abilities with a direct measure of daily function. Dement Geriatr Cogn Disord 22:83–86, 2006

Weiner MF, Davis B, Martin-Cook K, et al: A direct functional measure to help ascertain optimal level of residential care. Am J Alzheimers Dis Other Demen 22:355–359, 2007

Wells CE: Pseudodementia. Am J Psychiatry 136:895–900, 1979

Welsh KA, Butters N, Mohs RC, et al: The Consortium to Establish a Registry for Alzheimer's Disease (CERAD), part V: a normative study of the neuropsychological battery. Neurology 44:609–614, 1994

Wilkins AJ, Shallice T, McCarthy R: Frontal lesions and sustained attention. Neuropsychologia 25:359–365, 1987

Wilkinson GS, Robertson GJ: Wide Range Achievement Test 4 Professional Manual. Lutz, FL, Psychological Assessment Resources, 2006

Yesavage J, Brink T, Rose T: Development and validation of a geriatric depression screening scale: a preliminary report. J Psychiatr Res 17:37–49, 1983

Further Reading

Attix DK, Welsh-Bohmer: Geriatric Neuropsychology: Assessment and Intervention. New York, Guilford Press, 2005

Morris R, Becker JT: Cognitive Neuropsychology of Alzheimer's Disease. New York, Oxford University Press, 2004

Snyder PJ, Nussbaum PD, Robins DL: Clinical Neuropsychology: A Pocket Handbook for Assessment, 2nd Edition. Washington, DC, American Psychological Association, 2006

Zillmer E, Spiers MV, Culbertson WC: Principles of Neuropsychology, 2nd Edition. Belmont, CA, Wadsworth, 2008

4

Neuroimaging

Norman L. Foster, M.D.

Rational Use of Neuroimaging in Dementia Care

Evaluating a patient with cognitive impairment is complex and intellectually demanding. Diagnosis involves formulating and resolving a series of questions to determine the cause of symptoms and establish a care plan. Questions arise incrementally and are modified as information accumulates from the patient's history and examination. Obtaining further historical information or performing a more detailed and extensive examination can answer some of these questions. Other questions are best approached with the aid of laboratory tests and imaging. In every case, results must be interpreted accurately and testing used appropriately. Ideal utilization of neuroimaging involves an-

Supported in part by National Institutes of Health grants R01-AG22394 and U01-AG024904 (the Alzheimer's Disease Neuroimaging Initiative).

swering questions that cannot otherwise be resolved. Neuroimaging does not simplify dementia evaluations; it supplies additional information.

Asking the Right Questions With Imaging

Two steps are involved in evaluating suspected dementing illness. The first is to recognize suspicious complaints and symptoms and to decide if they indicate significant cognitive deficits. Brain imaging contributes little to this effort. If a patient has significant cognitive impairment, the second step is to determine its cause. At this point, neuroimaging plays a crucial role. It provides important evidence of a dementing disease, and results sometimes are so characteristic that the cause is identified. Diagnosis cannot be based on brain imaging alone, but detecting specific abnormalities or documenting a lack of abnormality can support or refute a particular diagnosis.

Diagnostic questions that imaging can help answer are listed in Table 4–1. Several disorders often contribute to an individual patient's cognitive impairment; consequently, the clinician must address each diagnostic question in turn. Depending on the clinical history and examination, all questions are not equally important, a fact that should govern the types of imaging ordered and their priority. Fortunately, a single neuroimaging study usually addresses several clinical questions simultaneously. However, when the information from a single scanning modality is insufficient, additional imaging may be necessary. Neuroimaging is particularly valuable in difficult and atypical cases. It may be the only way to conclusively disentangle multiple dementing disorders.

Choosing the Best Imaging Modality

Clinical neuroimaging employs structural and molecular methods. Structural methods produce images from absorption of X rays using computed tomography (CT) or from measuring magnetic susceptibility of protons using magnetic resonance imaging (MRI). Molecular methods count emissions from radioactive isotopes that produce either positrons, in positron emission tomography (PET), or gamma rays, in single-photon emission computed tomography (SPECT). Structural and molecular methods provide different and complementary information. Structural imaging is best at showing brain anatomy and the characteristics of tissue. Molecular imaging is best at showing brain chemistry and function. Although some MRI methods partially reflect brain

Table 4–1. Diagnostic questions in dementia most relevant to neuroimaging

Structural imaging most valuable	Molecular imaging most valuable
Is there a mass lesion?	What is the pattern of hypometabolism?
Is there cerebrovascular disease?	Is there loss of dopaminergic neurons?
Is there ventricular enlargement?	Are there amyloid plaques?
Is there generalized volume loss?	
Is there focal volume loss?	

function, they either are not generally available for clinical use or have uncertain clinical utility in patients with dementia. Molecular imaging provides some information about brain anatomy, but this information can only be inferred after disentangling biochemical data.

Framing the patient's problems as a series of specific clinical questions determines which imaging study is most likely to be helpful (Table 4–1). Structural neuroimaging with a noncontrast CT scan or magnetic resonance image should be performed as part of the initial evaluation of patients with a suspected dementing disease. Focal neurological findings should raise suspicion of a structural lesion, but CT and MRI are justified even when there are no focal findings because of a high prevalence of unsuspected abnormalities in patients with significant cognitive deficits. The role of molecular imaging in dementia evaluations is not as firmly established. The biochemical changes revealed by PET and SPECT often can be inferred from the clinical history and examination or from the patient's response to medication. Nevertheless, when diagnostic uncertainty remains, molecular imaging can be useful.

Determining the Relevance of Imaging Findings

To be useful, imaging results require integration with the clinical context. Physicians ordering imaging studies need to convey to the radiologist or nuclear medicine specialist the diagnostic questions that need to be answered. Even with this information, a radiologist cannot determine fully how findings relate to a patient's symptoms. The clinician needs a detailed understanding of the individual and his or her symptoms to judge whether image abnormalities are clinically relevant.

Clinicians often benefit from personally reviewing a scan. The location of lesions should be consistent with symptoms, and the size and number of lesions should correspond roughly with symptoms. Furthermore, radiologists may be able to estimate the age of individual lesions and thus aid the comparison of imaging findings with a patient's clinical course. Whether the localization and timing of clinical symptoms and imaging findings coincide is a reliable guide for deciding if scan abnormalities are clinically important.

Concerns About the Use of Neuroimaging in Dementia Evaluation

Many concerns have been expressed about the appropriate use of neuroimaging in patients with suspected dementing illness. Although these same concerns are relevant to the use of any diagnostic test, they seem to arise more often and are expressed more vigorously with evaluations of dementia than with those of other disorders. Table 4–2 summarizes potential errors and misuses of imaging to be taken into account when the clinician is considering imaging studies.

Structural Neuroimaging

Dementing illnesses frequently alter brain structure. CT and MRI facilitate diagnosis of tumors, stroke, and other focal destructive and mass lesions. They also are superior to radionuclide cisternography in identifying hydrocephalus.

Choosing CT or MRI

CT and MRI provide similar but not identical information about brain anatomy (Figure 4–1). CT provides better anatomical information about bone and intracranial calcifications. Because X rays are linear, CT scans accurately represent the location of brain lesions. Thus, CT is preferable in head trauma and for surgical applications. For dementia, the advantages of CT over MRI usually are outweighed by the former's limitations.

MRI offers greater resolution and contrast than CT and therefore can be used to precisely delineate gray matter and identify white matter hyperintensities in the aging brain. MRI also provides high-resolution coronal and sagittal views of the brain so that small brain areas important in cognition, such as the hippocampi and mamillary bodies, are more readily seen. Furthermore,

Table 4–2. Potential errors and misuses of imaging

Utilization errors

Overuse—Repeating studies or obtaining imaging studies using methods unlikely to contribute to a diagnosis, increasing costs without additional clinical benefit

Underuse—Failure to utilize the imaging modality that could provide critical information for diagnosis

Omission—Failure to incorporate significant imaging findings in diagnosis

Overdependence—Using imaging results to decide if the patient has dementia when clinical assessment alone is adequate, or using imaging results to make a diagnosis without utilizing other relevant clinical data

Interpretation errors

Overinterpretation—Assigning a cause of dementia based on clinically insignificant imaging findings

Misinterpretation—Failing to recognize the presence of clinically significant lesions, causing errors in radiographic diagnosis

Inconsistent interpretation—variability between radiologists or from patient to patient in the description or clinical significance ascribed to identical imaging findings

Technical errors

Lack of reliability   Inconsistent acquisition or processing of imaging data, causing misinterpretation

Artifact—Failure to prevent or identify image acquisition or analysis errors that prevent the accurate interpretation of scans

MRI can be performed repeatedly without the risks of radiation exposure. For these reasons, MRI is preferable to CT for dementia evaluations.

Technical Considerations

MRI produces images with maximized sensitivity to specific tissue characteristics by varying the timing and repetition of radio frequency pulse sequences and signal acquisition parameters (see Figure 4–1). T_1-weighted images are most useful for defining anatomic structures. T_2-weighted and spin-echo images are best suited for detecting white matter lesions. Some protocols are especially valuable in dementia evaluations. Fluid-attenuated inversion recovery (FLAIR) images highlight white matter abnormalities seen in T_2-weighted images while suppressing signal in cerebrospinal fluid (CSF); this enhances visual contrast

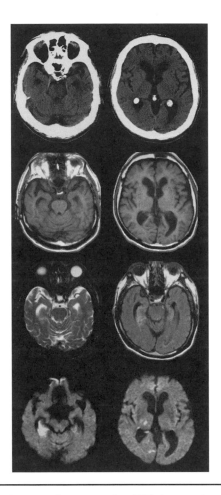

Figure 4–1.   Computed tomography (CT) images *(top row)* and magnetic resonance images from an 82-year-old patient comparing the ability of CT and four magnetic resonance imaging (MRI) sequences (T_1- *[row 2]* and T_2-weighted *[row 3, left]*, fluid-attenuated inversion recovery [FLAIR] *[row 3, right]*, and diffusion-weighted *[row 4]*) to demonstrate acute strokes in the right hippocampus and thalamus.

Source.   Reprinted from Foster NL: "Neuroimaging," in *The American Psychiatric Publishing Textbook of Alzheimer Disease and Other Dementias.* Edited by Weiner MF, Lipton AM. Washington, DC, American Psychiatric Publishing, 2009, pp. 105–136. Copyright 2009, American Psychiatric Publishing. Used with permission.

and helps distinguish widened capillary spaces from white matter pathology. Diffusion-weighted imaging (DWI) is sensitive to subtle changes in brain water content and diffusivity and is used for diffusion tensor imaging (DTI) and tractography. The degree of water content and diffusivity evolves after ischemic injury, so DWI can be used to estimate the age of vascular lesions. DWI also is the most sensitive method for detecting spongiform pathology. Pulse sequences designed to highlight paramagnetic properties of hemoglobin are the basis for functional MRI (fMRI) and can identify microhemorrhages associated with amyloid angiopathy and normal aging. Gradient echo imaging is the most widely used protocol for identifying hemorrhage. There is less experience with susceptibility-weighted imaging, but it appears to be even more sensitive (Haacke et al. 2007).

The most common contraindication for MRI is the presence of ferromagnetic implants or foreign bodies. Sometimes unexpected small metal particles from distant trauma cause only minor interference. When history is difficult to obtain, X-ray scout films must be obtained before proceeding with MRI. Although patients with artificial joints generally can be scanned safely, MRI is hazardous with pacemakers, some mechanical valves, and metal-containing sutures and surgical devices. Tattoos with metal-containing dyes can cause skin burns in high-field (>1.5-T) scanners. Furthermore, dental work and foreign objects, including jewelry, can cause severe image distortions and artifacts and should be removed when possible. Another problem, especially for those with claustrophobia, is the confining space of MRI. Imaging is most effective when the gap between patient and magnet is minimized, so small-bore scanners are preferred. Some less confining "open" scanners are available and can be appropriate in certain situations. The time required for MRI also is longer than for CT. As a consequence, MRI may require sedation or CT may be preferred for patients who have claustrophobia, have a movement disorder, or are less able to cooperate.

Diagnostic Questions Best Answered by Structural Neuroimaging

Is There a Space-Occupying Lesion?

The most obvious use of structural imaging is to identify a space-occupying or mass lesion. Focal neurological deficits such as hemiparesis, visual field cut, or aphasia warrant investigation with CT or MRI. Brain tumors, subdural hematomas, and brain abscesses are easily recognized. Most mass lesions in patients with dementia are identified when a brain scan is obtained to evaluate a focal neurological complaint. The most conspicuous exception is in elderly individuals for whom evaluations are delayed or incomplete. A CT scan or magnetic resonance image is needed when disruptive behavioral or personality changes occur de novo in middle or late adulthood. Frontal mass lesions often cause dementia and behavioral disturbance with few obvious focal neurological signs, and behavioral symptoms in these patients initially may be misinterpreted as purely psychiatric.

Mass lesions also are especially likely when dramatic dementia symptoms develop over less than a year. Although it may seem obvious that a glioma, central nervous system lymphoma, or subdural hemorrhage can cause rapidly evolving cognitive problems, obtaining an accurate history about the timing of symptom onset sometimes is very difficult.

Is There Cerebrovascular Disease?

The high likelihood of a stroke and other cerebrovascular diseases is a major rationale for structural neuroimaging in dementia evaluations. Although traditionally a single cause of dementia is sought, cerebrovascular disease frequently contributes to the severity of dementia when another dementing disease also is present. MRI is quite sensitive to cerebrovascular disease, so the major clinical challenge is to determine the significance of lesions that are found. Approximately 30% of the elderly have silent lacunar and cortical infarcts without clinical manifestations (Longstreth et al. 1998). Ideally, clinical relevance can be determined by correlating symptoms with the timing and location of the lesions. For example, in a dementia patient with prominent language disturbance, vascular lesions would be expected to preponderantly involve the left hemisphere. Careful review of all imaging data and comparing findings with different MRI sequences increase the sensitivity of identifying vascular lesions and estimating their age (see Figure 4–1). Nevertheless, relating imaging abnormalities to dementia can be difficult. History may be inadequate, and strokes often are asymptomatic. Substantial motor and sensory recovery may obscure the signs of stroke by the time cognition is evaluated.

The extent of vascular lesions is critical to their clinical relevance. A larger number of strokes and more extensive white matter abnormalities increase the probability of causing dementia. Too often clinical reports fail to distinguish minimal from extensive and confluent white matter abnormalities. The high sensitivity of MRI to changes in water content makes it easy to overestimate the clinical significance of deep white matter hyperintensities. White matter abnormalities are common in elders and should be evaluated critically because not all are pathological (Fazekas et al. 1993). Enlarged perivascular spaces cause increased signal on T_2-weighted images, but can be distinguished by low signal with FLAIR imaging (Figure 4–2). Neurodegenerative disease can cause white matter abnormalities from Wallerian degeneration to be indistinguishable from small vessel disease. Although no clear guide exists indicating how much abnormality is needed for clinical significance, criteria for vascular dementia established at the International Workshop of the National Institute of Neurological Disorders and Stroke and the Association Internationale pour la Recherche et l'Enseignement en Neurosciences (NINDS-AIREN) require involvement of at least 25% of white matter (Román et al. 1993).

Location of vascular lesions also is important. Even small thalamic infarcts can cause cognitive impairment. Likewise, cognition may be more affected when white matter hyperintensities involve cholinergic projection pathways (Bocti et al. 2005). Cholinergic fibers originate in the nucleus basalis of Meynert and fan out as they ascend, following a medial cingulate gyrus pathway and a lateral pathway through the external capsule and claustrum into the centrum semiovale adjacent to the gray-white junction (Figure 4–3).

Evidence of cerebrovascular disease on neuroimaging is insufficient to exclude Alzheimer disease (AD). Alzheimer pathology is often the primary factor for cognitive decline in older individuals with concurrent cerebrovascular injury. When a patient has extensive vascular lesions, AD can be identified confidently when gradual cognitive decline occurs without change in vascular lesions. Gradient echo MRI showing cortical microhemorrhages typical of cerebral amyloid angiopathy also provides indirect evidence of AD (Viswanathan and Chabriat 2006).

Although MRI is best for identifying vascular lesions, PET with ^{18}F-labeled fluorodeoxyglucose (FDG-PET) can help determine their cognitive consequences. Stroke often causes metabolic abnormalities that are more extensive than structural lesions due to loss of distant efferent nerve terminals. For example, a stroke damaging only the thalamus can cause ipsilateral cerebral cortical and contralateral cerebellar hypometabolism. These remote metabolic effects are clinically significant, and their localization reflects the types of cognitive deficits observed. Cerebral cortical hypometabolism is the best predictor of whether subcortical lacunar stroke will cause dementia (Kwan et al. 1999).

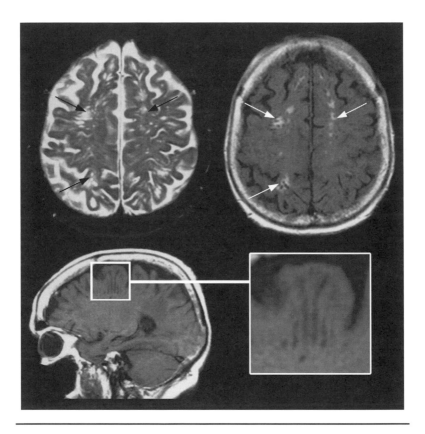

Figure 4–2. Magnetic resonance images demonstrating white matter hyperintensities due to enlarged perivascular spaces.

A T_2-weighted image *(top row, left)* shows multiple areas of increased signal in the white matter. A fluid-attenuated inversion recovery (FLAIR) magnetic resonance image *(top row, right)* reveals that many of these hyperintensities have a central area of low signal due to suppression of cerebrospinal fluid in perivascular spaces *(arrows).* Distinct features also are apparent in T_1-weighted sagittal images *(bottom row).* Perivascular spaces are linear, running perpendicular to the brain surface following penetrating vessels *(inset on right).* Areas of decreased signal in posterior periventricular areas have a patchy distribution characteristic of small vessel disease.

Source. Reprinted from Foster NL: "Neuroimaging," in *The American Psychiatric Publishing Textbook of Alzheimer Disease and Other Dementias.* Edited by Weiner MF, Lipton AM. Washington, DC, American Psychiatric Publishing, 2009, pp. 105–136. Copyright 2009, American Psychiatric Publishing. Used with permission.

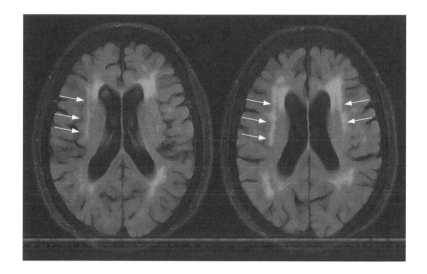

Figure 4–3. Axial fluid-attenuated inversion recovery (FLAIR) images in a 75-year-old woman demonstrating the distribution of white matter hyperintensities affecting ascending cholinergic tracts *(arrows)*.

Source. Reprinted from Foster NL: "Neuroimaging," in *The American Psychiatric Publishing Textbook of Alzheimer Disease and Other Dementias.* Edited by Weiner MF, Lipton AM. Washington, DC, American Psychiatric Publishing, 2009, pp. 105–136. Copyright 2009, American Psychiatric Publishing. Used with permission.

Is There Ventricular Enlargement?

Ventricular enlargement can be an important indicator of a dementing disease, particularly if the enlargement is progressive. The presence of ventricular enlargement often is determined subjectively, but a simple alternative is to calculate the ratio of the maximal width of frontal horns to the maximal width of the inner skull, which normally is <0.30. Ventricular enlargement can be caused by abnormalities in CSF flow or loss of brain volume (hydrocephalus ex vacuo). Disorders of CSF dynamics are uncommon causes of dementia but are reliably identified with CT and MRI. Either obstructive or communicating hydrocephalus increases intracranial pressure and manifests with headache and cognitive deficit. In obstructive hydrocephalus, the ventricular system balloons proximal to blockage of CSF flow. This obstruction commonly occurs at the cerebral aqueduct, causing disproportionate enlargement of third and lateral ventricles. Aqueductal flow of CSF can be measured precisely with MRI. MRI also can identify changes in periventricular brain water due to transependymal flow of CSF.

Structural imaging is essential in identifying normal-pressure hydrocephalus (NPH) (Table 4–3). Ventricular CSF flow is unobstructed in NPH so there is similar enlargement of all ventricles. The major challenge is to demonstrate that ventricular enlargement is not entirely attributable to cerebral atrophy. Consequently, ventricular enlargement should be disproportionately greater than sulcal enlargement. SPECT imaging also is supportive of the diagnosis of NPH when radionuclide injected by lumbar puncture into the subarachnoid space fails to clear after 48–72 hours.

Hydrocephalus ex vacuo is very common in AD and other neurodegenerative dementias. In these diseases, all ventricles expand roughly proportionate to enlargement of sulci. Unfortunately, relating the enlargement of ventricular volume to size of sulcal spaces remains purely subjective. However, when sulci are prominent, loss of brain volume is the likely cause of ventricular enlargement and warrants further analysis to determine the pattern of volume loss.

Is There Generalized or Focal Volume Loss?

Loss of brain volume is seen in AD and many other neurodegenerative diseases and is the most consistently reported structural imaging abnormality in dementia. However, age is a significant determinant of brain volume. Brain atrophy on average is greater in patients with AD than in normal elders, but significant overlap between individuals limits the diagnostic value of brain atrophy (Gado et al. 1982). When serial scans are available, diffuse progressive enlargement of CSF spaces over 1–2 years is easier to identify and suggests AD. However, repeated scans add little information to changes in cognition observed over the same time interval. Quantitative and focused approaches are more reliable. One method is to measure total brain volume using scans with uniform characteristics in all three dimensions. A second method is to consider the volume of specific brain regions.

Typical clinical MRI studies acquire images that have greater resolution in one plane than in others. However, it is possible to acquire so-called isovoxel images consisting of image elements that are contiguous and of equal size in all dimensions. This permits better delineation of boundaries between CSF, brain,

Table 4–3. Structural imaging abnormalities in probable normal-pressure hydrocephalus

Required findings

1. Ventricular enlargement not entirely attributable to cerebral atrophy or congenital enlargement (Evan's index >0.3 or comparable measure)

2. No macroscopic obstruction to CSF flow

3. At least one of the following:

   a. Enlargement of the temporal horns of the lateral ventricles not entirely attributable to hippocampus atrophy

   b. Callosal angle of 40 degrees or more

   c. Evidence of altered brain water content, including periventricular signal changes on CT and MRI not attributable to microvascular ischemic changes or demyelination

4. An aqueductal or fourth ventricular flow void on MRI

Other findings considered supportive

1. A brain imaging study performed before onset of symptoms showing smaller ventricular size or without evidence of hydrocephalus

2. Radionuclide cisternogram showing delayed clearance of radiotracer over the cerebral convexities after 48–72 hours

3. Cine MRI study or other technique showing increased ventricular flow rate

4. A SPECT-acetazolamide challenge showing decreased periventricular perfusion that is not altered by acetazolamide

Note. CSF = cerebrospinal fluid; CT = computed tomography; MRI = magnetic resonance imaging; SPECT = single-photon emission computed tomography.
Source. Adapted from Relkin et al. 2005.

and skull and more accurate measurement of brain volume. Voxel-based morphometry, a computer-assisted approach, is able to distinguish groups of patients with AD from individuals without dementia (and even patients with mild cognitive impairment). However, the diagnostic sensitivity and specificity of this approach in individual patients have not yet been studied adequately.

Changes in the volume of specific brain regions can be determined reliably with both subjective and quantitative methods. Pathology is so localized in some dementing diseases that focal atrophy often is easily recognized. Caudate atrophy is characteristic of Huntington disease and most evident with coronal images. Progressive supranuclear palsy (PSP) causes midbrain and pontine atrophy that frequently is apparent on sagittal MRI and can be used to distinguish PSP from other parkinsonian syndromes (Cosottini et al. 2007). If focal atrophy is evident, it can help confirm a suspected diagnosis, but sensitivity may not be high early in the course of the illness. Because brain size varies significantly with gender and age, these factors need to be taken into account.

The earliest pathological changes in AD occur in the entorhinal cortex, amygdala, and hippocampus (Braak and Braak 1991). Consequently, it is not surprising that MRI shows medial temporal volume loss in AD. Coronal views best visualize the hippocampus and should be obtained routinely in the evaluation of dementia. The resolution of MRI also allows assessment of specific structures within the medial temporal lobe. Hippocampal size is readily apparent on coronal magnetic resonance images, and visual assessment has good sensitivity and specificity in distinguishing AD from normal aging. Medial temporal lobe atrophy also can help identify which patients with mild cognitive impairment will progress to dementia (Visser et al. 2002).

Frontotemporal dementia (FTD) also causes focal atrophy involving superior frontal and anterior temporal cortex. Sometimes focal atrophy in these regions is evident on visual assessment. Because brains have considerable individual variation, focal abnormalities are more clearly pathological when they become more evident over time (Figure 4–4). Automated measurement of frontal and temporal volume and measurements of cortical thickness show distinctive abnormalities that correspond to clinical FTD syndromes (Du et al. 2007). In progressive nonfluent aphasia, atrophy is asymmetric, primarily involving language regions. Quantitative measures of focal atrophy distinguish groups of FTD patients from both normal elderly individuals and patients with AD. It is also important to note that FTD causes hippocampal and amygdalar atrophy (Boccardi et al. 2002). Thus, medial temporal atrophy is probably an unreliable way to distinguish AD from FTD.

Molecular Neuroimaging

Molecular imaging reveals the distribution of tracer quantities of radioactively labeled drugs designed to participate in metabolism, interact with enzymes and transporters, occupy cellular receptors, or bind cellular and extracellular pro-

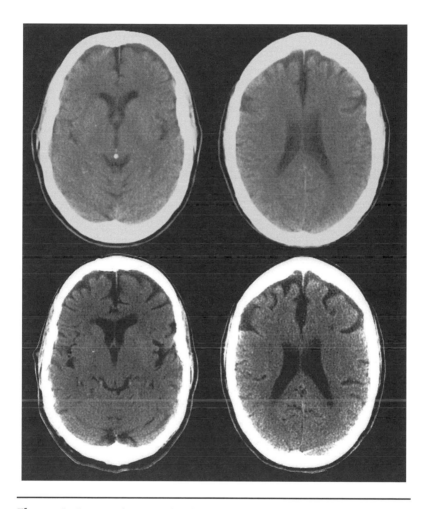

Figure 4–4.   Axial T_1-weighted magnetic resonance images, at time of initial assessment *(top row)* and 6 years later *(bottom row),* showing progressive focal frontal atrophy.

Source.   Reprinted from Foster NL: "Neuroimaging," in *The American Psychiatric Publishing Textbook of Alzheimer Disease and Other Dementias.* Edited by Weiner MF, Lipton AM. Washington, DC, American Psychiatric Publishing, 2009, pp. 105–136. Copyright 2009, American Psychiatric Publishing. Used with permission.

teins. This imaging can assess the characteristic biochemical signatures of dementing illnesses as they evolve. Each tracer has unique properties, but only a few molecular imaging strategies have reached clinical practice. Cerebral blood flow and metabolism usually are equivalent in dementing illnesses and are the most established molecular imaging methods.

Choosing PET or SPECT

The difference between PET and SPECT is the radioactive isotopes the two methods use. The positron-emitting isotopes used in PET (fluorine-18 and carbon-11) are easier to insert into drugs and naturally occurring substances without altering biological activity than are the large, single-photon–emitting isotopes commonly used in SPECT (technetium-99m and iodine-131). This difference makes it much easier to interpret and develop quantitative tracer kinetic models for PET than for SPECT. Furthermore, because positron annihilations produce two gamma rays oriented in opposite directions, PET provides more accurate localization and better spatial resolution than does SPECT, which relies on single-photon (gamma) emissions.

These theoretical differences have practical importance. The most commonly used SPECT tracers measure cerebral perfusion, whereas the most commonly used PET tracers measure glucose metabolism. Although glucose metabolism usually parallels cerebral perfusion, glucose uptake is more closely linked to neuronal activity. PET has diagnostic accuracy superior to that of SPECT in differentiating AD from vascular dementia (Messa et al. 1994). The subsequent discussion of molecular imaging therefore will focus primarily on PET methods.

Technical Considerations

Changes in the biological processes measured with molecular imaging can be independent of structural change or reflect structural changes. Consequently, CT or MRI results are critical for accurately interpreting molecular imaging scans. Many PET scanners now incorporate a CT scanner to help meld structural and molecular images. Unlike structural imaging studies, interpretation of PET and SPECT scans must take into account many factors that can affect the activity and distribution of radioligands, including cerebral blood flow and metabolism, patient medication, ambient room conditions, patient attributes such as open or closed eyes, and perhaps what the patient is thinking.

Both current and recent medication use may affect the binding of neurotransmitter ligands. Therefore, for molecular imaging, the conditions during scanning and medication use must be carefully recorded and controlled.

To decrease subject-to-subject variability, molecular imaging data are commonly "normalized" or adjusted by comparison to an average value in an image or a specified brain region. When this is done, it is possible to determine the value in one brain region relative to another but not the absolute rate of biochemical reactions. Nevertheless, the relative distribution of radiotracers has proven adequate for evaluating most disease changes. For glucose metabolism in dementia, there is no ideal region for normalization, but the pons seems to be best suited because pontine glucose metabolism is best preserved in AD (Minoshima et al. 1995).

Diagnostic Questions Best Answered by Molecular Neuroimaging

What Is the Pattern of Cerebral Hypometabolism?

Glucose is normally the brain's sole energy source, and glucose uptake primarily mirrors synaptic activity. FDG-PET images reflect brain activity over the 20–30 minutes following radioisotope injection. The patient's response to a task can be examined by having the patient perform it repeatedly over this uptake phase of the study. However, for clinical studies, individuals usually are asked to rest quietly in a darkened room. In normal individuals, cerebral metabolism is greatest in the basal ganglia, thalamus, cerebellum, and cerebral cortex; less in the brain stem; and lowest in white matter (Figure 4–5). Glucose metabolic rates in the cerebral cortex are reasonably uniform. When eyes are open, the visual cortex is activated and has higher glucose uptake.

Dementing diseases cause a global decline in glucose metabolism, with characteristic and distinctive patterns of regional predominance (Table 4–4).

Although the underlying disease determines the overall pattern of hypometabolism, individual differences in the regional intensity of the pattern are consistent with individual differences in clinical symptoms. For example, patients with prominent language disturbance primarily have hypometabolism in the dominant hemisphere, those with prominent visuospatial disturbance primarily have hypometabolism in the nondominant hemisphere, and patients with behavior disturbance have frontal hypometabolism.

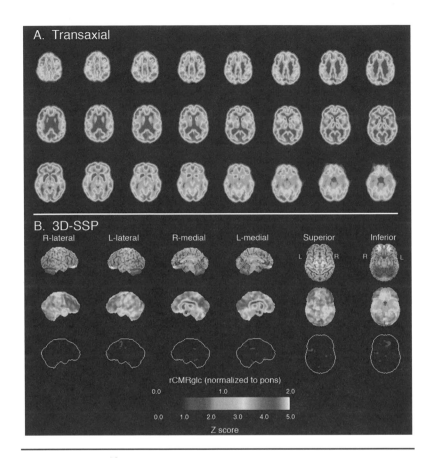

Figure 4–5. [^{18}F]Fluorodeoxyglucose positron emission tomography images from a cognitively normal elderly individual displayed as transaxial *(A)* and three-dimensional stereotactic surface projection (3D-SSP) *(B)* metabolic and statistical maps *(see color plate 1)*.

FDG-PET scans produce up to 128 transaxial images, here truncated to the most relevant brain slices for easier display. Relative rates of glucose metabolism, in this case relative to pons, are displayed using a color scale shown below the images, with hotter colors representing higher rates of glucose metabolism. Scan data were summarized and displayed in uniform space by 3D-SSP, an analysis software program.

Source. Reprinted from Foster NL: "Neuroimaging," in *The American Psychiatric Publishing Textbook of Alzheimer Disease and Other Dementias.* Edited by Weiner MF, Lipton AM. Washington, DC, American Psychiatric Publishing, 2009, pp. 105–136. Copyright 2009, American Psychiatric Publishing. Used with permission.

Table 4–4. Typical patterns of regional cerebral glucose metabolism in common dementing diseases

Disease	Pattern of glucose hypometabolism
Alzheimer disease	Symmetric or asymmetric bilateral temporoparietal and posterior cingulate, lesser frontal association cortex, sparing of primary sensorimotor and visual cortex
Vascular dementia	Multifocal cortical and subcortical, correlating with structural imaging lesions
Parkinson disease with dementia and dementia with Lewy bodies	Symmetric or asymmetric bilateral temporoparietal, posterior cingulate, and visual cortex; lesser frontal association cortex; sparing of primary sensorimotor cortex
Huntington disease	Caudate nucleus and lesser frontal association cortex
Progressive supranuclear palsy	Caudate nucleus, putamen, thalamus, pons, primarily superior and anterior frontal cortex; cerebellum spared
Corticobasal degeneration	Asymmetric frontal, temporal, and parietal cortex and thalamus contralateral to limb apraxia

The most established clinical use of FDG-PET is to distinguish AD from FTD. FDG-PET is helpful in this situation because AD and FTD have starkly contrasting patterns of hypometabolism. The use of FDG-PET to distinguish AD from FTD has been studied by Foster et al. (2007). In this study, visual interpretation of FDG-PET was based on the simple rule that FTD causes greater hypometabolism in anterior cingulate, anterior temporal, and frontal regions than in posterior cingulate and posterior temporoparietal cortex, whereas AD causes the opposite pattern. Adding FDG-PET to clinical evaluation increased diagnostic accuracy, with a specificity of 97.6% and a sensitivity of 86%.

FDG-PET provides objective evidence of a neurodegenerative disease when medical history is ambiguous or informants are unavailable or unreliable. The pattern of hypometabolism may reveal important additional information when patients have an atypical clinical presentation, or when diagnostic features are shared by two or more disorders. Cerebral hypometabolism in AD has a typical sequence of regional involvement but varies from patient to patient. Hypometabolism is first seen in the posterior cingulate gyrus. It then spreads to also affect the association cortex in the parietal and posterior temporal lobes (Figure 4–6). Eventually hypometabolism involves prefrontal cortex and most of the brain. Although the relative decrease in metabolism in posterior association cortex as compared with anterior association cortex remains throughout the course of AD, this discrepancy becomes harder to recognize as frontal regions become progressively more affected. As the surrounding frontal and parietal association cortex becomes more hypometabolic, the relative preservation of the primary sensorimotor cortex surrounding the central sulcus becomes increasingly evident. The occipital lobe, including the primary visual cortex, also is relatively spared. The caudate, putamen, and thalamus are spared relative to the cerebral cortex but are hypometabolic when compared with those of normal individuals of similar age (Foster et al. 1988). The cerebellum and brain stem are little affected in sporadic AD (Minoshima et al. 1995).

The initial involvement of the posterior cingulate gyrus in AD is perhaps unexpected, but considerable evidence now indicates that metabolic declines are greater in the posterior cingulate cortex and lateral temporal cortex because synaptic projections from the hippocampus and medial temporal cortex are damaged.

Clinical criteria for AD have relatively poor specificity, and misdiagnoses are common (Blacker et al. 1994). Visual interpretation of FDG-PET scans has higher diagnostic accuracy than clinical evaluation alone when autopsy diagnosis is used as the gold standard (Silverman et al. 2001).

FTD causes glucose hypometabolism predominantly in anterior brain regions, including the frontal cortex, anterior cingulate cortex, and anterior temporal regions (Foster et al. 2005). As symptoms progress, deficits become more pervasive, but anterior regions remain predominantly affected and primary motor-sensory and visual cortex and posterior association cortex are relatively spared. Several clinical phenotypes of FTD are recognized (see Chapter 9, "Frontotemporal Dementia and Other Tauopathies") and cause corresponding variations in this overall pattern of glucose hypometabolism. Patients with severe behavior disturbances tend to have predominant right hemisphere hypometabolism, whereas those with progressive aphasia exhibit more hypometabolism in the dominant hemisphere (Figure 4–7). Hypometabolism in some patients is mostly in the anterior temporal cortex, whereas in others it is almost entirely limited to the frontal cortex (Foster et al. 2005).

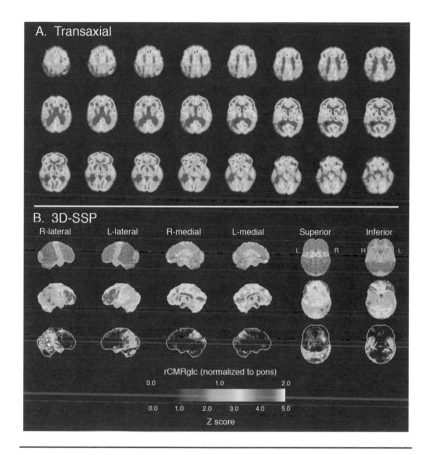

Figure 4–6. [^{18}F]Fluorodeoxyglucose positron emission tomography images from a patient with Alzheimer disease displayed as transaxial *(A)* and three-dimensional stereotactic surface projection (3D-SSP) *(B)* metabolic and statistical maps *(see color plate 2).*

Source. Reprinted from Foster NL: "Neuroimaging," in *The American Psychiatric Publishing Textbook of Alzheimer Disease and Other Dementias.* Edited by Weiner MF, Lipton AM. Washington, DC, American Psychiatric Publishing, 2009, pp. 105–136. Copyright 2009, American Psychiatric Publishing. Used with permission.

Dementia with Lewy bodies (DLB) and Parkinson disease with dementia (PDD) both show a pattern of glucose hypometabolism similar to that of AD, with the added characteristic of occipital hypometabolism, whether or not Alzheimer pathology is also present (Ishii et al. 1998). Current clinical criteria for DLB have good specificity yet poor sensitivity, and patients with pathologically confirmed DLB often have been misdiagnosed as having AD (Weiner et al. 2003). Imaging with a dopaminergic marker may be particularly valuable in distinguishing AD from DLB (see subsection "Is There Loss of Dopaminergic Neurons?" below) but cannot distinguish DLB from PDD. Although clinical presentation and clinical criteria differ, the pathological findings in these two disorders are indistinguishable.

Distinctive patterns of glucose hypometabolism also have been identified in PSP and corticobasal degeneration. In most cases, the characteristic motor symptoms of these conditions are generally sufficient for diagnosis, but on occasion, the pattern of hypometabolism may be helpful. FDG-PET findings differ in PSP and DLB and in PSP and PDD even though these illnesses have similar abnormalities on dopaminergic imaging. PSP causes glucose hypometabolism in the caudate nucleus, putamen, thalamus, pons, and cerebral cortex (Foster et al. 1988). Declines in glucose metabolism are most prominent in the superior and anterior portions of the frontal cortex in a manner that is now better understood as causing a pattern typical of tauopathies (see Chapter 9, "Frontotemporal Dementia and Other Tauopathies"). Glucose metabolism in the cerebellar cortex in PSP is normal. This finding can be helpful in distinguishing PSP from cerebellar degenerations, because gait ataxia is a common early complaint in both. Corticobasal degeneration is characterized by significant metabolic hemispheric asymmetry, just as clinical symptoms are typically very asymmetric. Nearly the entire affected hemisphere, including frontal, temporal, and parietal regions, is involved. However, in addition to the asymmetry in the cerebral cortex, there is ipsilateral thalamic hypometabolism, while the striatum seems relatively spared (Eidelberg et al. 1991). Although corticobasal degeneration, FTD, and PSP share tau pathology, they have different clinical symptoms and patterns of glucose hypometabolism.

FDG-PET is a measure of synaptic activity, which is affected early in neurodegenerative diseases. Synaptic changes have been best shown in AD, where synaptic failure precedes axonal loss and neuronal death (Selkoe 2002). How early changes in metabolism appear is unknown, but groups of individuals

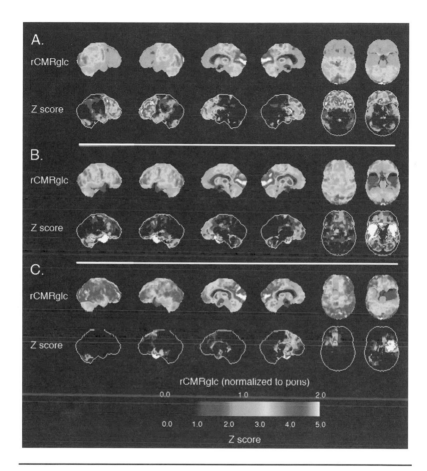

Figure 4–7. [18F]Fluorodeoxyglucose positron emission tomography images from three patients with frontotemporal dementia displayed as three-dimensional stereotactic surface projection metabolic and statistical maps, two with bifrontal hypometabolism *(A, B)* and the third with asymmetric predominantly temporal hypometabolism *(C) (see color plate 3).*

Source. Reprinted from Foster NL: "Neuroimaging," in *The American Psychiatric Publishing Textbook of Alzheimer Disease and Other Dementias.* Edited by Weiner MF, Lipton AM. Washington, DC, American Psychiatric Publishing, 2009, pp. 105–136. Copyright 2009, American Psychiatric Publishing. Used with permission.

presumed to be at high risk for AD based on the apolipoprotein E4 genotype show metabolic changes long before symptoms appear, particularly in the posterior cingulate gyrus (Small et al. 2000). Furthermore, several studies have shown that FDG-PET helps distinguish individuals with memory disturbance who later will develop AD. Many nondemented individuals with mild cognitive impairment show a pattern of cerebral glucose metabolism identical to that of patients with AD. Moreover, patients with mild cognitive impairment are much more likely to develop AD over the subsequent few years if they exhibit Alzheimer patterns of glucose hypometabolism (Anchisi et al. 2005).

Is There Loss of Dopaminergic Neurons?

Dopaminergic function is affected in many dementing illnesses, including DLB, PDD, and PSP. Furthermore, rigidity frequently develops in moderate and late AD. The presence of parkinsonian features provides important clinical evidence of these disorders, but the sensitivity of clinical diagnosis is relatively low. Molecular imaging provides a more objective and quantitative measure of dopaminergic function. Tracers are available to evaluate the integrity of dopaminergic neurons at several sites. Uptake of dopa, the dopamine precursor, can be measured with $[^{18}F]$fluorodopa. Radiotracers are available that bind to the vesicular monoamine transporter 2, which is responsible for storage of dopamine in synaptic vesicles, and to the dopamine transporter (DAT), which facilitates reuptake of dopamine into axons (Brooks et al. 2003). The SPECT DAT tracer $[^{123}I]$-β-CIT has received approval from the U.S. Food and Drug Administration for clinical use to visualize DAT distribution within the striatum. This measure of dopaminergic pathology can help differentiate DLB, which uniformly has loss of striatal dopaminergic terminals, from AD, which does not (Walker et al. 2007). After an initial uptake phase, remaining ligand is limited primarily to the striatum (site of dopaminergic projection axons from the substantia nigra). Both the amount of and the morphological shape of binding can be helpful diagnostically; normal distribution appears in a "comma" shape, but with loss of dopamine neurons, posterior and caudal binding diminish, causing a "full stop" or circular pattern (Figure 4–8). In a prospective study of dementia patients with and without DLB who had acceptable $[^{123}I]$-β-CIT scans, diagnostic accuracy compared with consensus diagnosis based on the scan alone was 85% for probable DLB, with a sensitivity of 77% and specificity of 90% (McKeith

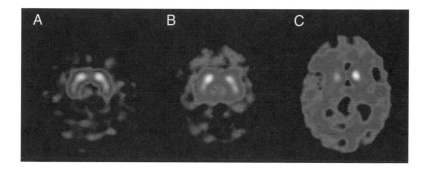

Figure 4–8. Single-photon emission computed tomography scans showing binding to dopamine uptake sites in the striatum from a cognitively normal individual *(A)*, an 83-year-old patient with Alzheimer disease *(B)*, and an 81-year-old patient with probable DLB *(C) (see color plate 4)*.
Source. Reprinted from Foster NL: "Neuroimaging," in *The American Psychiatric Publishing Textbook of Alzheimer Disease and Other Dementias.* Edited by Weiner MF, Lipton AM. Washington, DC, American Psychiatric Publishing, 2009, pp. 105–136. Copyright 2009, American Psychiatric Publishing. Used with permission. Images are provided courtesy of GE Healthcare.

et al. 2007). This compares favorably to the average sensitivity of 49% for the clinical diagnosis of probable DLB when compared with autopsy diagnosis. Consequently, [^{123}I]-β-CIT appears valuable for increasing the detection of DLB (the specificity, but not the sensitivity, of the clinical criteria for probable DLB is already high).

Use of drugs must be examined when interpreting scans of dopamine function. For example, bupropion and a number of other drugs affect [^{123}I]-β-CIT scans. Short-term use of levodopa or dopamine agonists and antagonists acting on postsynaptic dopamine receptors does not affect the scans. Therefore, it should be possible for the assessment team to identify DLB in patients receiving neuroleptic drugs without knowing for certain that parkinsonian symptoms are spontaneous.

Are There Amyloid Plaques?

Fibrillar amyloid-β protein can be visualized with ^{11}C tracer Pittsburgh compound B (PIB). This tracer is a derivative of thioflavin T, easily crosses the blood-brain barrier, and appears to bind only to fully formed plaques (Klunk et al. 2004). PIB binding is much more evident in the cerebral cortex in patients with AD, whereas binding is similar in white matter and cerebral cortex in normal individuals (Figure 4–9). Amyloid imaging complements FDG-PET findings. Increased PIB binding can be seen when FDG-PET scans are normal. Some normal elderly individuals and some patients with DLB also show increased PIB binding consistent with pathological studies (Rowe et al. 2007). The presence of increased PIB binding in nondemented elderly individuals and in patients with mild cognitive impairment raises the question whether these findings will predict later development of AD (Forsberg et al. 2008). Furthermore, PIB binding is seen in some patients.

$[^{18}F]$Florbetapir (AV-45), another amyloid imaging ligand appropriate for PET, will soon become clinically available based on convincing evidence that images reflect brain pathology (Clark et al. 2011). The binding characteristics of this and several other $[^{18}F]$amyloid-binding compounds in development are similar to those of ^{11}C-PIB. However, the longer half-life of ^{18}F will considerably improve the logistics and availability of amyloid imaging and thus have the potential to revolutionize diagnosis.

The precise role that amyloid imaging should play in diagnosis is evolving, especially in view of proposed new criteria for AD. These criteria change the paradigm for diagnosis through the use of CSF and imaging biomarkers to establish the highest degree of diagnostic certainty (Dubois et al. 2007).

Special Situations

Rapidly Progressive Dementia

Structural imaging is essential and MRI is clearly preferable to CT when evaluating a patient with rapidly progressive dementia. MRI is often valuable in detecting multiple, small, disseminated lesions due to metastases or vasculitis and in recognizing emboli following open-heart surgery, endocarditis, cardiac thrombus, or a peripheral venous thrombus reaching the brain through a patent foramen ovale.

Another advantage of MRI is its ability to detect prion diseases. Creutzfeldt-Jakob disease (CJD) and other prion diseases very commonly cause focal increased signal on DWI, FLAIR imaging, and proton-weighted MRI, and to a lesser extent on T_2-weighted imaging (Finkenstaedt et al. 1996). Diffusion

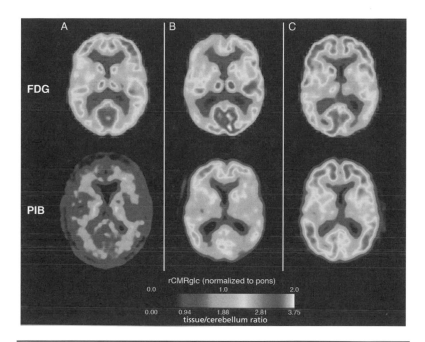

Figure 4–9. Transaxial [^{18}F]fluorodeoxyglucose positron emission tomography (FDG-PET) *(top row)* and Pittsburgh Compound B (PIB)–PET *(bottom row)* images from a cognitively normal elderly individual *(A)* and two patients with Alzheimer disease *(B, C) (see color plate 5)*.

Source. Reprinted from Foster NL: "Neuroimaging," in *The American Psychiatric Publishing Textbook of Alzheimer Disease and Other Dementias.* Edited by Weiner MF, Lipton AM. Washington, DC, American Psychiatric Publishing, 2009, pp. 105–136. Copyright 2009, American Psychiatric Publishing. Used with permission.

imaging appears most sensitive. It is important to recognize that CT scans and routine T_1-weighted magnetic resonance images may be normal in CJD. It therefore may be necessary to specifically request diffusion-weighted and FLAIR images and to focus the attention of the radiologist on the suspected regions of interest, since the typical abnormalities of prion disease may not be recognized because of its low prevalence.

MRI diffusion changes are probably caused by gliosis and microscopic spongiform vacuolation. MRI abnormalities in typical, sporadic CJD most often appear as bilateral, symmetric, increased signal in the putamen and caudate nuclei (Schroter et al. 2000). There also can be focal abnormalities in the cerebral cortex that have a distinctive ribbonlike appearance (Figure 4–10). By contrast, FLAIR and diffuse abnormalities in stroke involve both gray and white matter. The location of MRI changes in CJD can be symmetric or asymmetric, reflects the distribution of prion pathology, and correlates with patient symptoms (Mittal et al. 2002). In new-variant CJD, acquired from exposure to bovine spongiform encephalopathy, increased signal typically occurs in the pulvinar of the thalamus.

Early-Onset and Familial Dementia

Dementia occurring before age 60 requires closer consideration of diseases that are uncommon later in life. Traumatic injury, brain tumors, HIV, and other sexually transmitted infections are more likely causes in younger patients. FTD is nearly as common as AD in this age group. Early-onset dementia also is more often inherited. Some familial dementing disorders have distinctive imaging findings.

Cerebral autosomal dominant arteriopathy with subcortical infarcts and leukoencephalopathy (CADASIL) causes progressive dementia beginning in the third to sixth decades of life. This disease may go unrecognized for many years and may be first identified only after the typical features are seen on brain scanning. MRI shows lacunar infarcts, and microhemorrhages that become more numerous over time. The most distinctive imaging feature of CADASIL involves areas of hyperintensity in the anterior temporal lobes (Figure 4–11).

Familial AD also may have unusual clinical and imaging findings. Some presenilin 1 mutations cause spastic paraparesis and can be associated with less dense cotton-wool plaques. In such cases, AD pathology may involve areas that are usually spared, such as the primary motor cortex (Moretti et al. 2004). Likewise, some presenilin 1 mutations are associated with cerebellar amyloid plaques. Cerebellar glucose metabolism is usually normal in AD, but in familial cases there may be cerebellar hypometabolism (Murrell et al. 2001).

Evolving Symptoms

When dementing diseases progress, imaging can help in understanding unexpected symptoms. In neurodegenerative diseases, symptoms evolve gradually and follow a typical course characteristic for each disorder. Sometimes, however,

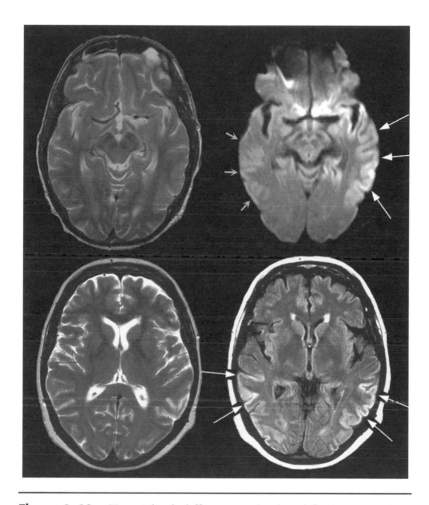

Figure 4–10. T_2-weighted, diffusion-weighted, and fluid-attenuated inversion recovery (FLAIR) magnetic resonance images from two patients with Creutzfeldt-Jakob disease.

In one patient, a T_2-weighted image *(top row, left)* shows no abnormality, whereas the diffusion-weighted image *(top row, right)* shows increased signal in the left temporal lobe *(large arrows)* that is not seen on the right *(small arrows)*. In the other patient, a T_2-weighted image *(bottom row, left)* also fails to show any abnormalities, although the FLAIR image *(bottom row, right)* shows increased signal in the temporoparietal cortical ribbon bilaterally *(large arrows)*.

Source. Reprinted from Foster NL: "Neuroimaging," in *The American Psychiatric Publishing Textbook of Alzheimer Disease and Other Dementias.* Edited by Weiner MF, Lipton AM. 2009. Copyright 2009, American Psychiatric Publishing. Used with permission.

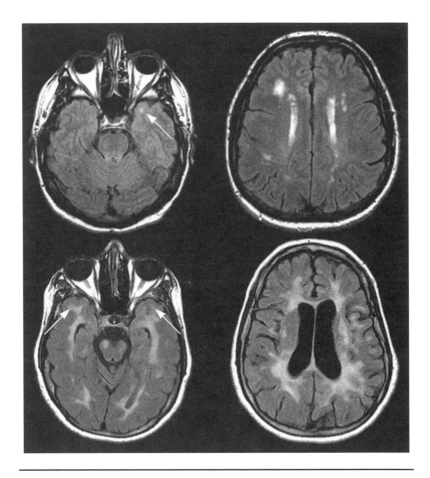

Figure 4–11.   Transaxial magnetic resonance images from patients with cerebral autosomal dominant arteriopathy with subcortical infarcts and leukoencephalopathy (CADASIL).

(Top row) Magnetic resonance image from a young patient with NOTCH3 mutation but minimal clinical symptoms shows a few areas of white matter hyperintensity, including a characteristic lesion at the gray-white junction in the anterior temporal lobe *(left, see arrow)*. *(Bottom row)* Older symptomatic CADASIL patient with dementia with even more extensive and confluent white matter abnormalities in anterior temporal lobes bilaterally *(left, see arrows)*. The image on the right shows confluent white matter hyperintensities involving most of the periventricular white matter.

Source.   Reprinted from Foster NL: "Neuroimaging," in *The American Psychiatric Publishing Textbook of Alzheimer Disease and Other Dementias*. Edited by Weiner MF, Lipton AM. 2009. Copyright 2009, American Psychiatric Publishing. Used with permission.

the cause of dementia may be brought into question when the course of a patient's illness differs from that predicted by the clinical diagnosis (see Figure 4–4). For example, patients with AD are not expected to develop sudden hemiparesis or aphasia. If this occurs, MRI is likely to show a cerebral infarct, subdural hematoma, or intracerebral hemorrhage. If apathy, inattention, perseveration, or loss of verbal fluency becomes more pronounced than memory loss in a patient thought to have AD, then FDG-PET is appropriate. The correct diagnosis could be FTD instead. FDG-PET showing bilateral temporoparietal hypometabolism or abnormal amyloid imaging may help confirm AD when cognitive deficits worsen in a patient with vascular dementia, even though no new vascular lesions are seen with MRI.

Patients with cognitive impairment due to neurological disease almost uniformly have abnormal FDG-PET scans, whereas those with cognitive complaints for other reasons usually have normal scans. FDG-PET scans are abnormal even when symptoms of AD are mild. Thus, a normal pattern of glucose metabolism may provide additional assurance that the initial diagnosis was in error when a patient thought to have AD fails to get worse. FDG-PET also may be useful in differentiating neurodegenerative disease from cognitive impairment due to psychiatric illness, medication side effects, or malingering.

Emerging Neuroimaging Methods

Neurotransmitter Imaging

Many molecular probes have been developed to examine neurotransmitter function. Cholinergic function is of particular interest in AD, which damages cholinergic neurons. Molecular imaging can reveal how cholinergic deficits develop over time and their relationship to symptoms and patient characteristics. The radioactively labeled vesamicol analogue IBVM binds to the presynaptic vesicular acetylcholine transporter and can serve as an in vivo marker of presynaptic cholinergic terminal density (Kuhl et al. 1996). Molecular imaging using the probe demonstrates that as with glucose metabolism, there is a generally uniform distribution of cholinergic terminals throughout the neocortex in normal individuals. In patients with AD, IBVM binding is decreased.

Accurately measuring cholinergic receptors is more challenging. However, significant alterations in muscarinic receptors do not occur in AD (Zubieta et al. 2001). Perhaps the most intriguing observations have been made using a

PET radioligand that binds to cholinesterase, such as ^{11}C-PMP. Although cholinesterase is not a precise indicator of cholinergic neurons, both PET and postmortem studies find a similar characteristic decrease of cholinesterase in AD (Kuhl et al. 1999). Peripheral red blood cell assays have typically been used to assess the potency of cholinesterase inhibitor drugs, even though inhibition in the central nervous system is most relevant. PET studies with ^{11}C-PMP showed that there could be a considerable discrepancy between central and peripheral cholinesterase inhibition after acute treatment with donepezil (Kuhl et al. 2000).

Functional Magnetic Resonance Imaging

fMRI utilizes the principle of BOLD contrast, or blood oxygenation level dependency of magnetic resonance signals, to assess local blood flow in response to a task or in the resting state. It exploits the observation that increased neuronal activity causes a transient increase in blood flow and temporarily decreases deoxyhemoglobin concentration. Under normal conditions, BOLD contrast in the brain reflects microvascular or venous blood.

Although fMRI has been used primarily to examine the anatomical correlates of cognitive function in normal individuals, an increasing number of studies have examined differences in normal elderly individuals and those with mild memory impairment and dementia (Bookheimer et al. 2000).

Diffusion Tensor Imaging

DTI applies advanced processing to diffusion-weighted magnetic resonance images to provide a measure of white matter integrity. Diffusion of protons in white matter is constrained by the direction of fiber tracts. By calculating vectors of diffusion, DTI can calculate and display the directional tendency of proton diffusion. Tissue that displays random diffusion of protons is called *isotropic;* tissue with restricted or bounded diffusion of protons is *anisotropic.* In DTI, the extent that directionality is coherent commonly is measured by calculating fractional anisotropy (FA), which ranges from 0, indicating random diffusion of protons, to 1, indicating highly constrained and linear diffusion. Areas such as the corpus callosum, with highly coherent white matter tracts favoring unidirectional flow, appear on the images as high signal (high FA). Loss of myelin causes loss of isotropy and loss of signal. Using this method, DTI can measure the local disruption of fiber tracts. Traumatic injury, infarction, and axonal loss from neurodegeneration can all cause axonal disruption, but DTI can distinguish among these possibilities using current techniques.

White matter tracts connecting limbic structures and areas of the brain that myelinate later in development are most susceptible to disruption in AD (Medina et al. 2006). Abnormalities can also be detected in carriers of familial AD mutations before dementia develops (Ringman et al. 2007).

Magnetic Resonance Spectroscopy

Magnetic resonance spectroscopy (MRS) uses an MRI scanner but provides no structural information. Instead, spectra are derived from targeted volumes of brain by measuring a few cubic centimeters and necessarily including both gray and white matter. Magnetic resonance spectra are generated from naturally occurring, biologically important elements such as ^{1}H and ^{31}P (Sanders 1995). MRS data are displayed as peaks representing the signals that different compounds produce.

Spectra of ^{1}H are derived from targeted volumes of brain, and the heights of peaks are used to measure the relative amounts of N-acetylaspartate (a presumed neuronal marker), phosphocreatine (a metabolic marker), choline and myoinositol (presumed glial markers), and, in some pathological states, lactate. MRS spectra of ^{31}P, covering different frequencies, can be used to determine the relative abundance of inorganic phosphorus, adenosine triphosphate (a metabolic marker), phosphocreatine, phosphomonoesters, and phosphodiesters. There also is the potential to measure ^{13}C-labeled compounds such as glucose and acetate and infer rates of metabolism (Ross et al. 2003).

New Neuroimaging Applications

Monitoring of Disease Progression and Drug Development

Neuroimaging could be used to monitor disease progression and response to therapy. Cerebral atrophy and synaptic failure increase as dementia progresses in neurodegenerative disease, and these can be observed with MRI and FDG-PET. Drugs can be radiolabeled to study their distribution and pharmacokinetics.

Imaging can be used to assess the effects of drugs on neurotransmitter function. The use of imaging to improve the accuracy of diagnosis in clinical trials could be expanded from MRI to include FDG-PET and amyloid imaging. Imaging could help detect the earliest evidence of disease and identify subjects for earlier treatment.

MRI is already incorporated as an outcome measure of treatment response in clinical drug trials (Grundman et al. 2001). Only a few longitudinal studies have been reported of FDG-PET in AD (Alexander et al. 2002), but others are under way.

Personalized Medicine: Risk and Prognosis

Dementing diseases affect individual patients in remarkably different ways. One patient with AD may be agitated, whereas another with the same dementia severity is withdrawn. Personalized medicine identifies the exact cause of disease early and selects the best treatment, by taking into account the individual patient's unique physiology and response to the illness. This approach uses individual differences to better target treatments.

Imaging could significantly advance the personalized approach to care. FDG-PET and amyloid imaging might detect impending dementia in those at genetic risk and accurately predict dementia in those with memory impairment (Small et al. 2000). Molecular imaging can identify individual variability in the distribution of pathology, and this information can be used to tailor individualized therapies.

AD can cause focal and asymmetric clinical syndromes. Likewise, individuals with AD can have FDG-PET scans that appear remarkably different while still remaining recognizable variations on a distinctive pattern of hypometabolism. The cause of this metabolic variability is unknown, but prognosis and response to treatment may be affected.

Key Clinical Points

- Neuroimaging should be used to answer specific clinical questions.
- Neuroimaging cannot determine if dementia is present.
- Magnetic resonance imaging (MRI) is the preferred structural imaging method for dementia, unless contraindicated.

- MRI is sensitive in identifying vascular lesions, but clinical relevance must be considered.
- The pattern of cerebral hypometabolism reflects clinical symptoms.
- The pattern of cerebral hypometabolism can help distinguish Alzheimer disease from frontotemporal dementia.
- Amyloid deposition can be imaged with positron emission tomography; the prognostic implications are not yet clear.

References

Alexander GE, Chen K, Pietrini P, et al: Longitudinal PET evaluation of cerebral metabolic decline in dementia: a potential outcome measure in Alzheimer's disease treatment studies. Am J Psychiatry 159:738–745, 2002

Anchisi D, Borroni B, Franceschi M, et al: Heterogeneity of brain glucose metabolism in mild cognitive impairment and clinical progression to Alzheimer disease. Arch Neurol 62:1728–1733, 2005

Blacker D, Albert MS, Bassett SS, et al: Reliability and validity of NINCDS-ADRDA criteria for Alzheimer's disease. The National Institute of Mental Health Genetics Initiative. Arch Neurol 51:1198–1204, 1994

Boccardi M, Pennanen C, Laakso MP, et al: Amygdaloid atrophy in frontotemporal dementia and Alzheimer's disease. Neurosci Lett 335:139–143, 2002

Bocti C, Swartz RH, Gao F-Q, et al: A new visual rating scale to assess strategic white matter hyperintensities within cholinergic pathways in dementia. Stroke 36:2126–2131, 2005

Bookheimer SY, Strojwas MH, Cohen MS, et al: Patterns of brain activation in people at risk for Alzheimer's disease. N Engl J Med 343:450–456, 2000

Braak H, Braak E: Neuropathological staging of Alzheimer-related changes. Acta Neuropathol 82:239–259, 1991

Brooks DJ, Frey KA, Marek KL, et al: Assessment of neuroimaging techniques as biomarkers of the progression of Parkinson's disease. Exp Neurol 184 (suppl 1):S68–S79, 2003

Clark CM, Schneider JA, Bedell BJ, et al: Use of florbetapir-PET for imaging beta-amyloid pathology. JAMA 305:275–283, 2011

Cosottini M, Ceravolo R, Faggioni L, et al: Assessment of midbrain atrophy in patients with progressive supranuclear palsy with routine magnetic resonance imaging. Acta Neurol Scand 116:37–42, 2007

Du AT, Schuff N, Kramer JH, et al: Different regional patterns of cortical thinning in Alzheimer's disease and frontotemporal dementia. Brain 130:1159–1166, 2007

Dubois B, Feldman HH, Jacova C, et al: Research criteria for the diagnosis of Alzheimer's disease: revising the NINCDS-ADRDA criteria. Lancet Neurol 6:734–746, 2007

Eidelberg D, Dhawan V, Moeller JR, et al: The metabolic landscape of cortico-basal ganglionic degeneration: regional asymmetries studied with positron emission tomography. J Neurol Neurosurg Psychiatry 54:856–862, 1991

Fazekas F, Kleinert R, Offenbacher H, et al: Pathologic correlates of incidental MRI white matter signal hyperintensities. Neurology 43:1683–1689, 1993

Finkenstaedt M, Szudra A, Zerr I, et al: MR imaging of Creutzfeldt-Jakob disease. Radiology 199:793–798, 1996

Forsberg A, Engler H, Almkvist O, et al: PET imaging of amyloid deposition in patients with mild cognitive impairment. Neurobiol Aging 29:1456–1465, 2008

Foster NL, Gilman S, Berent S, et al: Cerebral hypometabolism in progressive supranuclear palsy studied with positron emission tomography. Ann Neurol 24:399–406, 1988

Foster NL, Koeppe RE, Giordani BJ, et al: Variations of the phenotype in frontotemporal dementias, in Genotype-Proteotype-Phenotype Relationships in Neurodegenerative Diseases: Research and Perspectives in Alzheimer's Disease. Edited by Cummings J, Hardy J, Poncet M, et al. Berlin, Springer-Verlag, 2005, pp 139–152

Foster NL, Heidebrink JL, Clark CM, et al: FDG-PET improves accuracy in distinguishing frontotemporal dementia and Alzheimer's disease. Brain 130:2616–2635, 2007

Gado M, Hughes CP, Danziger W, et al: Volumetric measurements of the cerebrospinal fluid spaces in demented subjects and controls. Radiology 144:535–538, 1982

Grundman M, Sencakova D, Jack CR, et al: Use of brain MRI volumetric analysis in a mild cognitive impairment trial to delay the diagnosis of Alzheimer's disease, in Drug Discovery and Development for Alzheimer's Disease 2000. Edited by Fillet H, O'Connell A. New York, Springer, 2001, pp 24–32

Haacke EM, DelProposto ZS, Chaturvedi S, et al: Imaging cerebral amyloid angiopathy with susceptibility-weighted imaging. AJNR Am J Neuroradiol 28:316–317, 2007

Ishii K, Imamura T, Sasaki M, et al: Regional cerebral glucose metabolism in dementia with Lewy bodies and Alzheimer's disease. Neurology 51:125–130, 1998

Klunk WE, Engler H, Nordberg A, et al: Imaging brain amyloid in Alzheimer's disease with Pittsburgh Compound-B. Ann Neurol 55:306–319, 2004

Kuhl DE, Minoshima S, Fessler JA, et al: In vivo mapping of cholinergic terminals in normal aging, Alzheimer's disease, and Parkinson's disease. Ann Neurol 40:399–410, 1996

Kuhl DE, Koeppe RA, Minoshima S, et al: In vivo mapping of cerebral acetylcholinesterase activity in aging and Alzheimer's disease. Neurology 52:691–699, 1999

Kuhl DE, Minoshima S, Frey KA, et al: Limited donepezil inhibition of acetylcholinesterase measured with positron emission tomography in living Alzheimer cerebral cortex. Ann Neurol 48:391–395, 2000

Kwan LT, Reed BR, Eberling JL, et al: Effects of subcortical cerebral infarction on cortical glucose metabolism and cognitive function. Arch Neurol 56:809–814, 1999

Longstreth WT Jr, Bernick C, Manolio TA, et al: Lacunar infarcts defined by magnetic resonance imaging of 3660 elderly people: the Cardiovascular Health Study. Arch Neurol 55:1217–1225, 1998

McKeith I, O'Brien J, Walker Z, et al: Sensitivity and specificity of dopamine transporter imaging with 123I-FP-CIT SPECT in dementia with Lewy bodies: a phase III, multicentre study. Lancet Neurol 6:305–313, 2007

Medina D, DeToledo-Morrell L, Urresta F, et al: White matter changes in mild cognitive impairment and AD: a diffusion tensor imaging study. Neurobiol Aging 27:663–672, 2006

Messa C, Perani D, Lucignani G, et al: High-resolution technetium-99m-HMPAO SPECT in patients with probable Alzheimer's disease: comparison with fluorine-18-FDG PET. J Nucl Med 35:210–216, 1994

Minoshima S, Frey KA, Foster NL, et al: Preserved pontine glucose metabolism in Alzheimer's disease: a reference region for functional brain analysis. J Comput Assist Tomogr 19:541–547, 1995

Mittal S, Farmer P, Kalina P, et al: Correlation of diffusion-weighted magnetic resonance imaging with neuropathology in Creutzfeldt-Jakob disease. Arch Neurol 59:128–134, 2002

Moretti P, Lieberman AP, Wilde EA, et al: Novel insertional presenilin 1 mutation causing Alzheimer disease with spastic paraparesis. Neurology 62:1865–1868, 2004

Murrell JR, Miravalle L, Foster NL, et al: Early-onset familial Alzheimer's disease (AD) from the first American report: a presenilin-1 (PS1) mutation found in descendants. J Neuropathol Exp Neurol 60:543, 2001

Relkin N, Marmarou A, Klinge P, et al: Diagnosing idiopathic normal-pressure hydrocephalus. Neurosurgery 57 (3, suppl):S1–S3; discussion ii–v, 2005

Ringman JM, O'Neill J, Geschwind D, et al: Diffusion tensor imaging in preclinical and presymptomatic carriers of familial Alzheimer's disease mutations. Brain 130:1767–1776, 2007

Román GC, Tatemichi TK, Erkinjuntti T, et al: Vascular dementia: diagnostic criteria for research studies. Report of the NINDS-AIREN International Workshop. Neurology 43:250–260, 1993

Ross B, Lin A, Harris K, et al: Clinical experience with 13C MRS in vivo. NMR Biomed 16:358–369, 2003

Rowe CC, Ng S, Ackermann U, et al: Imaging beta-amyloid burden in aging and dementia. Neurology 68:1718–1725, 2007

Sanders JA: Magnetic resonance spectroscopy, in Functional Brain Imaging. Edited by Orrison WW, Lewine JD, Sanders JA, et al. St Louis, MO, Mosby, 1995, pp 419–467

Schroter A, Zerr I, Henkel K, et al: Magnetic resonance imaging in the clinical diagnosis of Creutzfeldt-Jakob disease. Arch Neurol 57:1751–1757, 2000

Selkoe DJ: Alzheimer's disease is a synaptic failure. Science 298:789–791, 2002

Silverman DH, Small GW, Chang CY, et al: Positron emission tomography in evaluation of dementia: regional brain metabolism and long-term outcome. JAMA 286:2120–2127, 2001

Small GW, Ercoli LM, Silverman DH, et al: Cerebral metabolic and cognitive decline in persons at genetic risk for Alzheimer's disease. Proc Natl Acad Sci U S A 97:6037–6042, 2000

Visser PJ, Verhey FR, Hofman PA, et al: Medial temporal lobe atrophy predicts Alzheimer's disease in patients with minor cognitive impairment. J Neurol Neurosurg Psychiatry 72:491–497, 2002

Viswanathan A, Chabriat H: Cerebral microhemorrhages. Stroke 37:550–555, 2006

Walker Z, Jaros E, Walker RW, et al: Dementia with Lewy bodies: a comparison of clinical diagnosis, FP-CIT SPECT imaging and autopsy. J Neurol Neurosurg Psychiatry 78:1176–1181, 2007

Weiner MF, Hynan LS, Parikh B, et al: Can Alzheimer's disease and dementias with Lewy bodies be distinguished clinically? J Geriatr Psychiatry Neurol 16:245–250, 2003

Zubieta JK, Koeppe RA, Frey KA, et al: Assessment of muscarinic receptor concentrations in aging and Alzheimer's disease with [11C]NMPB and PET. Synapse 39:275–287, 2001

Further Reading

Herholz K, Herscovitch P, Heiss W-D: NeuroPET: PET in Neuroscience and Clinical Neurology. New York, Springer, 2004

McRobbie DW, Moore EA, Graves MJ, et al: MRI From Picture to Proton, 2nd Edition. New York, Cambridge University Press, 2007

Talairach J, Tournoux P: Co-Planar Stereotaxic Atlas of the Human Brain: 3-Dimensional Proportional System: An Approach to Cerebral Imaging. New York, Thieme Medical, 1988

5

Alzheimer Disease

David S. Geldmacher, M.D.

Epidemiology

Alzheimer disease (AD) affects more than 5 million people in the United States and is the most common cause of dementia in the country. The economic burden of caring for patients with dementia is reported as more than $170 billion annually in the United States, exceeding the costs of more common illnesses such as diabetes and arthritis. The number of cases is expected to exceed 13 million in the United States by 2050, with much of the growth attributable to the aging of the population (Hebert et al. 2003).

Clinically diagnosed AD, alone or in combination with other illnesses, accounts for up to 90% of reported dementia cases. Up to two-thirds of those cases also have concomitant pathologies, especially cerebrovascular lesions and Lewy bodies, that might contribute to the symptomatic expression of the dementia (Lim et al. 1999).

Many risk factors have been reported. The strongest associations are with age, family history, and apolipoprotein E genotype. The apolipoprotein E4 allele *(APOE4)* is associated with increased risk, with a dose-related effect on overall risk and earlier age at onset. Approximately 12 other gene loci are associated with small increases in risk for sporadic AD, but the specific abnormalities and the mechanisms by which they enhance risk remain unknown (Bertram et al. 2007).

Other putative risk factors for sporadic, late-onset disease include depression, cardiovascular disease (including hypertension), diabetes mellitus, elevated low-density lipoprotein cholesterol level, elevated plasma homocysteine level, low educational achievement, lack of intellectual activity, lack of physical activity, lack of social interaction, lack of leisure activities, and excessive response to stress, as manifest in elevated plasma cortisol levels. Mixed data have been reported on the effect of hormone replacement therapy in postmenopausal women. Some epidemiological studies suggest that hormone replacement therapy lowers risk, but evidence from clinical trials has indicated that it may exacerbate risk for cognitive decline and dementia in women (Shumaker et al. 2004).

Clinical History and Course of Illness

The defining features of AD are progressive deficits in memory and other aspects of cognition. The deficits result in reduced ability to perform daily activities, and most patients with AD will become totally dependent on others unless they die of other causes first. The deficits result from synaptic dysfunction and neuronal loss that follow a predictable distribution in the brain. Dysfunction in hippocampus, limbic cortex, and polymodal association cortex results in the characteristic clinical pattern of AD and assists in its clinical differentiation from other dementing illnesses, which have different anatomical patterns of neuronal dysfunction.

In this section, I address separately losses in domains such as memory, praxis, visual processing, and executive dysfunction; however, it is important to remember that intact human cognition is a seamless and interdependent whole. Parsing cognitive function into specific domains reflects the conveniences of taxonomy and testing rather than physiological reality.

Cognitive Symptoms

The DSM-IV-TR criteria for diagnosis of AD require evidence of impairment in memory, as well as one other cognitive domain, such as language, praxis, visual processing, or executive function (American Psychiatric Association 2000) (see Table 1–3 in Chapter 1, "Neuropsychiatric Assessment and Diagnosis"). Factor analysis of cognitive testing in 663 patients with probable AD revealed that memory, language, and praxis are the principal cognitive deficits (Talwalker 1996), but this study did not include careful assessment of executive function. More recent studies have found executive dysfunction in a majority of patients (Stokholm et al. 2006). Other focal cognitive deficits associated with temporoparietal lesions, such as spatial disorientation, acalculia, and left-right disorientation, also develop in many patients (Table 5–1).

Memory

Memory dysfunction is usually the first symptom recognized in individuals with AD. It is detectable by neuropsychological tests even in preclinical phases of the disease (Jacobs et al. 1995). The typical memory impairment involves difficulties with learning new information but relative preservation of remote factual information.

AD-related memory change is often described as "short-term memory loss." Recent memories are impaired because new information cannot be adequately stored for later recall. As a result, affected persons initially have difficulty remembering recent events. The span of the "short term" increases over time as the interval since the last period of normal memory function becomes longer. Declarative memory is most impaired in AD. This fact-oriented memory system allows individuals to store and recall specific information and experiences. Procedural memory (knowing how to perform a task) is often better preserved, contributing to the superficial appearance of normality in mild AD. Emotionally toned memories are often better maintained as well. For many individuals, subtle deficits in learning occur prior to overt memory symptoms, but familiar settings, old habits, and preserved social skills mask the problem.

The character of memory loss changes over time. In the mild and moderate stages of the illness, recall of material learned before the onset of memory dysfunction often appears to be preserved. Detailed evaluation of patients reveals that subtle deficits in recall of remote occurrences are frequently present, partic-

Table 5–1. Domains of cognitive impairment in Alzheimer disease

Memory	Visual processing
Deficits in learning	Poor object or person recognition
Semantic knowledge failure	Spatial confusion
Repetitiveness	Impaired directed attention
Orientation	Executive dysfunction
Distorted time sense	Poor planning
Language	Poor judgment
Anomia and word finding difficulty	Impairment on complex tasks
Poor speech content	Disinhibition
Impaired prosody	
Praxis	
Ideomotor apraxia	
Limb-kinetic apraxia	

ularly for specifics like dates and the sequence of events (Storandt et al. 1998). In the late stage, memory dysfunction extends to complete failure of recall for previously well-remembered information, such as the names of the patient's own spouse or children.

Orientation

Although it is often considered a separate cognitive domain, orientation to time and place represents specific types of memory; orientation to person is different. A continuous process of updating memory systems with the passage of time and changes in location is required to maintain orientation. Orientation to time is most vulnerable, but patients often dismiss deficiencies in this ability by stating that the day or date is not important to them, or that they have not looked at the newspaper or television. For healthy older adults, frequent reference to these external resources is generally not required to maintain time and day orientation. More relative concepts of time can also be distorted, such that persons with AD may be unable to recount the hour of the day or the time passed since a recent holiday. As the illness progresses, orientation to place becomes more disrupted. This may result in becoming lost in familiar settings while driving or walking. Spatial disorientation later becomes apparent on a smaller scale, like the home environment. Family members often report this as confusion or difficulty in locating rooms. Spatial disorientation is often worse under conditions of low light, and can be particularly troublesome for families when the patient cannot find the bathroom. Loss of orientation to self is not typical except in profound AD, but language or response disturbances may prevent more mildly affected individuals from identifying themselves on questioning.

Language

Language impairments are a prominent part of the clinical picture. They usually begin as word finding difficulty in spontaneous speech, which may later become severe enough to interrupt the flow of speech and mimic dysfluent aphasia. Initially, patients may complain of frequent tip-of-tongue experiences. Circumlocution becomes common. Some healthy adults have verbal idiosyncrasies or mannerisms that have a similar pattern. It is therefore useful to confirm with family members that the worrisome verbal expression pattern is a change.

Language usually becomes progressively vague. It frequently lacks specifics, because patients substitute generic words or broad categories in place of more explicit nouns. Pronouns (*he, she, they*) are often used in place of proper nouns. There is also an increased use of automatic phrases and clichés, particularly when the patient is pressed for detailed information. Prosody (the normal rhythm, melody, and emotional intonation of speech) is affected in many patients, particularly in more severe stages. Reading skills and verbal comprehension worsen as the disease progresses. In late stages, global aphasia or muteness (aphemia) is common. When present, disrupted communication patterns contribute to strain in caregiving relationships.

Praxis

Nearly all patients will eventually develop apraxia in more severe stages of the disease. Ideomotor apraxia (difficulty in translating an idea into the proper spatially directed action) is most common. This disorder results in reduced ability to manage clothing fasteners or eating utensils. Some patients will lose the conceptual basis of tool use; this is closely related to the loss of semantic knowledge underlying the language and memory problems (Chainay et al. 2006). Another common manifestation of apraxia in more advanced disease is the inability to position parts of the body in space. This deficit is a form of limb-kinetic apraxia and can lead to problems in dressing. It also contributes to difficulties in positioning the body, such as when getting into a car.

Higher Visual Function

Disorders of higher visual processing are common and can be the presenting symptoms in a variant of AD known as *posterior cortical atrophy.* The dysfunction is evident at the level of basic visual processing, including impaired sensitivity to movement and visual contrast. Deficits in depth perception are also observed. Visual processing difficulties can be grouped into three main categories: impaired recognition (agnosia), impaired spatial processing, and impaired visual attention. These domains are differentially affected in individual patients. Impaired recognition becomes evident as agnosia, or the inability to recognize familiar objects. This should be differentiated from anomia, in which the object is recognized but cannot be named. The inability to recognize faces (prosopagnosia) may also evolve, typically in more advanced cases. Problems in spatial processing contribute to spatial disorientation, such as becoming lost in an otherwise familiar environment. Deficits in directed attention become evident in impaired visual exploration, which has important implications for functional tasks, such as driving, that require active scanning of the environment. When severe, spatial processing and directed attention deficits lead to a visual disturbance known as Balint syndrome, an inability to integrate bits of the spatial environment into a coherent whole. As a result, patients have difficulty using vision to voluntarily direct their gaze toward items of interest or accurately guide hand and arm movements.

Executive or Frontal Lobe Function

Executive dysfunction, including problems with judgment, problem solving, planning, and abstract thought, affect a majority of patients, beginning early in the disease course (Stokholm et al. 2006). These behaviors require selecting tasks appropriately, sequencing their execution, and monitoring performance to ensure successful completion. Intact executive function also requires the suppression of inappropriate responses to the environment. Failures in this area of cognition manifest as failure to manage more complicated tasks, such as family finances or meal preparation. Socially inappropriate behavior, disinhibition, and poor task persistence may also emerge. The presence of executive dysfunction predicts the transition from more benign age-related cognitive changes to early dementia. Executive dysfunction may result in both positive symptoms with abnormally triggered behaviors and negative symptoms characterized by a failure to respond to a normally motivating circumstance.

Noncognitive and Behavioral Symptoms

Although not specifically included in the formal diagnostic criteria for AD, noncognitive and behavioral symptoms are important aspects of the clinical expression of the disease and sometimes the presenting complaints (Table 5–2). As the disease progresses, these problems often account for a larger proportion of the burden of care than cognitive dysfunction.

Apathy

Although many clinicians think of agitation as the typical behavioral symptom of AD, personality changes involving passivity and apathy are more frequent early in the illness. Apathy is separable from depression and represents an organic loss of motivation. It occurs in 25%–50% of patients. Apathy includes diminished initiative, reduced emotional expression, and decreased expressions of affection. Social withdrawal, mood changes, or depression has been found in more than 70% of AD cases, with a mean duration of more than 2 years prior to diagnosis (Jost and Grossberg 1996).

Unawareness of Deficits

Another common noncognitive problem in AD is unawareness of illness, which occurs in more than 50% of patients. It is often domain specific; a patient will acknowledge the presence of forgetfulness but deny any functional consequence of the impairment. In most cases, unawareness of deficits appears to represent a self-monitoring deficit of organic origin and should not be solely attributed to psychological denial. Unawareness of illness is a major impediment to early diagnosis and may reduce the effective implementation of management strategies. Anosognosia is also associated with the risk for dangerous behaviors in patients with dementia (Starkstein et al. 2007).

Psychosis

In contrast to unawareness and apathy, psychosis and agitation tend to occur later in the disease. Their emergence is associated with more rapid global decline. Estimates of the prevalence of psychotic features in AD vary widely and are

Table 5–2. Typical noncognitive and behavioral manifestations of Alzheimer disease

Apathy	Mood disorders
Poor initiation	Depression
Poor persistence	Anxiety
Anosognosia/unawareness of illness	Agitation
Psychosis	Nonspecific motor behaviors
Delusions	Wandering
Paranoia	Pacing
Misidentification	Verbal aggression
Hallucinations	Physical aggression
	Sundowning

prone to selection bias. Population-based estimates suggest the prevalence for delusions is about 20%; hallucination prevalence is about 15% (Bassiony and Lyketsos 2003). Delusions are often paranoid in character and may lead to accusations of theft, infidelity, and persecution. The delusion that caregivers or family members are impostors or that one's home is not one's real home is a common trigger for wandering or aggression. Hallucinations in AD are more common in the visual domain but sometimes have auditory components. Hallucinations are frequently of deceased parents or siblings, unknown intruders, and animals. (See also Chapter 12, "Treatment of Psychiatric Disorders in People With Dementia.")

Mood Disorders

Estimates of depression prevalence in dementia vary widely, and depression appears to increase with disease severity. Major depression was observed in about 20% of an AD sample with a mean Mini-Mental State Examination (MMSE) score of 18 (Zubenko et al. 2003). Patients with depression prior to the onset of cognitive decline are more likely to experience major depression during the course of their disease. Anxiety can also be expected in about 25% of patients by the time they reach moderate levels of cognitive impairment. Anxiety tends to be more prominent in the later phases of the illness, but some individuals with AD will experience prominent anxious symptoms early in their course. Catastrophic reactions are intense emotional outbursts of short duration and are associated with anxiety and characterized by abrupt onset of tearfulness, aggressive verbalizations or actions, and contrary behaviors. They are often reactions to environmental stressors, thwarted desires, or attempts at personal care. (See also Chapter 12, "Treatment of Psychiatric Disorders in People With Dementia.")

Agitation and Sundowning

Agitation is reported in 50%–60% of patients with AD. Agitation is not a specific symptom; it can be divided into several behavior classes, including physical aggression/assaultiveness, verbal aggression and outbursts, and nonaggressive physical behaviors (Cohen Mansfield and Deutsch 1996). Aggressive behaviors are most clearly linked to delusions and delusional misidentification. Verbal aggression is more common than physical assault. Men and patients with more advanced functional decline are more likely to demonstrate physical or verbal aggression. Aggressive behaviors usually follow an escalating pattern, with verbal outbursts preceding the physical acts. Many episodes of aggression are triggered by attempted caregiver assistance with personal care, especially bathing.

Wandering, pacing, and recurrent purposeless activities are typical nonaggressive motor behaviors. Wandering is sometimes associated with delusional misidentification; a wanderer may be trying to locate his or her "real" home or locate a "missing" loved one. Wandering has also been associated with poor visuospatial abilities, perhaps reflecting difficulty with incorporating visual information into a coherent spatial map. Dim lighting conditions and nighttime are therefore exacerbating factors for wandering. Risks resulting from wandering include getting lost outdoors and an increased likelihood of fractures. Pacing is somewhat more idiosyncratic, with fewer clearly associated neuropsychological features. The constant movement of pacing contributes to accelerated weight loss in some patients, which can be refractory to dietary interventions unless the locomotor activity is reduced. A more benign form of physical nonaggressive behavior is rummaging in drawers or closets. Rummagers appear to be searching for some item but are often unable to describe what it is. This frequent sorting of personal effects is also associated with delusions of theft.

Sundowning is the term commonly used to describe predictable increases in confusion and behavioral symptoms in the afternoon and evening hours.

It is reported in up to 25% of patients, especially in more advanced stages (Little et al. 1995). Sundowning is not a unitary symptom and often reflects diurnal variation in other symptoms rather than a specific pathophysiology.

Course of Illness

Most patients will pass through a recognizable phase of mild cognitive impairment prior to diagnosis. In mild cognitive impairment, similar deficits in cognition may be identifiable, particularly in the memory domain, but the impairments do not cause disability in usual social or occupational function.

Average survival for patients with AD is 4–6 years following diagnosis (Larson et al. 2004). Many individuals will have prominent symptoms for several years prior to diagnosis. Approximately half of patients will die of complications of global neurological dysfunction, such as immobility and malnutrition; the other half will die of other age-related diseases, such as stroke or cancer.

AD typically follows a relentlessly progressive course, although there may be periods of relative symptom stability. Symptoms tend to progress less rapidly in both early and late disease, with more rapid losses—especially in activities of daily living—in moderate disease.

The disease is commonly conceptualized as a series of "stages" to facilitate communication between providers; formal staging instruments are rarely used in clinical settings. Because the pathological expression of the illness follows a generally linear pattern, these stages do not have clear biological correlates. Typical clinical features of AD at different stages of the illness are listed in Table 5–3.

Mental Status Findings

The symptom pattern and distribution of pathology in AD dictate that cognition should be the major focus of the mental state examination when dementia is suspected. A well-conducted mental status examination should provide enough information to make a diagnosis by standard criteria. Differentiating other dementia types may require more extensive cognitive evaluation. The MMSE (Folstein et al. 1975) has become a de facto standard for assessing cognition in practice settings, particularly for the determination of dementia severity. Age- and education-adjusted norms for the MMSE have been published and should be used as the reference for acceptable performance (Crum et al.

Table 5–3.   Typical clinical features of Alzheimer disease, classified by dementia severity

Mild

   Impaired memory; may not be obvious to casual observer

   Losses in more complicated activities (e.g., meal planning, finances)

   Self-care preserved

   Passive personality change

   Subtle social withdrawal

   Little or no active behavioral manifestations

Moderate

   Obvious memory impairment

   Overt impairment in usual activities (e.g., using stove, telephone)

   Self-care failing (e.g., bathing, grooming)

   Behavioral difficulties typical (e.g., sundowning, paranoia)

   Social skills variable

   Needs supervision

Severe

   Memory fragments only

   May not recognize familiar people

   Loss of all complex activities

   Needs assistance with self-care

   Reduced mobility

1993). In addition, because the MMSE does not represent a comprehensive assessment of the cognitive impairments associated with AD, it should not be substituted for a thorough cognitive evaluation focusing on domains most commonly affected.

Global Assessments

By definition, the diagnosis of AD can be made only in the presence of a clear sensorium. Clouding of consciousness suggests a superimposed medical illness with delirium. Thought content is often impoverished, but its organization is linear and logical. Tangential thinking may be suspected, but this should be carefully evaluated to exclude circumlocution related to word finding difficulties. Loosening of associations is not typical. Psychosis occurs in a minority of individuals, usually in the setting of moderate or more advanced stages of the disease. Delusions with a paranoid character, particularly regarding theft of personal items, are most common. In many cases, these misperceptions are propagated by cognitive deficits. A typical pattern involves a patient forgetting where he or she has placed an item and becoming suspicious that it was stolen. This is often followed by progressively more elaborate hiding of personal effects in obscure locations, which are then also forgotten. Hallucinations are much less frequently noted during examination and occur most often in the context of low illumination and in severe dementia. Judgment declines with increasing dementia severity. Insight into impairments, especially losses in functional skills, is reduced in more than half of AD patients. Up to 50% of patients will have mood complaints consistent with major or minor depression (Lyketsos et al. 1997); euphoria and hypomania are rare. Affect is usually appropriate to the circumstances but may be blunted. Anxiety may be provoked by the unfamiliarity of the testing process and environment.

Cognitive Assessments

Learning and Memory

The patient should be asked to repeat and remember three unrelated words. Lists of semantically related words, such as *red, blue,* and *green,* or *butter, eggs,* and *coffee,* are less useful because remembering their theme can aid recall. If not being conducted as part of the MMSE, the three memory items can be repeated as often as necessary to ensure that the patient can repeat them all. Normal performance is to learn and repeat all three words with the first exposure. After a meaningful delay, generally 5 or more minutes of other mental state testing, the patient should be asked to recall the three words. Normal performance is to recall all three. For those that the patient cannot remember, further steps may be taken to clarify the nature of the memory impairment. The patient can be given a semantic clue, such as "One of the words was a kind of flower." Patients with AD are often not helped by semantic cues, whereas individuals with other memory problems, such as those associated with healthy aging, are more likely to benefit from cuing. Recognition memory can be assessed by asking the patient to select the memory item from a list of semantically related words.

The clinician can check remote memory by asking the patient to name the last five presidents. Alternatively, if a knowledgeable informant is available to confirm the information, patients might be asked to provide the date when they were married or widowed, the number of grandchildren they have, or details of their military service or employment history.

To assess nonverbal aspects of memory, the clinician can ask the patient to observe while the clinician identifies and hides an object in the examination room. The examiner might show a watch or stethoscope to the patient and place it in a drawer. After a few minutes of ongoing physical or cognitive examination, the clinician can ask the patient to recall what was hidden (object memory) and where (spatial memory). Because details are lost from remote memory, it may be useful to ask the patient to provide details of important historical events, such as the attacks on September 11, 2001, or to recall his or her own experiences on learning about the 1963 Kennedy assassination. It is impossible to know how accurately the patient recalls his or her experience, but adults with intact memories are usually able to give lucid and richly detailed recollections of how they received the news, how they reacted, whom they were with, and so forth. Those with poor memories will often be very vague or give temporally inappropriate replies (e.g., saying that they learned about the Pearl Harbor attack on television).

Orientation

Orientation to time, especially dates, is lost early in the course of the disease. Many patients with AD try to minimize aspects of disorientation. Excuses such as a reduced need to keep up with dates are common and are a cue that significant disorientation may be present. The MMSE provides extensive orientation testing. Additional inquiries about the approximate time of day, what meal might be expected next, or the last major holiday can augment the MMSE. Disorientation to self occurs only in advanced dementia. Its presence in the context of mild or moderate cognitive disability suggests delirium or a primary psychiatric disturbance.

Language

Assessment of language includes consideration of naming, comprehension, fluency and effort of speech, sentence repetition, reading, and writing. Language deficits are important in the evaluation for AD because nearly all healthy older adults have normal spontaneous language, except for momentary lapses in word finding, especially for proper names.

Impaired naming on examination often correlates with word finding difficulty in the spontaneous speech of the patient with AD. This impairment can be tested with everyday objects available to the examiner, such as a jacket, shoe, or watch. Parts of objects are more difficult to name than whole objects. Therefore, the patient might be asked to name, in addition to a jacket as a whole, the collar, lapel, sleeve, pocket, and cuff. Responses should be considered correct only if the patient provides a reasonable name for the item. Descriptions of appearance or function should be considered incorrect. Socioeconomic and cultural factors may influence naming of some items, but most individuals should name most of the items effortlessly.

Persons with AD typically have fluent speech that may seem empty, with reduced meaningful content. Except in advanced stages, comprehension is usually sufficient to understand basic conversation and follow simple examination-related commands. Comprehension for syntactically complex instructions is more vulnerable. It can be tested with a two-step command in which the word order does not reflect the order of the intended action (e.g., "Before pointing to the door, point to the ceiling"). This is somewhat more language intensive and less memory dependent than the three-step, syntactically straightforward command on the MMSE.

Praxis and Temporoparietal Function

A brief sequence of commands can be used to assess language comprehension, ideomotor praxis, and left-right orientation. The patient should be asked to carry out a different imagined action with each hand (e.g., using a hammer to hit a nail or a key to open a lock). A subsequent two-handed task, such as slicing bread, tests the patient's ability to integrate the actions of both hemispheres in a single, spatially specific task. These requests can be followed with commands that require the patient to correctly identify right and left, in reference to his or her own body (e.g., "Touch your right hand to your left ear") and the examiner's (e.g., "Point to my left hand with your left hand"). Most normal adults will perform these tasks effortlessly. Mildly affected patients most often perform poorly on the two-handed praxis test.

Visual and Spatial Processing

Many persons with AD have problems in processing perspective and apparent depth. This ability can be tested by having the patient copy a drawing of a cube or other simple three-dimensional figure. Normal performance is to accurately depict three sides and three dimensions. Even mildly affected patients may represent three visible surfaces with no attempt to show their three-dimensional relationship (Figure 5–1).

The integration of motor behavior in space can be further tested with a drawing task. The Clock Drawing Test (Figure 5–2) assesses multiple realms of cognition, including executive function (planning), spatial relationships, and semantic knowledge. Normal performance involves placing all numbers and the hands in the correct position (see Figures 1–4 and 1–5 in Chapter 1, "Neuropsychiatric Assessment and Diagnosis").

Executive Function

Word list fluency can provide useful information about executive function. In this test, the patient is asked to state as many words as he or she can that conform to a semantic category, such as animals or fruits, that is set by the examiner. This is a common neuropsychological test that can be abbreviated for use in a medical assessment. Patients who give fewer than 15 animal names in 1 minute have a high likelihood of dementia (Duff Canning et al. 2004).

Abstract Thought

The examiner can assess abstract reasoning by asking the patient to identify abstract similarities in word pairs, such as "How is a chair like a table?" or "How is an apple like a banana?" Persons with AD are apt to note the difference rather than a similarity. Alternatively, they are likely to identify a concrete rather than abstract similarity. Examples of concrete responses include that a chair and table "go together" or that both the apple and banana "have skin." Interpretation of proverbs is a useful but less desirable test of abstract thought because of cultural, educational, and generational biases.

Attention, Concentration, and Working Memory

To test attention, concentration, and working memory—three related parts of cognition—the examiner can ask the patient to add coins, specifically a penny, a dime, a nickel, and a quarter. For this task, the names of the coins must be used, because the working memory system is engaged throughout the subtly complicated process of translating the names to numerical values, performing stepwise addition, and reporting the answer in a unit different from what was

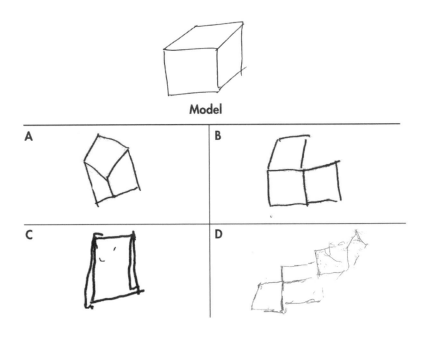

Figure 5–1.   Examples of abnormal cube copying in patients with Alzheimer disease.

The model figure is the "solid" cube. *(A)* Loss of three-dimensional aspects, with preserved representation of the three visible sides (MMSE=22). *(B)* Reduced representation of perspective (MMSE=20). *(C)* Lost representation of perspective/depth (MMSE=14). *(D)* Perseverative response (MMSE=12).

MMSE=Mini-Mental State Examination.

Source.   Reprinted from Geldmacher DS: "Alzheimer Disease," in *The American Psychiatric Publishing Textbook of Alzheimer Disease and Other Dementias.* Edited by Weiner MF, Lipton AM. Washington, DC, American Psychiatric Publishing, 2009, pp. 155–172. Copyright 2009, American Psychiatric Publishing. Used with permission.

provided. Patients without dementia are not overly threatened by this task because it involves familiar items and the everyday activity of adding pocket change. The task is also sufficiently familiar that a pencil and paper are not required for normal performance. The patient who asks for writing tools or who dismisses the task as something he or she would need to write down should raise

A

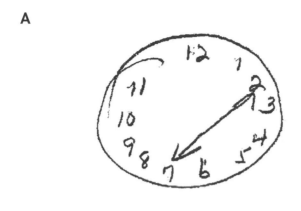

B

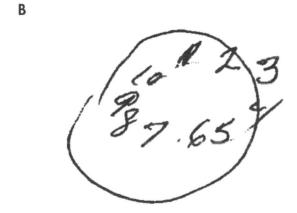

Figure 5–2. Freehand responses to the request "Draw the face of a clock." The drawings show *(A)* intact spatial organization but reduced semantic knowledge of hand configuration and placement for 2:35 (MMSE = 24) and *(B)* marked spatial disorganization (MMSE = 14).

MMSE = Mini-Mental State Examination.

Source. Reprinted from Geldmacher DS: "Alzheimer Disease," in *The American Psychiatric Publishing Textbook of Alzheimer Disease and Other Dementias.* Edited by Weiner MF, Lipton AM. Washington, DC, American Psychiatric Publishing, 2009, pp. 155–172. Copyright 2009, American Psychiatric Publishing. Used with permission.

suspicion of impairment. This pocket change addition task is useful as a cognitive screening tool because it can assess calculation simultaneously with working memory. The patient who answers "36 cents" can add numbers but has failed to include all four coins.

Other tests of working memory or related aspects of attention can be used if pocket change addition is inappropriate—for example, if the person is unfamiliar with the common names of U.S. coins. Alternatives include asking the patient to state the months of the year or days of the week in reverse order. These tests do not, however, incorporate the complexities of translation and addition of the coin-adding task.

Digit span is a common test of primary memory that also depends on attention. In this task, the patient is asked to repeat a string of random digits in the order that he or she heard them. Normal performance is to correctly repeat strings of five or more digits. Deficits may be more pronounced when patients are asked to repeat digits in reverse order. Normal performance in the reverse task is to reach a span at least two digits less than the forward span.

Physical and Neurological Findings

The general physical and neurological examinations remain normal through most of the course of AD. In later stages, extrapyramidal signs (e.g., rigidity) and gait disturbances may become prominent. The point prevalence of myoclonus in AD cohorts is about 5%. It typically worsens with increasing disease severity. Multifocal myoclonus may be difficult to distinguish from seizures in later-stage patients. Epileptic seizures can be expected to arise in 10%–20% of patients with AD, typically in later-stage disease (Mendez et al. 1994).

Laboratory and Imaging Findings

No specific laboratory or imaging test definitively identifies AD. The American Academy of Neurology evidence-based practice parameter for the diagnosis of AD recommends blood tests to exclude systemic illnesses as the cause of cognitive impairment (Table 5–4). These tests assess general metabolic and hematologic states, thyroid function, and vitamin B_{12} levels (Knopman et al. 2001). Syphilis serology tests are no longer considered part of the routine screening. Apolipoprotein E genotyping has been suggested to reduce the rate of false-positive diagnoses when used with clinical criteria (Mayeux et al. 1998), but it is not reimbursed by most insurers and its added value in clinical settings is questionable.

Imaging is recommended as a part of the routine assessment of patients with dementia symptoms. Computed tomography or magnetic resonance imaging (MRI) is useful to exclude structural lesions that may contribute to the dementia; these lesions include cerebral infarctions, neoplasm, extracerebral fluid collections, and hydrocephalus. Current evidence suggests that the presence of mesial temporal atrophy on MRI strongly supports the likelihood of AD when appropriate clinical features are present (Figure 5–3) (Wahlund et al. 2005). Positron emission tomography (PET) scans reveal temporoparietal hypometabolism in patients with AD (Hoffman et al. 2000). In the United States, Medicare has approved PET scanning for the specific indication of distinguishing AD from frontotemporal dementia.

Cerebrospinal fluid (CSF) examination is not a routine part of the dementia evaluation. Standard CSF tests have a low likelihood of influencing diagnosis in most people with dementia. CSF examination is more useful in cases with serological evidence of past syphilis, as well as in patients with immunosuppression or atypical dementia symptom patterns, such as young age at onset or very rapid progression. CSF assays for soluble amyloid-β (Aβ) and tau are commercially available. Some clinicians find them useful in cases of difficult differential diagnosis between Alzheimer and non-Alzheimer causes of dementia, but their utility in more routine clinical populations is unclear.

Electroencephalography is also not recommended as part of the routine evaluation for AD (Knopman et al. 2001). Electroencephalographic findings are nonspecific. They are frequently normal in early stages and evolve toward generalized slowing.

The definitive diagnosis of AD can only be made through autopsy (or biopsy) by identifying appropriate numbers of neuritic plaques and neurofibrillary tangles (NFTs) in specified regions of the brain. The pathological diagnosis requires the presence of a clinical history consistent with dementia, because some individuals with heavy AD pathological burden retain normal cognitive function (Snowdon 2003). Biopsy is not generally recommended for diagnosis. Because of variability in the distribution of plaques and tangles across individuals, a negative biopsy does not exclude AD, although a positive biopsy can confirm it. However, the current state of dementia therapeutics argues that biopsy results are not likely to alter treatment plans. Despite the absence of a reliable laboratory test to definitively identify AD, clinical diagnosis yields an accuracy of >90%, with good concurrence between community-based providers and experts (Mok et al. 2004).

Table 5–4.   Recommended testing for patients presenting with cognitive impairment

Screen for depression

Blood tests

    Comprehensive chemistry panel, including hepatic and renal function

    Complete blood count

    Thyroid function tests

    Vitamin B_{12} level

Brain imaging

    Computed tomography is generally sufficient for screening

Source.   Adapted from Knopman et al. 2001.

Pathology

On gross examination at autopsy, the brain is usually atrophic with enlarged ventricles and sulci (Figure 5–4). Total brain weight is invariably reduced, although significant overlap occurs with the range of brain weights for normal older adults. The hallmark pathological features of the disease remain the neuritic plaques and NFTs first described by Alzheimer (1907).

Neuritic Plaques

Neuritic plaques are extracellular and consist primarily of Aβ, an abnormal proteinaceous material, and cellular elements. Aβ is a ~4-kD peptide that consists of 39–43 amino acid fragments proteolytically derived from a transmembrane protein known as amyloid precursor protein (APP).

Plaques are microscopic, ranging in diameter from 15 to 100 μ, and are distributed in cortex and limbic nuclei (Figure 5–5). The highest concentration is found in the hippocampus. Plaques with a high proportion of distorted presynaptic neuronal elements—dystrophic neurites—are known as *neuritic plaques.* Neurites include intracellular elements of paired helical filaments, lysosomes, and mitochondria. Activated microglial cells are typically found in and around a dense core of extracellular amyloid, whereas fibrillary astrocytes may be seen at the periphery (Wisniewski and Wegiel 1991). "Diffuse" plaques lack the dense Aβ core and do not possess significant numbers of dystrophic neurites. Diffuse plaques are not clearly associated with neuronal loss and cognitive dysfunction.

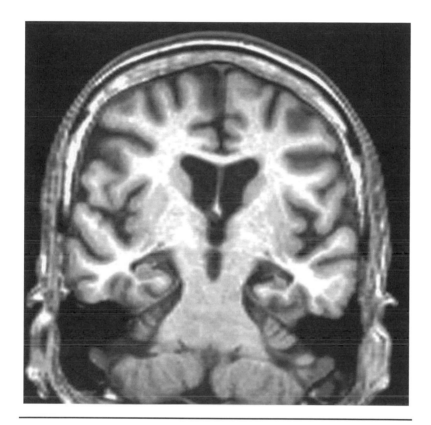

Figure 5–3.   Coronal T_1-sequence magnetic resonance image through the hippocampal region in a patient with mild Alzheimer disease and a MMSE score of 20.

Ambient cistern is widened between hippocampus and brain stem without concomitant dilatation of the temporal horn of the lateral ventricle.

MMSE = Mini-Mental State Examination.

Source.   Reprinted from Geldmacher DS: "Alzheimer Disease," in *The American Psychiatric Publishing Textbook of Alzheimer Disease and Other Dementias.* Edited by Weiner MF, Lipton AM. Washington, DC, American Psychiatric Publishing, 2009, pp. 155–172. Copyright 2009, American Psychiatric Publishing. Used with permission.

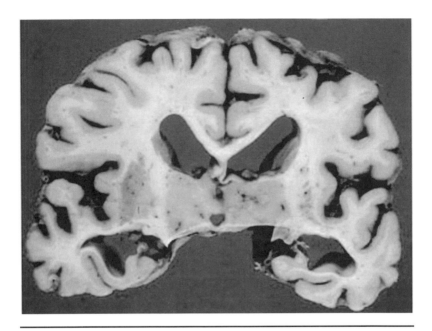

Figure 5–4.   Coronal pathological section of a patient with confirmed Alzheimer disease with hippocampal complex atrophy and dilatation of the temporal horn of the lateral ventricle *(see color plate 6).*
Source.   Reprinted from Geldmacher DS: "Alzheimer Disease," in *The American Psychiatric Publishing Textbook of Alzheimer Disease and Other Dementias.* Edited by Weiner MF, Lipton AM. Washington, DC, American Psychiatric Publishing, 2009, pp. 155–172. Copyright 2009, American Psychiatric Publishing. Used with permission.

Amyloid can also accumulate in cerebral blood vessels, a condition known as cerebral amyloid angiopathy; this leads to subcortical cerebrovascular disease evident on imaging and an increased risk for intracerebral hemorrhage. PET scan techniques can now visualize Aβ accumulations in the living brain.

Neurofibrillary Tangles

NFTs are the second classical finding in AD (Figure 5–6). NFTs are intracellular collections of abnormal filaments, which have a distinctive paired helical

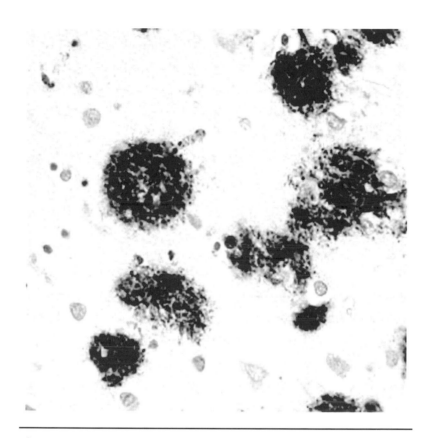

Figure 5–5. Photomicrograph of plaques in the cerebral cortex of a patient with Alzheimer disease *(see color plate 7).*
The section is immunostained for amyloid-β, which appears as dark extracellular granular material. The plaques are large compared with surrounding cellular nuclei.
Source. Reprinted from Geldmacher DS: "Alzheimer Disease," in *The American Psychiatric Publishing Textbook of Alzheimer Disease and Other Dementias.* Edited by Weiner MF, Lipton AM. Washington, DC, American Psychiatric Publishing, 2009, pp. 155–172. Copyright 2009, American Psychiatric Publishing. Used with permission

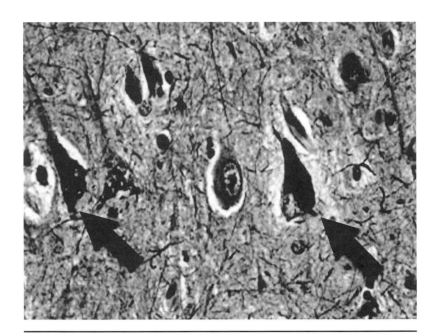

Figure 5–6.   High-power photomicrograph of Bielschowsky-stained neuro-fibrillary tangles *(see arrows)* in the cerebral cortex of a patient with Alzheimer disease *(see color plate 8).*
Tangles are intraneuronal and consist of collapsed cytoskeletal elements, including characteristic paired helical filaments. Tangle development interferes with normal neuronal function through loss of axonal transport and other vital homeostatic mechanisms.
Source.   Reprinted from Geldmacher DS: "Alzheimer Disease," in *The American Psychiatric Publishing Textbook of Alzheimer Disease and Other Dementias.* Edited by Weiner MF, Lipton AM. Washington, DC, American Psychiatric Publishing, 2009, pp. 155–172. Copyright 2009, American Psychiatric Publishing. Used with permission.

structure unique to AD. NFTs are found throughout the neocortex and limbic nuclei, and their density correlates with the degree of neuronal loss. They are also strongly represented in the basal forebrain, substantia nigra, raphe nuclei, and locus coeruleus. NFTs occupy large areas within the cell bodies of affected pyramidal neurons. This class of neurons is responsible for long axonal projections that facilitate inter- and intrahemispheric communication and appears especially sensitive to the effects of AD (Mann et al. 1985).

Synaptic Loss

Widespread cortical synaptic loss occurs and is the major determinant of cognitive disability in AD. Oligomers of Aβ are now implicated as direct synaptotoxins (Lacor et al. 2004). The deep layers of the temporal cortex and the hippocampus sustain the greatest degree of synaptic loss. In addition, synaptic inputs to the cortex are reduced up to 40% by the time of death. The amount of synaptic loss in the frontal cortex correlates well with cognitive impairment in AD (DeKosky and Scheff 1990). Substantial neuronal dropout also occurs in the basal forebrain nuclei (e.g., nucleus basalis of Meynert), which produce the neurotransmitter acetylcholine. The number of NFTs in these deep forebrain cholinergic nuclei closely relates to the degree of cognitive dysfunction in AD (Masliah and Terry 1993). A large proportion of synapses and neurons are also lost in the locus coeruleus and the raphe nuclei. Neurons in these brain stem nuclei produce monoamine neurotransmitters and distribute them in the cerebral cortex via long ascending axons. Losses of acetylcholine, serotonin, and norepinephrine inputs to cerebral cortex contribute to the expression of cognitive and behavioral symptoms.

Genetics

A very small proportion of AD cases (<5%) follow an autosomal dominant inheritance pattern. Individuals in such cases typically develop symptoms prior to age 55, with some experiencing symptoms as early as the fourth decade of life. Mutations on chromosomes 1, 14, and 21 are associated with up to 75% of all early-onset familial cases (Janssen et al. 2003). All of the known mutations result in excess production of Aβ. Another chromosome 21–related form of AD is found in individuals with trisomy 21 (Down syndrome) and rarely in their relatives (Schupf et al. 2001). Instead of a mutated gene, individuals with trisomy 21 possess three copies of APP, resulting in production of excess Aβ, which overwhelms normal clearance pathways, leading to increased Aβ deposition.

Genetic epidemiology suggests that sporadic late-onset AD is best considered a complex genetic disease, with both genetic and environmental contributions. Twin studies, for example, suggest a concordance of only 20% in monozygotic twin pairs (Breitner et al. 1995). APOE4 is the genetic factor most clearly associated with increased risk for sporadic late-onset disease (Bertram et al. 2007). APOE4 is a lipid-carrying protein encoded on chromosome 19 that also binds to circulating Aβ. Other alleles of the APOE4 gene convey less risk and may even be protective. Numerous other putative risk factor loci have been identified, including sites on chromosomes 2, 9, 10, 12, and 15, but the specific genetic defects and the mechanisms by which these genes exert risk remain unknown (Bertram et al. 2007).

Pathophysiology

Both APP and Aβ are normal neuronal protein products. Aβ is produced by the sequential proteolytic activities known as γ-secretase and β-secretase. β-Secretase is also known as β-site APP-cleaving enzyme 1 (APP-BACE1; Stockley and O'Neill 2007). Functionally, γ-secretase activity appears to result from a transmembrane protein complex rather than a single enzyme (Verdile et al. 2007). Following β-secretase cleavage of APP, the action of γ-secretase produces the Aβ peptide, which normally ranges from 38 to 43 amino acids in length. A third enzyme, known as α-secretase, is also involved in normal APP processing. The cleavage site for α-secretase lies within the Aβ sequence and results in nonamyloidogenic products.

In AD, either an increased proportion of Aβ is produced or there is reduced clearance of Aβ, or some combination of the two factors occurs. The 42–amino acid Aβ species is the most likely to associate into fibrils, which are the precursor to plaque formation. Fibrils aggregate into extracellular deposits in an insoluble β-pleated sheet configuration. Previously, parenchymal deposition of Aβ was assumed to be the crucial step in AD pathophysiology. There is growing evidence, however, that prefibrillar, diffusible oligomeric assemblies of Aβ are toxic to neurons and synapses, suggesting that the disease process is under way well prior to plaque formation (Lacor et al. 2004). This evidence is important because it raises the possibility of redefining the boundaries of the disease from both pathological and therapeutic perspectives.

The exact mechanism by which neuronal dysfunction and death occur in AD is unknown. Glycoproteins similar to APP are associated with cell surface interactions and nuclear signaling, which suggests that APP or its normal derivatives might play a role in maintaining synaptic function and neuronal health (Kamenetz et al. 2003). Aβ also is an activating trigger for microglial cells, leading them to produce several inflammatory cytokines, such as tumor necrosis factor–α, that have cytotoxic properties. Activation of microglia may contribute to a self-propagating cycle of local inflammation and neuronal dysfunction (Block et al. 2007). Although most models of AD pathophysiology place Aβ in a causative role, other approaches suggest oxidative stress or bioenergetic failure as a triggering factor in the amyloid cascade (Swerdlow and Khan 2004). It is possible that AD is a disorder with heterogeneous origins, with different primary mechanisms resulting in similar patterns of neuronal failure and pathological expression in different individuals.

Neurochemical Abnormalities

Acetylcholine

Acetylcholine is important for the cognitive functions of attention and memory. Clinical disease severity correlates with loss of cerebral cortical markers for acetylcholine metabolism (Bierer et al. 1995). Choline O-acetyltransferase, which is responsible for acetylcholine synthesis, and acetylcholinesterase, which degrades acetylcholine, are both depleted. The degree of cholinergic reduction in the cortex is closely associated with the amount of cellular loss in the basal forebrain nuclei, where the neurons that produce much of the cortical acetylcholine are located.

Monoamines

Deficiencies in norepinephrine and serotonin also contribute to both cognitive and noncognitive symptoms, especially anxiety and symptoms related to attention and mood. Norepinephrine is important for arousal, learning, and memory. The major site for norepinephrine production is the locus ceruleus in the brain stem, which undergoes significant cell loss in AD. AD is also associated with decreased markers of serotonin activity in the cortex and loss of serotonin-producing cells in the raphe nuclei of the brain stem (Lyness et al. 2003).

Intrinsic classical neurotransmitters, such as γ-aminobutyric acid (GABA), are also diminished, as are many cortically localized neuropeptides, such as somatostatin and corticotropin-releasing factor (Ellison et al. 1986; Panchal et al. 2004). The role of these changes in the clinical syndrome is unknown.

Glutamate and Other Transmitters

Conflicting evidence exists on the status of glutamate in the brain of a patient with AD. Glutamate is the major excitatory neurotransmitter of the cerebral cortex, and neuronal markers of glutamate activity are generally decreased, especially in temporal cortex (Ellison et al. 1986). However, some authors report that glutamate clearance from the synapse is diminished in more advanced disease. Residual synaptic glutamate is thought to result in overexcitation and dysfunction of postsynaptic neurons associated with excess calcium influx (Butterfield and Pocernich 2003). Direct human data on this hypothesis are limited. The role of these changes in the clinical syndrome is unknown.

Treatment

Optimal treatment involves both pharmacological and nonpharmacological approaches (Doody et al. 2001). Currently approved therapies include members of the acetylcholinesterase inhibitor and N-methyl-D-aspartate (NMDA) receptor antagonist classes. These are generally considered symptomatic therapies and have not been demonstrated to alter the underlying pathological process. Treatment of behavioral symptoms is also symptomatically oriented (see Chapter 13, "Pharmacological Treatment of Neuropsychiatric Symptoms"), and no drugs have been specifically approved for these symptoms. Details of treatment outcomes are discussed in Chapter 14, "Pharmacological Treatment of Alzheimer Disease and Mild Cognitive Impairment."

Key Clinical Points

- Alzheimer disease (AD), alone or in combination with other pathology, is the most common cause of dementia in people over age 65.
- Diagnosis of AD requires that the patient have impairment of memory and another cognitive domain, such as language, praxis, visual and spatial processing, or executive function.
- Noncognitive phenomena, including apathy and unawareness, are important contributors to the burden of AD.
- The general neurological examination of AD patients is usually normal, although myoclonus may be present.
- Criterion-based diagnosis is very accurate; imaging and cerebrospinal fluid testing techniques to definitively identify the presence of AD are rapidly emerging.

- The genetic basis of most cases of AD remains unknown, but the mechanism appears to differ from those underlying autosomal-dominant early-onset disease.
- Abnormalities in the processing of amyloid-β peptide contribute to the pathological expression of AD.
- Multiple neurotransmitter systems, especially regulatory pathways involving acetylcholine and the monoamines, are affected.

References

Alzheimer A: Über eine eigenartige Erkrankung der Hirnrinde. Allgemeine Zeitschrift für Psychiatrie und psychisch-gerichtliche Medizin 64:146–148, 1907 (English translation in: Arch Neurol 21:109–110, 1967)

American Psychiatric Association: Diagnostic and Statistical Manual of Mental Disorders, 4th Edition, Text Revision. Washington, DC, American Psychiatric Association, 2000

Bassiony MM, Lyketsos CG: Delusions and hallucinations in Alzheimer's disease: review of the Brain Decade. Psychosomatics 44:388–401, 2003

Bertram L, McQueen MB, Mullin K, et al: Systematic meta-analyses of Alzheimer disease genetic association studies: the AlzGene database. Nat Genet 39:17–23, 2007

Bierer LM, Haroutunian V, Gabriel S, et al: Neurochemical correlates of dementia severity in Alzheimer's disease: relative importance of the cholinergic deficits. J Neurochem 64:749–760, 1995

Block ML, Zecca L, Hong JS: Microglia-mediated neurotoxicity: uncovering the molecular mechanisms. Nat Rev Neurosci 8:57–69, 2007

Breitner JC, Welsh KA, Gau BA, et al: Alzheimer's disease in the National Academy of Sciences–National Research Council Registry of Aging Twin Veterans, III: detection of cases, longitudinal results, and observations on twin concordance. Arch Neurol 52:763–771, 1995

Butterfield DA, Pocernich CB: The glutamatergic system and Alzheimer's disease: therapeutic implications. CNS Drugs 17:641–652, 2003

Chainay H, Louarn C, Humphreys GW: Ideational action impairments in Alzheimer's disease. Brain Cogn 62:198–205, 2006

Cohen-Mansfield J, Deutsch LH: Agitation: subtypes and their mechanisms. Semin Clin Neuropsychiatry 1:325–339, 1996

Crum RM, Anthony JC, Bassett SS, et al: Population-based norms for the Mini-Mental State Examination by age and education level. JAMA 269:2386–2391, 1993

DeKosky ST, Scheff SW: Synapse loss in frontal cortex biopsies in Alzheimer's disease: correlation with cognitive severity. Ann Neurol 27:457–464, 1990

Doody RS, Stevens JC, Beck C, et al: Practice parameter: management of dementia (an evidence-based review). Report of the Quality Standards Subcommittee of the American Academy of Neurology. Neurology 56:1154–1166, 2001

Duff Canning SE, Leach L, Stuss D, et al: Diagnostic utility of abbreviated fluency measures in Alzheimer disease and vascular dementia. Neurology 62:556–562, 2004

Ellison DW, Beal MF, Mazurek MF, et al: A postmortem study of amino acid neurotransmitters in Alzheimer's disease. Ann Neurol 20:616–621, 1986

Folstein MF, Folstein SE, McHugh PR, et al: "Mini-mental state": a practical method of grading the cognitive state of patients for the clinician. J Psychiatr Res 12:189–198, 1975

Hebert LA, Sherr PA, Bienias JL, et al: Alzheimer disease in the U.S. population: prevalence estimates using the 2000 census. Arch Neurol 60:1119–1122, 2003

Hoffman JM, Welsh-Bohmer KA, Hanson M, et al: FDG PET imaging in patients with pathologically verified dementia. J Nucl Med 41:1920–1928, 2000

Jacobs DM, Sano M, Dooneief G, et al: Neuropsychological detection and characterization of preclinical Alzheimer's disease. Neurology 45:957–962, 1995

Janssen JC, Beck JA, Campbell TA, et al: Early onset familial Alzheimer's disease: mutation frequency in 31 families. Neurology 60:235–239, 2003

Jost BC, Grossberg GT: The evolution of psychiatric symptoms in Alzheimer's disease: a natural history study. J Am Geriatr Soc 44:1078–1081, 1996

Kamenetz F, Tomita T, Hsieh H, et al: APP processing and synaptic function. Neuron 37:925–937, 2003

Knopman DS, DeKosky ST, Cummings JL, et al: Practice parameter: diagnosis of dementia (an evidence-based review). Report of the Quality Standards Subcommittee of the American Academy of Neurology. Neurology 56:1143–1153, 2001

Lacor PN, Buniel MC, Chang L, et al: Synaptic targeting by Alzheimer's related amyloid-β oligomers. J Neurosci 24:191–200, 2004

Larson EB, Shadlen MF, Wang L, et al: Survival after initial diagnosis of Alzheimer disease. Ann Int Med 140:501–509, 2004

Lim A, Tsuang D, Kukull W, et al: Clinico-neuropathological correlation of Alzheimer disease in a community-based case series. J Am Geriatr Soc 47:564–569, 1999

Little JT, Satlin A, Sunderland T, et al: Sundown syndrome in severely demented patients with probable Alzheimer's disease. J Geriatr Psychiatry Neurol 8:103–106, 1995

Lyketsos CG, Steele C, Baker L, et al: Major and minor depression in Alzheimer's disease: prevalence and impact. J Neuropsychiatry Clin Neurosci 9:556–561, 1997

Lyness SA, Zarow C, Chui HC: Neuron loss in key cholinergic and aminergic nuclei in Alzheimer disease: a meta-analysis. Neurobiol Aging 24:1–23, 2003

Mann DMA, Yates PO, Marcyniuk B: Correlation between senile plaque and neurofibrillary tangle counts in cerebral cortex and neuronal counts in cortex and subcortical structures in Alzheimer's disease. Neurosci Lett 56:51–55, 1985

Masliah E, Terry RD: Role of synaptic pathology in the mechanisms of dementia of the Alzheimer's type. Clin Neurosci 1:192–198, 1993

Mayeux R, Saunders AM, Shea S, et al: Utility of the apolipoprotein E genotype in the diagnosis of Alzheimer's disease. N Engl J Med 338:506–511, 1998

Mendez MF, Catanzaro P, Doss RC, et al: Seizures in Alzheimer disease: clinicopathologic study. J Geriatr Psychiatry Neurol 7:230–233, 1994

Mok W, Chow TW, Zheng L, et al: Clinicopathological concordance of dementia diagnoses by community versus tertiary care clinicians. Am J Alzheimers Dis Other Demen 19:161–165, 2004

Panchal M, Rholam M, Brakch N: Abnormalities of peptide metabolism in Alzheimer disease. Curr Neurovasc Res 1:317–323, 2004

Schupf N, Kapell D, Nightingale B, et al: Specificity of the fivefold increase in AD in mothers of adults with Down syndrome. Neurology 57:979–984, 2001

Shumaker SA, Legault C, Kuller L, et al: Conjugated equine estrogens and incidence of probable dementia and mild cognitive impairment in postmenopausal women: Women's Health Initiative Memory Study. JAMA 291:2947–2958, 2004

Snowdon DA: Healthy aging and dementia: findings from the Nun Study. Ann Intern Med 139:450–454, 2003

Starkstein SE, Jorge R, Mizrahi R, et al: Insight and danger in Alzheimer's disease. Eur J Neurol 14:455–460, 2007

Stockley JH, O'Neill C: The proteins BACE1 and BACE2 and β-secretase activity in normal and Alzheimer's disease brain. Biochem Soc Trans 35:574–576, 2007

Stokholm J, Vogel A, Gade A, et al: Heterogeneity in executive impairment in patients with very mild Alzheimer's disease. Dement Geriatric Cogn Disord 22:54–59, 2006

Storandt M, Kaskie B, Von Dras DD, et al: Temporal memory for remote events in healthy aging and dementia. Psychol Aging 13:4–7, 1998

Swerdlow RH, Khan SM: A "mitochondrial cascade hypothesis" for sporadic Alzheimer's disease. Med Hypotheses 63:8–20, 2004

Talwalker S: The cardinal features of cognitive and noncognitive dysfunction and the differential efficacy of tacrine in Alzheimer disease patients. J Biopharm Stat 6:443–456, 1996

Verdile G, Gandy SE, Martins RN: The role of presenilin and its interacting proteins in the biogenesis of Alzheimer's beta amyloid. Neurochem Res 32:609–623, 2007

Wahlund LO, Almkvist O, Blennow K, et al: Evidence-based evaluation of magnetic resonance imaging as a diagnostic tool in dementia workup. Top Magn Reson Imaging 16:427–437, 2005

Wisniewski HM, Wegiel J: Spatial relationships between astrocytes and classical plaque components. Neurobiol Aging 12:593–600, 1991

Zubenko GS, Zubenko WN, McPherson S, et al: A collaborative study of the emergence and clinical features of the major depressive syndrome of Alzheimer's disease. Am J Psychiatry 160:857–866, 2003

Further Reading

Chai CK: The genetics of Alzheimer's disease. Am J Alzheimers Dis Other Demen 22:37–41, 2007

Geldmacher DS: Visuospatial dysfunction in neurodegenerative disease. Front Biosci 8:428–436, 2003

Walsh DM, Selkoe DJ: Aβ oligomers–a decade of discovery. J Neurochem 101:1172–1184, 2007

6

Mild Cognitive Impairment

Yonas E. Geda, M.D, M.Sc.

Ronald C. Petersen, Ph.D., M.D.

Because of the high prevalence of Alzheimer disease and other dementias and the high cost of their care, it is imperative to devise a means to prevent or delay the onset of dementing illnesses. Prevention research depends in large measure on identifying a high-risk group suitable for interventional studies. One such group is persons with mild cognitive impairment (MCI). MCI can be defined as the gray zone between normal cognitive aging and early dementia. Individuals with amnestic MCI show memory impairment greater than ex-

Preparation of this chapter was supported by grants K01 MH68351, U01 AG06786, P50 AG16574, and U01 AG10483 from the National Institutes of Health and the Robert Wood Johnson Foundation.

pected for their age, but otherwise function independently and do not meet the commonly accepted criteria for dementia (Petersen et al. 2005). Patients with amnestic MCI develop dementia at rates of 10%–15% per year, compared with rates of 1%–2% per year in the general population (Petersen et al. 1999).

History

Reisberg and colleagues were perhaps the first to use the term *mild cognitive impairment* (Reisberg et al. 2008). Using the Global Deterioration Scale (Reisberg et al. 1982), they defined MCI as a score of 3 on a 7-point scale (1=normal, 7=severe dementia). In 1986, the term *age-associated memory impairment* was proposed by an expert panel (Crook et al. 1986). In 1994, the International Psychogeriatric Association created the term *age-associated cognitive decline* (Levy 1994). The operational criteria referred to a variety of cognitive domains that are presumed to decline in normal aging, and included age- and education-adjusted normative values. Finally, the Clinical Dementia Rating scale (Morris 1993) includes a category of "questionable dementia," used to describe individuals with a score of 0.5. The Mayo Clinic criteria for MCI have incorporated advances made by use of theoretical constructs preceding it, and the category of amnestic MCI was also empirically validated in a prospective study (Petersen et al. 1999).

Progression of MCI to Dementia

Several studies have estimated the progression rate of MCI to dementia (Petersen et al. 1999, 2005). Findings vary depending on the study design and measurement instrument. For example, a group that recruited study participants by advertisement and then prospectively followed a cohort of subjects reported a conversion rate of 6% per year (Daly et al. 2000), in contrast to a clinical trial in which a conversion rate of 16% per year was reported (Petersen et al. 2005). Prior to that, researchers reported a conversion rate in the range of 10%–15% per year. Despite discrepancies between studies, all of them show that individuals with MCI develop dementia at a higher rate than the general population. Thus, MCI appears to be an optimal target for clinical trials.

One topic of debate is the "instability" of the MCI construct. French investigators reported a reversion rate from MCI to normal of as high as 40% over 2–3 years. However, their sole MCI criterion was performance on the Benton Visual Retention Test (Benton et al. 1983). An international consensus panel on MCI emphasized the importance of progressive decline rather than reliance on poor performance at any one point (Winblad et al. 2004).

Clinical Features

Elderly persons commonly present with memory concerns. Although such concerns could result from depression or concern about the normal changes of aging, they could also suggest an early dementing illness. A typical clinical scenario follows:

> A 72-year-old right-handed man with 12 years of education presented with concern over forgetfulness for recent events and future engagements. Family members and close friends had made similar observations. He had difficulty identifying the onset of these symptoms but felt that they had started insidiously and progressed gradually over a period of 2–3 years. He was living independently and had no difficulty carrying out activities of daily living, such as handling his own finances, cooking, and driving. He denied depression, stress, or significant medical issues.
> A clinical evaluation, including history, physical examination, and brief cognitive screening, suggested cognitive impairment, but not severe enough to warrant a diagnosis of dementia; hence, a tentative clinical diagnosis of MCI was made. Psychometric testing and a brain magnetic resonance imaging (MRI) study were ordered. Neuropsychological testing revealed memory impairment, particularly on measures of learning and delayed recall, greater than expected for age; other cognitive domains such as language and visuospatial skills were relatively intact. MRI revealed mild hippocampal atrophy.

The key finding from this patient's history is persistent, serious forgetfulness of insidious onset that gradually progressed over 2–3 years. All other cognitive domains (language, comportment–executive function, visuospatial skills) were intact. The individual did not have a decline in function. This was probably an early disease process involving information processing in the medial temporal lobes; the most likely diagnosis is amnestic MCI.

Subtypes

The original Mayo Clinic criteria for amnestic MCI are 1) a memory complaint, preferably corroborated by an informant; 2) impaired memory for age on psychometric testing; 3) normal general cognitive function; 4) intact activities of daily living; and 5) no dementia (Petersen et al. 2001). Although amnestic MCI is the most widely studied and empirically validated construct, an international consensus on MCI suggested three additional subtypes (Winblad et al. 2004).

Figure 6–1 depicts the diagnostic algorithm that can be used to arrive at a diagnosis of a particular MCI subtype. The process has two major steps: establishment of the diagnosis of MCI, followed by identification of the type and number of cognitive domains involved. The algorithm is initiated when a patient or informant reports cognitive complaints such as forgetfulness for recent events and future engagements. The clinician then determines that the patient neither has dementia nor has cognitive functioning normal for age. Once this is established, the next step is to make sure that there is no substantial decline in function detected by a careful history from the patient and corroborated by a collateral source. If the decline in function is not sufficient to warrant diagnosis of dementia, the physician assumes a diagnosis of MCI and proceeds to identify the number and types of cognitive domains impaired.

Neuropsychological testing can be helpful in classifying MCI subtypes. A diagnosis of *amnestic MCI—single domain* is assumed if the impairment involves only memory, whereas *amnestic MCI—multiple domain* pertains to impairments in memory plus at least one other cognitive domain, such as language, executive function, or visuospatial skills. Likewise, a diagnosis of *non-amnestic MCI—single domain* is assumed if the impairment is in a single nonmemory domain, whereas *non-amnestic MCI—multiple domain* refers to impairments in multiple nonmemory domains.

This diagnostic algorithm may be helpful in gaining more insight into the prodromal forms of various dementing illnesses, which may in turn have therapeutic implications. Medications for treatment of prodromal forms of dementia may very well be specific to the underlying etiology of the developing disorder.

The single- and multiple-domain amnestic MCI subtypes with presumed degenerative etiology are probably prodromal Alzheimer disease (Winblad et al. 2004). The non-amnestic subtypes with impairments in the nonmemory do-

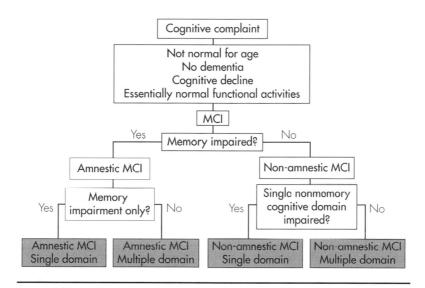

Figure 6–1.   Flowchart of decision process for diagnosing subtypes of mild cognitive impairment (MCI).

Source.   Reprinted from Geda YE, Negash S, Petersen RC: "Mild Cognitive Impairment," in *The American Psychiatric Publishing Textbook of Alzheimer Disease and Other Dementias.* Edited by Weiner MF, Lipton AM. Washington, DC, American Psychiatric Publishing, 2009, pp. 173–180. Copyright 2009, American Psychiatric Publishing. Used with permission.

mains have a higher likelihood of progressing to a non-Alzheimer dementia, such as dementia with Lewy bodies.

Neuropsychiatric Features

Relatively less work has been conducted on the neuropsychiatric aspect of MCI. This issue is logical to address because the medial temporal lobe and its connections with prefrontal and other structures play a critical role in both cognitive function and emotional behavior (Mesulam 1998). Findings from the first population-based investigation of the neuropsychiatric symptoms of MCI were reported by Lyketsos et al. (2002). Since then, similar studies have been done using samples largely derived from primary or tertiary care settings (Feldman et al. 2004). Psychiatric symptoms were examined in prodromal Alzheimer disease (Copeland et al. 2003) as well. Lyketsos et al. (2002) postulated that if MCI is a pre–Alzheimer disease state, the prevalence rate of neuropsychiatric symptoms in MCI should be intermediate between that of normal aging and dementia, and indeed some findings substantiate this hypothesis (Geda et al. 2004; Hwang et al. 2004).

Geda et al. (2006) prospectively followed 840 cognitively intact elders for a median period of 3.5 years (range=1–15 years) to the outcome of incident MCI. The authors observed that depression, as measured by the abbreviated Geriatric Depression Scale (Sheikh and Yesavage 1986), more than doubled the risk of transition from normal aging to incident MCI. They also observed a synergistic interaction between depression and the apolipoprotein E (APOE) genotype.

Geda et al. (2006) proposed four hypotheses to explain the association between depression and incident MCI. The first is an *etiological pathway*, through which depression leads to MCI by its effect on a neurobiological pathway in which increased secretion of corticosteroids or other "neurotoxic" biological factors lead to brain damage. An implication of this hypothesis is that treating depression may help to prevent MCI. The second hypothesis pertains to a *shared risk factor* or *confounding*, in which depression is noncausally associated with an independent risk factor for MCI (Szklo and Nieto 2000). The risk factor could be genetic, environmental, or both. This hypothesis points to a susceptibility gene variant or another nongenetic risk factor that increases the risk of depression and MCI independently. The third hypothesis is *reverse causality*, in which a person experiencing cognitive decline may develop depression as a reaction. The depressive symptoms may then "unmask" MCI in individuals with limited cognitive reserve. Thus, depression could be an early manifestation of preclinical MCI or a reaction to the initial symptoms of MCI. Lastly, there could be an *interaction*, in which depression is a risk factor for MCI only in the presence of a susceptibility gene variant or another nongenetic risk factor. Geda et al. found evidence, for example, of a synergistic interaction between the APOE genotype and depression. Of course, these four mechanisms (and other possible mechanisms) are not mutually exclusive. Future studies based on these possible mechanisms could prove useful in understanding the psychiatric variables in MCI, as well as in designing clinical trials that target psychiatric symptoms in the setting of MCI.

Neuroimaging

Although the cornerstone of MCI diagnosis is the history and clinical examination, neuroimaging can have an important role in clarifying MCI diagnosis (see Chapter 4, "Neuroimaging"). For example, MRI with visual qualitative and/or automated voxel-based morphometry may be helpful in predicting which MCI subjects will progress to dementia. Early MRI work was mainly limited to measurement of the hippocampal volume (Jack et al. 1999), but as imaging research has progressed, atrophy of the entorhinal cortex has been identified as an early marker of amnestic MCI and a predictor of future Alzheimer disease (Grundman et al. 2004; Korf et al. 2004). An important challenge in MRI research is variability in methods of measuring hippocampal volume, but DeCarli et al. (2007) found that subjective visual assessment of hippocampal volume can be useful.

Diffusion-weighted imaging is also a highly sensitive early indicator of abnormalities that may precede structural changes in the hippocampus. Proton magnetic resonance spectroscopy may also be a valuable tool in identifying the subtypes of MCI and tracking pathological processes responsible for cognitive decline (Kantarci et al. 2004).

Investigations using functional MRI (fMRI) have reported positive correlations between performance on memory tasks and activation of the medial temporal lobe or hippocampal gyrus. Increased activation of the right parahippocampal gyrus has been observed with increasing clinical impairment. This finding was interpreted as suggesting recruitment of additional networks and structures to compensate for the medial temporal dysfunction in these patients (Dickerson et al. 2004). Researchers in fMRI studies of MCI have reported increased activation or recruitment of several other structures, such as the frontal, temporal, anterior cingulate, and fusiform gyri. These activations have been interpreted as compensatory networks by some investigators (Yetkin et al. 2006). However, decreased activation has been observed in anterior frontal, prefrontal, precuneus, and posterior cingulate gyri as well (Dannhauser et al. 2005).

Other functional imaging techniques include single-photon emission computed tomography, a technique that measures regional cerebral blood flow, and positron emission tomography (PET), which provides a direct measure of brain metabolism. Reduced cerebral perfusion and glucose metabolism in temporoparietal regions, posterior cingulate gyrus, and hippocampus have been associated with progressive cognitive decline in MCI; however, these changes lack sensitivity and specificity (Chételat et al. 2003). Mosconi et al. (2005) investigated metabolic activity in the hippocampi of subjects with MCI using both region of interest (ROI) and voxel-based analysis (VBA). The results were consistent with those of previous reports showing hypometabolism in the hippocampi of subjects with MCI, but this was evident only with the ROI technique and not with VBA. The limitations of PET in terms of spatial resolution and the deformation of brain areas in VBA were proposed as likely explanations for the discrepant findings in this study and others.

Researchers at the University of Pittsburgh have developed a marker known as Pittsburgh compound B (PIB), which enables in vivo imaging of brain amyloid (Klunk et al. 2003, 2004). PIB led to tremendous enthusiasm in the research community with regard to its potential for detecting incipient or preclinical Alzheimer disease. Price et al. (2005) evaluated five normal control, five MCI, and five clinical Alzheimer disease cases using PIB. Case patients with Alzheimer disease and normal control subjects were easily separated on the basis of PIB retention, whereas the MCI case patients were either more similar to the Alzheimer patients or appeared normal rather than exhibiting the expected transitional or intermediate state of PIB retention. This finding may reflect that MCI is a heterogeneous condition. Incident MCI cases might resemble normal controls, whereas advanced MCI (prevalent MCI) cases might resemble Alzheimer disease.

Neuropathology

Do persons with MCI actually have Alzheimer disease at the time of their clinical diagnosis of MCI? This is a reasonable question because many of the biomarker and neuroimaging studies have implied that the Alzheimer disease process is well under way even at the MCI clinical stage. Two studies have addressed this issue. One study found that individuals who died while their clinical classification was amnestic MCI did not meet criteria for the neuropathological diagnosis of Alzheimer disease (Jicha et al. 2006). Most of the subjects studied appeared to have transitional pathology, implying that had they lived longer, they would have developed the full neuropathological picture of Alzheimer disease. The most common characteristics of these subjects were neurofibrillary pathology in the medial temporal lobe and diffuse amyloid deposition in the neocortex, but not sufficient neuritic plaque pathology to meet Alzheimer disease neuropathological criteria.

Another study followed subjects previously diagnosed with MCI who progressed to dementia (Petersen et al. 2006). This study revealed that only 80% of the subjects with amnestic MCI developed clinical and pathological Alzheimer disease. This finding indicates that although the amnestic MCI criteria are reasonably specific, they are not sufficient to permit the definitive diagnosis of Alzheimer disease at this stage. Some of the subjects went on to have other forms of dementia, such as dementia with Lewy bodies, frontotemporal dementia, or vascular dementia. Consequently, because it is important not to mislabel subjects as having Alzheimer disease, it is preferable to retain the diagnosis of MCI with its qualifications with regard to longitudinal outcome.

Treatment

No standard treatment is used for MCI, but numerous clinical trials are being undertaken with the aim of delaying the onset of dementia (Chertkow 2002). These trials have been reviewed comprehensively by Geda and Petersen (2001). Results of a large clinical trial involving 70 medical centers in North America were reported by Petersen et al. (2005). In this randomized, double-blind, placebo-controlled study, the objective was to assess the safety and efficacy of high-dose vitamin E (2,000 IU/day) and donepezil (10 mg/day), and the study was designed to have adequate power to detect a decrease in the conversion rate of MCI to Alzheimer disease from the anticipated 45% down to 30% over the course of 3 years. Among the 769 subjects who were randomly assigned, the annual conversion rate from MCI to Alzheimer disease was approximately 16% per year (48% over 3 years). Donepezil reduced the risk of progression to Alzheimer disease for the first 18 months of the trial but not afterward. Vitamin E had no therapeutic effect.

Key Clinical Points

- Amnestic mild cognitive impairment (MCI) seems to be an intermediate stage between normal aging and Alzheimer disease.

- Amnestic MCI is associated with biological markers such as decreased hippocampal volume and the accumulation of amyloid plaques in the brain.
- Other forms of MCI may be related to other types of brain pathology.
- Neuropsychiatric symptoms are more prevalent in MCI subjects than in age-matched control subjects.

References

Benton A, Hamsher K, Varney NR, et al: Contributions to Neuropsychological Assessment. New York, Oxford University Press, 1983

Chertkow H: Mild cognitive impairment. Curr Opin Neurol 15:401–407, 2002

Chételat G, Desgranges B, de la Sayette V, et al: Mild cognitive impairment: can FDG-PET predict who is to rapidly convert to Alzheimer's disease? Neurology 60:1374–1377, 2003

Copeland MP, Daly E, Hines V, et al: Psychiatric symptomatology and prodromal Alzheimer's disease. Alzheimer Dis Assoc Disord 17:1–8, 2003

Crook T, Bartus R, Ferris S, et al: Age-associated memory impairment: proposed diagnostic criteria and measures of clinical change. Report of a National Institute of Mental Health Work Group. Dev Neuropsychol 2:261–276, 1986

Daly E, Zaitchik D, Copeland M, et al: Predicting conversion to Alzheimer disease using standardized clinical information. Arch Neurol 57:675–680, 2000

Dannhauser TM, Walker Z, Stevens T, et al: The functional anatomy of divided attention in amnestic mild cognitive impairment. Brain 128:1418–1427, 2005

DeCarli C, Frisoni GB, Clark CM, et al: Qualitative estimates of medial temporal atrophy as a predictor of progression from mild cognitive impairment to dementia. Arch Neurol 64:108–115, 2007

Dickerson BC, Salat DH, Bates JF, et al: Medial temporal lobe function and structure in mild cognitive impairment. Ann Neurol 56:27–35, 2004

Feldman H, Scheltens P, Scarpini E, et al: Behavioral symptoms in mild cognitive impairment. Neurology 62:1199–1201, 2004

Geda YE, Petersen RC: Clinical trials in mild cognitive impairment, in Alzheimer's Disease and Related Disorders. Edited by Gauthier S, Cummings J. London, Martin Dunitz, 2001, pp 69–83

Geda YE, Smith GE, Knopman DS, et al: De novo genesis of neuropsychiatric symptoms in mild cognitive impairment (MCI). Int Psychogeriatr 16:51–60, 2004

Geda YE, Knopman DS, Mrazek DA, et al: Depression, apolipoprotein E genotype, and the incidence of mild cognitive impairment: a prospective cohort study. Arch Neurol 63:435–440, 2006

Grundman M, Petersen RC, Ferris SH, et al: Mild cognitive impairment can be distinguished from Alzheimer disease and normal aging for clinical trials. Arch Neurol 61:59–66, 2004

Hwang TJ, Masterman DL, Ortiz F, et al: Mild cognitive impairment is associated with characteristic neuropsychiatric symptoms. Alzheimer Dis Assoc Disord 18:17–21, 2004

Jack CR Jr, Petersen RC, Xu YC, et al: Prediction of AD with MRI-based hippocampal volume in mild cognitive impairment. Neurology 52:1397–1403, 1999

Jicha GA, Parisi JE, Dickson DW, et al: Neuropathologic outcome of mild cognitive impairment following progression to clinical dementia. Arch Neurol 63:674–681, 2006

Kantarci K, Petersen RC, Boeve BF, et al: 1H MR spectroscopy in common dementias. Neurology 63:1393–1398, 2004

Klunk WE, Engler H, Nordberg A, et al: Imaging the pathology of Alzheimer's disease: amyloid imaging with positron-emission tomography. Neuroimaging Clin N Am 13:781–789, 2003

Klunk WE, Engler H, Nordberg A, et al: Imaging brain amyloid in Alzheimer's disease using Pittsburgh Compound-B. Ann Neurol 55:306–319, 2004

Korf ES, Wahlund LO, Visser PJ, et al: Medial temporal lobe atrophy on MRI predicts dementia in patients with mild cognitive impairment. Neurology 63:94–100, 2004

Levy R: Aging-associated cognitive decline. Int Psychogeriatr 6:63–68, 1994

Lyketsos CG, Lopez O, Jones B, et al: Prevalence of neuropsychiatric symptoms in dementia and mild cognitive impairment: results from the Cardiovascular Health Study. JAMA 288:1475–1483, 2002

Mesulam MM: From sensation to cognition. Brain 121:1013–1052, 1998

Morris J: The Clinical Dementia Rating (CDR): current version and scoring rules. Neurology 43:2412–2414, 1993

Mosconi L, Tsui WH, De Santi S, et al: Reduced hippocampal metabolism in MCI and AD: automated FDG-PET image analysis. Neurology 64:1860–1867, 2005

Petersen RC, Smith GE, Waring SC, et al: Mild cognitive impairment: clinical characterization and outcome. Arch Neurol 56:303–308, 1999

Petersen RC, Doody R, Kurz A, et al: Current concepts in mild cognitive impairment. Arch Neurol 58:1985–1992, 2001

Petersen RC, Thomas RG, Grundman M, et al: Vitamin E and donepezil for the treatment of mild cognitive impairment. N Engl J Med 352:2379–2388, 2005

Petersen RC, Parisi JE, Dickson DW, et al: Neuropathologic features of amnestic mild cognitive impairment. Arch Neurol 63:665–672, 2006

Price JC, Klunk WE, Lopresti BJ, et al: Kinetic modeling of amyloid binding in humans using PET imaging and Pittsburgh Compound-B. J Cereb Blood Flow Metab 25:1528–1547, 2005

Reisberg B, Ferris SH, de Leon MJ, et al: The Global Deterioration Scale for assessment of primary degenerative dementia. Am J Psychiatry 139:1136–1139, 1982

Reisberg B, Ferris SH, Kluger A, et al: Mild cognitive impairment (MCI): a historical perspective. Int Psychogeriatr 20:18–31, 2008

Sheikh JI, Yesavage JA: Geriatric Depression Scale (GDS): recent evidence and development of a shorter version, in Clinical Gerontology: A Guide to Assessment and Intervention. New York, Haworth Press, 1986, pp 165–173

Szklo M, Nieto F: Epidemiology: Beyond the Basics. Gaithersburg, MD, Aspen, 2000

Winblad B, Palmer K, Kivipelto M, et al: Mild cognitive impairment: beyond controversies, towards a consensus. Report of the International Working Group on Mild Cognitive Impairment. J Intern Med 256:240–246, 2004

Yetkin FZ, Rosenberg RN, Weiner MF, et al: FMRI of working memory in patients with mild cognitive impairment and probable Alzheimer's disease. Eur Radiol 16:193–206, 2006

Further Reading

Busse A, Hensel A, Gühne U, et al: Mild cognitive impairment: long-term course of four clinical subtypes. Neurology 67:2176–2185, 2006

Winblad B, Palmer K, Kivipelto M, et al: Mild cognitive impairment: beyond controversies, towards a consensus. Report of the International Working Group on Mild Cognitive Impairment. J Intern Med 256:240–246, 2004

7

Vascular Cognitive Disorder

Cassandra E.I. Szoeke, Ph.D., F.R.A.C.P., M.B.B.S.,
B.Sc. (Hons.)

Stephen Campbell, F.R.A.C.P., M.Ch.B.S., B.Sc.

Edmond Chiu, A.M., M.B.B.S., D.P.M., F.R.A.N.Z.C.P.

David Ames, B.A., M.D., F.R.C.Psych., F.R.A.N.Z.C.P.

The term *vascular cognitive disorder* is used in this chapter to represent the diversity of vascular changes that can lead to cognitive impairment. A key factor with this form of cognitive impairment is that vascular changes are to some extent preventable. Therefore, early detection and accurate diagnosis, with initiation of appropriate treatments and risk factor control, can have a significant impact on patient outcomes.

History

Although initial research on dementia routinely attributed cognitive damage to arteriosclerosis and chronic cerebral ischemia, the discovery of Alzheimer disease changed this view, and the importance of vascular cognitive disorders was then largely ignored. Once Alzheimer disease was seen as the major cause of dementia, the criteria formulated to assess this disease became the basis of all dementia diagnosis (American Psychiatric Association 1994; World Health Organization 1993). The subsequent focus on memory impairment as the defining event leading to a diagnosis of dementia has eclipsed the significance of damage to other cognitive domains of equal functional importance.

Dementia after stroke was reported by Thomas Willis in the seventeenth century. In 1899, arteriosclerosis and senile dementia were delineated as distinct syndromes, with older patients thought more likely to have vascular dementia (Holstein 1997). However, later histological studies in older patients with dementia that revealed predominantly Alzheimer disease pathology temporarily diminished the view that vascular disease played a significant role in these patients (Nolan et al. 1998). A renewed interest in vascular etiologies occurred in the late 1960s, when a strong association between hypertension, arteriosclerosis, and dementia was reported (Román 2003). Hachinski and colleagues described multi-infarct dementia in 1974. More recently, the association between vascular disease and characteristic findings seen in patients with Alzheimer disease was recognized. An improved understanding of the metabolic, chemical, and neurogenic control of cerebral blood flow and metabolism, as well as advances made in neuroimaging, has led to a resurgence of interest in vascular cognitive disorder.

Diagnostic Criteria

Vascular cognitive disorder encompasses vascular dementia, vascular cognitive impairment without dementia, and mixed Alzheimer and cerebrovascular dementias. Just as strokes located within different regions of the brain can produce highly variable symptoms, lesions of different types and at different locations vary enormously in the cognitive deficits that result. Stroke physicians have recognized a number of syndromes, which have specific outcomes, treatment options, and prognoses. Likewise, a similar mechanism of damage can result in a range of deficits in cognitive, behavioral, and executive functions, and therefore an appropriate syndromal classification can have important implications for management.

Development of Diagnostic Criteria

A variety of terms and scales have been used. The term *dementia of the cerebrovascular type* was limited by its exclusion of cardiac or hypotensive causes of cerebral ischemia. The term *multi-infarct dementia* was accompanied by a scale to aid in diagnosis (Hachinski et al. 1975). Although the Hachinski model made clear distinctions between Alzheimer disease and multi-infarct vascular cognitive disorder, it did not account well for those individuals with cognitive change from one single event or from progressive, insidious small-vessel damage.

Dementia is defined in DSM-IV-TR (American Psychiatric Association 2000) as a syndrome of acquired intellectual deficits that results in significant impairment of social or occupational functioning. Criteria from DSM-IV-TR, the International Classification of Diseases (ICD-10; World Health Organization 1993), and the International Workshop of the National Institute of Neurological Disorders and Stroke and the Association Internationale pour la Recherche et l'Enseignement en Neurosciences (NINDS-AIREN; Román et al. 1993) require the presence of memory impairment. Although the early involvement of the medial temporal lobes in Alzheimer disease leads to almost universal early involvement of memory, memory may be only slightly impaired in cerebrovascular disease.

The most widely used diagnostic criteria for vascular dementia have been the NINDS-AIREN consensus criteria, presented in Table 7–1. These are based on the ICD-10 dementia diagnosis but address pathological subtypes of vascular dementia syndromes and take into account the fact that the clinical course is not necessarily "stepwise" but is potentially static, remitting, or progressive. These criteria also address specific clinical findings and the importance of neuropsychological assessment, with an emphasis on deficits in cognitive domains other than memory, in contrast to classical Alzheimer dementia. These criteria established the importance of brain imaging showing a temporal relationship between the appearance of a new cortical stroke or progression of white matter disease and change in cognitive function. This was the first criteria set to include neuroimaging with specific criteria to describe location and severity of lesions (Román et al. 1993). Using these criteria, a diagnosis can be reached of *probable* (memory impairment+ another cognitive domain+cerebrovascular disease imaging evidence with clear association to decline) or *possible* (memory impairment+another cognitive domain+cerebrovascular disease without imaging evidence or clear association to decline) vascular dementia.

None of the current criteria include individuals with intact memory whose executive dysfunction is severe enough to impair daily functioning. Neither do they include those with vascular cognitive impairment or mild vascular cognitive disorder, although these patients are at risk of significant progression and comorbidity from their vascular risk factors and are most likely to benefit from identification, early intervention, and therapy.

Comparison of Scales and Diagnostic Criteria

Unfortunately, the NINDS-AIREN criteria have a low sensitivity (Chui et al. 2006). The Hachinski scoring paradigm (Hachinski et al. 1975) has been a reliable means of identifying patients with vascular dementia. Of the scales available, the Hachinski scale has the highest interrater reliability, the DSM-IV (American Psychiatric Association 1994) criteria have the best sensitivity (50%), and the NINDS-AIREN criteria have the highest specificity (97%) (Chui et al. 2000). In addition to assessment of the clinical performance of these criteria, postmortem studies comparing clinical diagnosis with pathological findings have been conducted. Gold et al. (1997) examined 113 autopsy-confirmed cases of dementia and found that the Hachinski scale had 88% specificity and the NINDS-AIREN criteria had 80% specificity. The highest sensitivity (63%) was achieved by the State of California Alzheimer's Disease Diagnostic and Treatment Centers (AD-DTC) criteria (Amar et al. 1996). Although the NINDS-AIREN criteria have adequate specificity for vascular dementia (93% for probable, 84% for possible), they have poor sensitivity (20% for probable, 55% for possible) (Gold et al. 2002), indicating that a large proportion of cases of vascular dementia are not detected by the current classification system. Another limitation of these criteria is in their application. When the DSM-IV, NINDS-AIREN, and ADDTC criteria were all used to classify a large subset of patients with incident dementia from the Cardiovascular Health Study, the different criteria identified entirely different subjects (Lopez et al. 2005). Similar results were seen with a study of nearly 1,900 patients enrolled in the Canadian Study of Health and Aging, in which a tenfold difference was seen in the incidence of vascular dementia, depending on the classification used (Erkinjuntti et al. 2007).

The greatest limitation of the NINDS-AIREN criteria is their reliance on imaging. Strict application of the imaging criteria to poststroke patients showed no

Table 7–1. NINDS-AIREN criteria for the diagnosis of vascular dementia

A. The clinical diagnosis of *probable* vascular dementia requires:

1. *Dementia* as defined by DSM criteria.

2. *Cerebrovascular disease,* including focal neurological signs consistent with stroke (with or without history of stroke), and brain imaging evidence of CVD including *multiple large vessel infarcts or a single strategically placed infarct* (angular gyrus, thalamus, basal forebrain, or anterior or posterior communicating territories), as well as *multiple basal ganglia* and *white matter lacunes,* or *extensive periventricular white matter lesions,* or combinations of these.

3. *A relationship between cognitive disorder and stroke,* suggested by one or more of the following: (a) onset within 3 months following a stroke; (b) abrupt deterioration in cognitive functions; or (c) fluctuating, stepwise progression of cognitive deficits.

B. Clinical features consistent with *probable* vascular dementia include early gait disturbance; unsteadiness and frequent, unprovoked falls; early urinary frequency, urgency, and other urinary symptoms not explained by urologic disease; pseudobulbar palsy; and personality and mood changes, abulia, depression, emotional incontinence, or other subcortical deficits including psychomotor retardation and impaired executive function.

C. Clinical diagnosis of *possible* vascular dementia requires DSM dementia and focal neurologic signs in patients without imaging evidence of CVD; or without clear temporal relationship between dementia and stroke; or in persons with subtle onset and variable course (plateau or improvement) of cognitive deficits and evidence of relevant CVD.

D. Criteria for diagnosis of *definite* vascular dementia are (a) clinical criteria for *probable* vascular dementia; (b) CVD demonstrated from biopsy or autopsy; (c) neurofibrillary tangles and neuritic plaques not exceeding those expected for age; and (d) absence of other clinical or pathological disorder capable of producing dementia.

Note. CVD=cardiovascular dementia; NINDS-AIREN=National Institute of Neurological Disorders and Stroke and the Association Internationale pour la Recherche et l'Enseignement en Neurosciences.
Source. Reprinted from Román GC, Tatemichi TK, Erkinjuntti T, et al.: "Vascular Dementia: Diagnostic Criteria for Research Studies. Report of the NINDS-AIREN International Workshop." *Neurology* 43:250–260, 1993. Used with permission.

difference in findings between those with and those without dementia, with a greater degree of hippocampal atrophy being the only distinguishing feature of those with dementia (Ballard et al. 2004). This finding raises the possibility that some cases of poststroke dementia may represent an "unmasking" of preexisting Alzheimer pathology.

In addition to the low sensitivity of current diagnostic criteria, the criteria fail to detect cases of mixed vascular and Alzheimer pathology. It is surprising that although up to a 40% overlap exists between vascular and neurodegenerative dementias (Kalaria and Ballard 1999), no diagnostic criteria include mixed-type dementia. Gold et al. (2002) estimated that up to 50% of mixed dementia cases are classified as "pure" vascular cognitive disorder. Even the reliability of autopsy studies has to be questioned, given that the incidence can vary from 0% to 55% (Zekry et al. 2002). The complexity of multifactorial pathology is increased by the ability of vascular lesions in the centers involved in memory (basal ganglia, thalamus, or deep white matter) to significantly worsen the symptoms of Alzheimer disease (Snowdon et al. 1997).

Subtypes

Vascular cognitive disorder is cognitive impairment with evidence on imaging, history, or clinical examination of cerebrovascular disease that is judged to be responsible for the cognitive impairment. Memory impairment, if present, is characteristically of the non-amnestic type (e.g., inefficiency in both initial registration and recall of information, with recall of established memory often similarly affected). The term *vascular cognitive impairment* is used when a patient has cognitive decline with intact functional ability. The term *vascular dementia* is used when the severity of cognitive deficits is sufficient to impair the patient's ability to live independently.

The reported subtypes of dementia discussed in the following subsections overlap with pathophysiological systems, with classification based on the underlying etiology. The three main contributions to dementia of the vascular type are localized infarction, microvascular disease, and concurrent atrophy.

Subcortical Ischemic Vascular Cognitive Disorder

The most common form of vascular cognitive disorder is thought to be subcortical vascular damage. Given that lacunar stroke represents 20%–30% of symptomatic stroke, this subtype of vascular cognitive disorder is likely to be highly prevalent in the aging population. The hypothesis is that these small lacunes produce a loss of subcortical neurons or that the disconnection of neurons from the cortical neuronal pathways causes the constellation of dysexecutive syndrome, slowed cognition and motor processing speed, and attentional impairment. Memory deficits generally consist of impaired recall of both recent and distant information, with relatively intact recognition. Neuroimaging reveals lacunar infarcts and deep white matter changes.

This pattern of cerebral damage is caused by diffuse small-vessel disease. Clinical features depend on the location of lacunar lesions and often include frontal lobe signs (especially impairment of executive function), global cognitive decline, and affective symptoms. These features have been linked to cerebral blood flow abnormalities in frontal areas and basal ganglia (Yang et al. 2002), and patients with this pattern of damage are at high risk of developing secondary depression.

Multi-Infarct Vascular Cognitive Disorder

Patients with multi-infarct vascular cognitive disorder have evidence of strokes or white matter infarcts on structural imaging. The development of focal neurological signs on examination or evidence of an increased burden of cerebral ischemia on brain imaging is temporally associated with the cognitive decline. This subtype is often described as having a stepwise decline.

Vascular Cognitive Disorder Due to Strategic Infarcts

In patients with vascular cognitive disorder due to strategic infarcts, the degree of cognitive decline is out of keeping with the overall vascular burden. Infarcts are strategically placed so as to interfere maximally with memory and cognition, as in cases of anterior cerebral artery infarct, parietal lobe infarcts, cingulate gyrus infarction, and especially thalamic infarction.

Diffuse White Matter Disease

In addition to cognitive decline, patients with vascular cognitive disorder characteristically have diffuse white matter disease *(leukoaraiosis)* on neuroimaging. Several large studies have reported the correlation of leukoaraiosis and cognitive decline (Longstreth et al. 2005; van den Heuvel et al. 2006). The syndrome of Binswanger disease is a specific subtype of diffuse subcortical leukoencephalopathy caused by thickening of the walls of the small arteries and fibrinoid necrosis of the larger vessels within the brain (Ramos-Estébanez and Rebello Alvarez-Amandi 2000). The associated vasculopathy, aneurysm formation, and stenosis in the leptomeningeal and cortical vessels cause damage to the subcortical white matter.

Vascular Cognitive Disorder Due to Hemorrhagic Lesions (Amyloid Angiopathy)

Amyloid angiopathy involves the accumulation of amyloid within the walls of cerebral blood vessels. This can cause bleeding and interruption of cerebral blood flow. Hereditary conditions, such as hereditary cystatin C amyloid angiopathy, have been described. These patients have recurrent cerebral hemorrhages before age 40 years.

Inflammatory Vascular Disease

Rare arteriopathies can cause multiple infarcts and vascular cognitive disorder. These arteriopathies include inflammatory arteriopathies, such as polyarteritis nodosa and temporal arteritis, and noninflammatory arteriopathies, such as moyamoya disease and fibromuscular dysplasia.

Hypoperfusion

Hypoperfusion due to large-vessel or cardiac disease can affect the watershed areas of the brain. It can be seen in states of low cardiac output, such as severe congestive heart failure or decreased cerebral flow from any other cause.

Mixed Dementia (Alzheimer and Vascular)

A diagnosis of mixed dementia is based on history and typical neuropsychological findings of Alzheimer disease and evidence of cerebrovascular disease, either clinically or based on neuroimaging evidence of ischemic lesions.

Epidemiology

A Swedish study reported a lifetime risk of developing vascular dementia of 34.5% for men and 19.4% for women (Hagnell et al. 1992). Vascular dementia may be the second most common dementia, with 10%–20% of people with late-onset dementia having evidence of this type (Rocca et al. 1991), but the high prevalence of vascular lesions in patients diagnosed with Alzheimer disease has led many to suggest that in fact, mixed Alzheimer–vascular dementia is the most common type of dementia in developed countries (del Ser et al. 1990). Although the risk of developing both Alzheimer-type and vascular dementias increases with age, it increases more steeply for Alzheimer disease. Under age 75 years, men are at higher risk for vascular-type and women are at higher risk for Alzheimer-type dementia; in older age, the sex difference is less pronounced (Jorm and Jolley 1998). Dementia is common in those who have had strokes, either immediately or with delayed onset.

The overlap between vascular cognitive disorder and ischemic stroke has been the source of much phenotypic confusion. Ischemic stroke was initially divided into large- and small-vessel disease, whereas vascular cognitive impairment was initially divided into cortical and subcortical types, although more recently these diagnostic criteria have been revised (Kidwell and Warach 2003). The location of the infarct is the most significant determinant of poststroke dementia. After age 65, one-third of people who have had a stroke will develop symptoms of dementia (Esiri et al. 1999).

Genetics

Monogenic conditions represent only a minority of cases of vascular cognitive disorder. The angiopathies are important genetic disorders predisposing individuals to both stroke and vascular cognitive disorder. Certain familial forms of dementia related to homocystinuria and types of amyloidosis have been described (Adam et al. 1982). In vascular dementia, no significant difference has been found in concordance rates among monozygotic and dizygotic twin pairs (Bergem et al. 1997), suggesting that environmental factors play a large role. Population-based genetic screening has not been successful in discovering a clear genetic risk factor for developing vascular cognitive disorder. Studies have examined whether there is an association between vascular dementia and apolipoprotein E polymorphisms, but the findings have been conflicting (Gorelick 1997).

Some rare genetic disorders result in cerebral ischemic damage, the best described being cerebral autosomal dominant arteriopathy with subcortical infarcts and leukoencephalopathy (CADASIL; Chabriat et al. 2009) (see Chapter 4, Figure 4–11) and autosomal dominant hereditary cerebral hemorrhage with amyloidosis (Bornebroek et al. 1996; Nishitsuji et al. 2007; Wang et al. 1997).

CADASIL is a rare autosomal dominant condition localized to chromosome arm 19q12 that affects small vessels supplying the deep white matter. Leukoaraiosis has evidence for genetic risk, with twin studies revealing a heritability of 71% and genomewide scanning showing strong linkage on chromosome 4p (DeStefano et al. 2006). The area on 4p has no previously identified stroke risk factor genes, but is known to contain aging- and mitochondria-related genes.

Etiology

An important consideration in the etiology of vascular cognitive disorder is its relationship with aging. In advanced age, the reduction in cognitive reserve means that a smaller lesion can result in clinically significant cognitive impairment. In addition, other factors associated with aging, such as vitamin deficiency leading to hyperhomocysteinemia (vitamin B_{12}, folic acid) and end-organ dysfunction (particularly cardiac), can predispose to dementia. Vascular disease can cause both focal and diffuse effects on the brain. Whereas focal disease is most likely to result from large-vessel pathology secondary to thrombotic or embolic vascular occlusions, hypertension is the main cause of diffuse disease from small-vessel pathology.

Brain parenchymal damage of vascular origin can occur from ischemia, hemorrhage, or edema. The main types of damage result from one or a combination of single strategic infarcts, multiple infarcts, lacunes, small-vessel disease, or diffuse white matter disease. The areas of the brain that when damaged cause cognitive impairment are the white matter of the cerebral hemispheres and the deep gray nuclei (striatum and thalamus). There are complex feedback loops in the pathophysiology of vascular cognitive disorder. Hypertension, diabetes, and cardiac disease predispose to vascular events. Although the various subtypes of vascular lesion can coexist, the etiology of each is addressed separately below.

Macrovascular Disease

Risk factors for macrovascular cerebrovascular disease include increasing age, hypertension, cigarette smoking, hyperlipidemia, diabetes, atrial fibrillation, and hyperhomocysteinemia. Other risk factors include decreased physical activity, obesity, use of oral contraceptives, increased plasma fibrinogen, and a hypercoagulable state (activated protein C or S deficiency, antiphospholipid antibodies) (Kakafika et al. 2007; Muscal and Brey 2007).

Chronic atrial fibrillation, aneurysms of the left ventricle, and poor left ventricular contraction increase risk of stroke by promoting thrombus formation in the chambers of the heart. Large-artery atherosclerotic disease within the carotids or vertebrobasilar systems or an embolic source from the aortic arch can cause macrovascular stroke. There are rarer sources of emboli, such as paradoxical emboli (via a patent foramen ovale), paradoxical emboli (from an atrial myxoma), or infective emboli (from endocarditis).

Small-Vessel or Penetrating Artery Disease

Small-vessel disease results in arterial wall changes, expansion of the Virchow-Robin spaces, perivascular parenchymal rarefaction, and gliosis. In addition, it can cause discrete small deep infarcts (lacunes) due to occlusion of long-perforating arterial branches. These infarcts are most commonly due to chronic hypertension with secondary hypertrophy of the media of the arteriolar wall and subsequent deposition of fibrinoid material within the vessel wall. An alternative rarer source of this pathology is microscopic emboli from a central source, or small-vessel arteritis. These lacunae are found more typically in the internal capsule, deep gray nuclei, and white matter.

Chronic altered blood flow within small intracranial vessels can lead to diffuse white matter damage, also termed *leukoaraiosis*. Leukoaraiosis greater than 25% is considered to be pathological (Ball 1989). Subcortical vascular dementia is a diffuse small-vessel disease with minimal or absent infarction and with homogeneous pathological and clinical features.

Neurotransmitters

Cholinergic (Mesulam et al. 2003), serotonergic, and hypothalamic-pituitary-adrenocortical axis abnormalities (Gottfries et al. 1994) have been implicated in the altered cognition in vascular cognitive disorder. Other neurotransmitters, including dopamine, glutamate, and γ-aminobutyric acid (GABA), have shown some evidence of involvement. The high degree of mixed pathology complicates the ability to determine the contribution of vascular and Alzheimer pathology to these changes.

Animal studies suggest that vascular disruption is associated with cholinergic denervation (Moser et al. 2006). There is also feedback with neurotransmitters having a known role in modulating cerebral blood flow. For this reason, cholinesterase inhibitors have been used with some reported success (Wilkinson et al. 2003). The changes in cholinergic markers in vascular dementia are not as significant as those in Alzheimer disease (Jia et al. 2004); an effect was found only in cholinergic terminal markers, not on receptor numbers. This has been confirmed in a study of 42 autopsy cases, in which specimens from subjects with Alzheimer disease and patients with mixed dementia had greater cholinergic deficit than did tissue from subjects with vascular dementia (Perry et al. 2005). Trials demonstrating that partial N-methyl-D-aspartate (NMDA) channel blockade by memantine is efficacious (Orgogozo et al. 2002) further reinforce that neurotransmitters have a role in vascular cognitive disorder.

Overlap With Alzheimer Disease

Using DSM-IV criteria, population-based studies have shown that mixed dementia and vascular dementia are equally common (Knopman et al. 2003). In addition to finding overlap between Alzheimer and vascular dementias, studies have found similar overlaps with dementia with Lewy bodies and vascular change (Barber et al. 1999), indicating that vascular pathology may affect outcome in many disorders with cognitive decline. The commonality of risk factors between Alzheimer disease and vascular disease could be the co-occurrence of two common conditions or the result of common etiological factors. The amyloid-β plaque protein of Alzheimer disease is known to deposit within the blood vessels of the aging brain, and can produce an angiopathy characterized by microinfarcts and hemorrhages. Amyloid angiopathy is present in more than half of patients with Alzheimer disease and is almost universal in those with Down syndrome (Vinters 1987). The amyloid-β molecule could also have vasogenic actions through reactive oxygen species (Niwa et al. 2001). Complex interactions between vascular and Alzheimer pathology have been suggested. For example, amyloid angiopathy may enhance the formation and/or compromise the elimination of amyloid-β and phosphorylated tau. Cells with inadequate blood supply may themselves be predisposed to create these protein by-products.

Whether or not vascular dementia and Alzheimer disease share common etiologies, lacunar infarcts in the basal ganglia, thalamus, and deep white matter appear to greatly increase the risk for symptomatic Alzheimer disease (Snowdon et al. 1997). The presence of macrovascular strokes has been reported to double the rate of progression of dementia in Alzheimer disease (Heyman et al. 1998).

Assessment

History and Clinical Examination

The presence of cerebrovascular risk factors and focal neurological findings with onset in temporal relation to cognitive decline suggest a vascular etiology. History should therefore include family history and personal history of hypertension, smoking, hyperlipidemia, diabetes, arrhythmias, and evidence of other vascular pathologies such as cardiovascular and peripheral vascular disease. The classic stepwise progression of changes is characteristic of multi-infarct dementia. Specific characteristics in the history are associated with certain vascular cognitive disorders. For example, Binswanger disease has an average onset in the fourth to seventh decades of life. Most patients with this disease have coexistent hypertension. Progression usually is slow, over a period of years, and includes deficits in cognition, mood and behavioral changes, and motor dysfunction. Early features are often mood and behavioral changes and early-onset urinary incontinence and gait abnormalities (Binswanger 1884). CADASIL, described earlier, affects persons in the third and fourth decades; these patients have more severe cerebrovascular disease and are less likely to have hypertension.

Assessments used to determine the degree of cognitive impairment are described in Chapter 2, "Medical and Neurological Evaluation and Diagnosis," and Chapter 3, "Neuropsychological Assessment." The most commonly used scale, the Mini-Mental State Examination (Folstein et al. 1975), assesses vascular cognitive impairment poorly. Improvement in the bedside tools for assessment of cognition is under way. Assessment of mood is also important; a scale such as the Geriatric Depression Scale (Jongenelis et al. 2007) can be used.

All patients should undergo routine laboratory testing, as indicated in Chapter 2. In some situations, echocardiography, Holter monitoring, and carotid duplex scanning may be indicated.

Neuroimaging

The use of magnetic resonance imaging (MRI) to describe both the severity and location of disease is a cornerstone of the NINDS-AIREN criteria. With the increased use of computed tomography and MRI, the number of patients diagnosed with "silent" vascular brain injury has increased.

Large epidemiological imaging studies have shown that one-third of older individuals had evidence of lacunar strokes (Longstreth et al. 1998), and although these did predispose to further strokes (Longstreth et al. 2001), their association with cognitive changes is not proven. No clear relationship has been shown between vascular lesion load and the presence of dementia (Ballard et al. 2004), and epidemiological imaging studies have shown that "silent lesions" are a common finding in healthy individuals (Longstreth et al. 2001).

Functional imaging techniques such as positron emission tomography (PET) (Kerrouche et al. 2006) and single-photon emission computed tomography (SPECT) also have utility in differentiating vascular-type from Alzheimer-type dementia. SPECT shows a pattern of multiple, asymmetric perfusion deficits in multi-infarct dementia. PET shows that in subcortical vascular dementia, oxygen extraction fraction is maintained despite reduced perfusion.

Neuropsychological Assessment

Neuropsychological testing (see also Chapter 3) is an essential part of the clinical assessment. To distinguish vascular from Alzheimer dementia, characteristic changes are sought in the different cognitive domains. Specifically, changes in attention, speed of information processing, and executive functioning are characteristic of vascular cognitive disorder. Given the nature of vascular disease, patients with vascular cognitive disorder can have patchy neuropsychological deficits. They tend to have better recall than patients with Alzheimer disease but have poor verbal fluency and often more perseverative behavior. Neuropsychological findings vary depending on the site and extent of vascular damage; deep white matter disease is reflected by reduced speed of processing, as well as impaired dexterity and executive function.

Association With Psychiatric Disorders

The behavioral and psychiatric symptoms of dementia are addressed in Chapter 12, "Treatment of Psychiatric Disorders in People With Dementia," and their management is discussed in Chapter 13, "Pharmacological Treatment of Neuropsychiatric Symptoms." Evidence suggests that the severity of depression in vascular cognitive disorder relates to the severity of frontal lobe damage (Alexopoulos 2003). Examination of patients with known vascular dementia revealed that over 70% had clinically significant anxiety and 20% had evidence of depression on standardized validated measures (Ballard et al. 2000). Although psychological symptoms are common in dementias of all types, both anxiety and depression were statistically more likely in patients with vascular dementia than in those with Alzheimer-type dementia.

Treatment

Stroke prevention prevents vascular dementia (Goldstein 2006). Therefore, addressing all the risk factors for stroke and using treatments to prevent cerebrovascular disease are encouraged. Cardiovascular risk factors should be treated, not only to delay progression of cognitive impairment but also to prevent the development of vascular comorbidity. Thus, medication and lifestyle interventions to treat hypertension, hyperlipidemia, and diabetes are important. Diet is important, with recommendations for low-fat intake and appropriate levels of folate and B vitamins, because increased homocysteine levels, which are a key risk factor for stroke, are associated with low levels of folate and B vitamins (Smith 2006). Antiplatelet agents, anticoagulants, endarterectomy, and stenting all have a place in the management of vascular disorders.

Neurotransmitter Modulators

Cholinesterase inhibitors and NMDA receptor antagonists have shown promise as treatments for patients with vascular cognitive impairment. Cholinesterase inhibitors have had modest positive results in controlled trials (Erkinjuntti 2002). The NMDA receptor antagonist memantine has been shown in two controlled trials to produce a small beneficial effect on cognition but no improvement on global measures of function (McShane et al. 2006; Orgogozo et al. 2002).

Outcome

No relationship has been found in vascular dementia between cognitive progression and rate of atrophy detected by neuroimaging (O'Brien et al. 2001). The Canadian Study of Health and Aging showed that 2.6% of participants had vascular cognitive impairment and that 1.5% met criteria for vascular dementia. At 5-year follow-up of patients with vascular cognitive impairment without dementia, all who were still alive had progressed to a diagnosis of dementia (Wentzel et al. 2001). Prospective studies have confirmed this high rate of conversion from vascular cognitive impairment to dementia (Meyer et al. 2002). For this reason, targeting this group for preventive treatment is important.

Conclusion

As the population ages, the incidence of vascular disease will increase and therefore the contribution of vascular change to cognitive decline will rise. Recent work on vascular disease has allowed new options for treatment. Although the benefits in trials of cholinesterase inhibitors in vascular dementia have been modest and clinical applications are not yet clearly delineated, the research has been limited by the inclusion of only subjects with late-stage disease and with entry criteria requiring significant memory impairment. New work with treatment in earlier vascular cognitive impairment with clear diagnostic criteria, in addition to primary and secondary prevention with optimization of cardiovascular risk, holds promise for reducing the burden of disease within the community.

Key Clinical Points

- Diagnostic criteria for vascular cognitive disorder need to be refined.
- Significant overlap exists between vascular cognitive disorder and Alzheimer disease and possibly other dementias.
- Vascular dementia has a poor prognosis if untreated.
- Identification and treatment of vascular risk factors are essential.
- Psychiatric comorbidity is common and should be detected and treated.

References

Adam J, Crow TJ, Duchen LW, et al: Familial cerebral amyloidosis and spongiform encephalopathy. J Neurol Neurosurg Psychiatry 45:37–45, 1982
Alexopoulos GS: Vascular disease, depression, and dementia. J Am Geriatr Soc 51:1178–1180, 2003

Amar K, Wilcock GK, Scott M, et al: The diagnosis of vascular dementia in the light of the new criteria. Age Ageing 25:51–55, 1996

American Psychiatric Association: Diagnostic and Statistical Manual of Mental Disorders, 4th Edition. Washington, DC, American Psychiatric Association, 1994

American Psychiatric Association: Diagnostic and Statistical Manual of Mental Disorders, 4th Edition, Text Revision. Washington, DC, American Psychiatric Association, 2000

Ball MJ: "Leukoaraiosis" explained. Lancet 1:612–613, 1989

Ballard C, Neill D, O'Brien J, et al: Anxiety, depression and psychosis in vascular dementia: prevalence and associations. J Affect Disord 59:97–106, 2000

Ballard CG, Burton EJ, Barber R, et al: NINDS AIREN neuroimaging criteria do not distinguish stroke patients with and without dementia. Neurology 63:983–988, 2004

Barber R, Scheltens P, Gholkar A, et al: White matter lesions on magnetic resonance imaging in dementia with Lewy bodies, Alzheimer's disease, vascular dementia, and normal aging. J Neurol Neurosurg Psychiatry 67:66–72, 1999

Bergem AL, Engedal K, Kringlen E, et al: The role of heredity in late-onset Alzheimer disease and vascular dementia: a twin study. Arch Gen Psychiatry 54:264–270, 1997

Binswanger O: Die Abgrenzung der allgemeinen progressiven Paralyse, I–III. Berliner klinische Wochenschrift 48:1103–1105, 1137–1139, 1180–1186, 1884

Bornebroek M, Haan J, Maat-Schieman ML, et al: Hereditary cerebral hemorrhage with amyloidosis–Dutch type (HCHWA-D), I: a review of clinical, radiologic and genetic aspects. Brain Pathol 6:111–114, 1996

Chabriat H, Joutel A, Dichgans M, et al: CADASIL. Lancet Neurol 8:643–653, 2009

Chui HC, Mack W, Jackson JF, et al: Clinical criteria for the diagnosis of vascular dementia: a multicenter study of comparability and interrater reliability. Arch Neurol 57:191–196, 2000

Chui HC, Zarow C, Mack WJ, et al: Cognitive impact of subcortical vascular and Alzheimer's disease pathology. Ann Neurol 60:677–687, 2006

del Ser T, Bermejo F, Portera A, et al: Vascular dementia: a clinicopathological study. J Neurol Sci 96:1–17, 1990

DeStefano A, Atwood L, Massaro JM, et al: Genome-wide scan for white matter hyperintensity: the Framingham Heart Study. Stroke 37:77–81, 2006

Erkinjuntti T: Diagnosis and management of vascular cognitive impairment and dementia. J Neural Transm Suppl 63:91–109, 2002

Erkinjuntti T, Ostbye T, Steenhuis R, et al: The effect of different diagnostic criteria on the prevalence of dementia. N Engl J Med 337:1667–1674, 2007

Esiri MM, Nagy Z, Smith MZ, et al: Cerebrovascular disease and threshold for dementia in the early stages of Alzheimer's disease. Lancet 354:919–920, 1999

Folstein MF, Folstein SE, McHugh PR: "Mini-mental state": a practical method for grading the cognitive state of patients for the clinician. J Psychiatr Res 12:189–198, 1975

Gold G, Giannakopoulos P, Montes-Paixao Júnior C, et al: Sensitivity and specificity of newly proposed clinical criteria for possible vascular dementia. Neurology 49:690–694, 1997

Gold G, Bouras C, Canuto O, et al: Clinicopathological validation study of four sets of clinical criteria for vascular dementia. Am J Psychiatry 159:82–87, 2002

Goldstein L: Primary prevention of ischemic stroke: a guideline. Stroke 37:1583–1633, 2006

Gorelick PB: Status of risk factors for dementia associated with stroke. Stroke 28:459–463, 1997

Gottfries CG, Blennow K, Karlsson I, et al: The neurochemistry of vascular dementia. Dementia 5:163–167, 1994

Hachinski VC, Lassen NA, Marshall J: Multi-infarct dementia: a cause of mental deterioration in the elderly. Lancet 2:207–210, 1974

Hachinski V, Iliff LD, Zilhka A, et al: Cerebral blood flow in dementia. Arch Neurol 32:632–637, 1975

Hagnell O, Franck A, Gräsbeck A, et al: Vascular dementia in the Lundby study, 1: a prospective, epidemiological study of incidence and risk from 1957 to 1972. Neuropsychobiology 26:43–49, 1992

Heyman A, Fillenbaum G, Welsh-Bohmer KA, et al: Cerebral infarcts in patients with autopsy-proven Alzheimer's disease: CERAD, part XVIII. Consortium to Establish a Registry for Alzheimer's Disease. Neurology 51:159–162, 1998

Holstein M: Alzheimer's disease and senile dementia, 1885–1920: an interpretive history of disease negotiation. J Aging Stud 11:1–13, 1997

Jia JP, Jia JM, Zhou WD, et al: Differential acetylcholine and choline concentrations in the cerebrospinal fluid of patients with Alzheimer's disease and vascular dementia. Chin Med J (Engl) 117:1161–1164, 2004

Jongenelis K, Gerritsen DL, Pot AM, et al: Construction and validation of a patient- and user-friendly nursing home version of the Geriatric Depression Scale. Int J Geriatr Psychiatry 22:837–842, 2007

Jorm AF, Jolley D: The incidence of dementia: a meta-analysis. Neurology 51:728–733, 1998

Kakafika AI, Liberopoulos EN, Mikhailidis DP: Fibrinogen: a predictor of vascular disease. Curr Pharm Des 13:1647–1659, 2007

Kalaria RN, Ballard C: Overlap between pathology of Alzheimer disease and vascular dementia. Alzheimer Dis Assoc Disord 13 (suppl 3):S115–S123, 1999

Kerrouche N, Herholz K, Mielke R, et al: 18FDG PET in vascular dementia: differentiation from Alzheimer's disease using voxel-based multivariate analysis. J Cereb Blood Flow Metab 26:1213–1221, 2006

Kidwell CS, Warach S: Acute ischemic cerebrovascular syndrome: diagnostic criteria. Stroke 34:2995–2998, 2003

Knopman DS, Parisi JE, Boeve BF, et al: Vascular dementia in a population-based autopsy study. Arch Neurol 60:569–575, 2003

Longstreth WT Jr, Bernick C, Manolio TA, et al: Lacunar infarcts defined by magnetic resonance imaging of 3660 elderly people: the Cardiovascular Health Study. Arch Neurol 55:1217–1225, 1998

Longstreth WT Jr, Diehr P, Beauchamp NJ, et al: Patterns on cranial magnetic resonance imaging in elderly people and vascular disease outcomes (letter). Arch Neurol 58:2074, 2001

Longstreth WT Jr, Arnold AM, Beauchamp NJ Jr, et al: Incidence, manifestations, and predictors of worsening white matter on serial cranial magnetic resonance imaging in the elderly: the Cardiovascular Health Study. Stroke 36:56–61, 2005

Lopez OL, Kuller LH, Becker JT, et al: Classification of vascular dementia in the Cardiovascular Health Study Cognition Study. Neurology 64:1539–1547, 2005

McShane R, Areosa Sastre A, Minakaran N: Memantine for dementia. Cochrane Database of Systematic Reviews 2006, Issue 2. Art. No.: CD003154. DOI: 10.1002/14651858.CD003154.pub5.

Mesulam M, Siddique T, Cohen B: Cholinergic denervation in a pure multi-infarct state: observations on CADASIL. Neurology 60:1183–1185, 2003

Meyer JS, Xu G, Thornby J, et al: Is mild cognitive impairment prodromal for vascular dementia like Alzheimer's disease? Stroke 33:1981–1985, 2002

Moser KV, Stöckl P, Humpel C: Cholinergic neurons degenerate when exposed to conditioned medium of primary rat brain capillary endothelial cells: counteraction by NGF, MK-801 and inflammation. Exp Gerontol 41:609–618, 2006

Muscal E, Brey RL: Neurological manifestations of the antiphospholipid syndrome: risk assessments and evidence-based medicine. Int J Clin Pract 61:1561–1568, 2007

Nishitsuji K, Tomiyama T, Ishibashi K, et al: Cerebral vascular accumulation of Dutch-type Abeta42, but not wild-type Abeta42, in hereditary cerebral hemorrhage with amyloidosis, Dutch type. J Neurosci Res 85:2917–2923, 2007

Niwa K, Porter VA, Kazama K, et al: A beta-peptides enhance vasoconstriction in cerebral circulation. Am J Physiol Heart Circ Physiol 281:H2417–H2424, 2001

Nolan KA, Lino MM, Seligmann AW, et al: Absence of vascular dementia in an autopsy series from a dementia clinic. J Am Geriatr Soc 46:597–604, 1998

O'Brien JT, Paling S, Barber R, et al: Progressive brain atrophy on serial MRI in dementia with Lewy bodies, AD, and vascular dementia. Neurology 56:1386–1388, 2001

Orgogozo J, Rigaud A, Stoffler A, et al: Efficacy and safety of memantine in patients with mild to moderate vascular dementia: a randomized, placebo-controlled trial (MMM300). Stroke 33:1834–1839, 2002

Perry E, Ziabreva I, Perry R, et al: Absence of cholinergic deficits in "pure" vascular dementia. Neurology 64:132–133, 2005

Ramos-Estébanez C, Rebollo Alvarez-Amandi MR: Binswanger disease: a common type of vascular dementia [in Spanish]. Rev Neurol 31:53–58, 2000

Rocca WA, Hofman A, Brayne C, et al: The prevalence of vascular dementia in Europe: facts and fragments from 1980–1990 studies. EURODEM–Prevalence Research Group. Ann Neurol 30:817–824, 1991

Román GC: Vascular dementia: a historical background. Int Psychogeriatr 15 (suppl 1):S11–S13, 2003

Román GC, Tatemichi TK, Erkinjuntti T, et al: Vascular dementia: diagnostic criteria for research studies. Report of the NINDS-AIREN International Workshop. Neurology 43:250–260, 1993

Smith AD: Prevention of dementia: a role for B vitamins? Nutr Health 18:225–226, 2006

Snowdon DA, Greiner LH, Mortimer JA, et al: Brain infarction and the clinical expression of Alzheimer disease. The Nun Study. JAMA 277:813–817, 1997

van den Heuvel DM, ten Dam VH, de Craen AJ, et al: Increase in periventricular white matter hyperintensities parallels decline in mental processing speed in a non-demented elderly population. J Neurol Neurosurg Psychiatry 77:149–153, 2006

Vinters HV: Cerebral amyloid angiopathy: a critical review. Stroke 18:311–324, 1987

Wang ZZ, Jensson O, Thorsteinsson L, et al: Microvascular degeneration in hereditary cystatin C amyloid angiopathy of the brain. APMIS 105:41–47, 1997

Wentzel C, Rockwood K, MacKnight C, et al: Progression of impairment in patients with vascular cognitive impairment without dementia. Neurology 57:714–716, 2001

Wilkinson D, Doody R, Helme R, et al: Donepezil in vascular dementia: a randomized, placebo-controlled study. Neurology 61:479–486, 2003

World Health Organization: The ICD-10 Classification of Mental and Behavioural Disorders: Diagnostic Criteria for Research. Geneva, World Health Organization, 1993

Yang DW, Kim BS, Park JK, et al: Analysis of cerebral blood flow of subcortical vascular dementia with single photon emission computed tomography: adaptation of statistical parametric mapping. J Neurol Sci 203–204:199–205, 2002

Zekry D, Hauw JJ, Gold G, et al: Mixed dementia: epidemiology, diagnosis, and treatment. J Am Geriatr Soc 50:1431–1438, 2002

Further Reading

Amarenco P, Lavallee P, Touboul PJ: Statins and stroke prevention. Cerebrovasc Dis 17 (suppl 1):81–88, 2004

Casserly I, Topol E: Convergence of atherosclerosis and Alzheimer's disease: inflammation, cholesterol, and misfolded proteins. Lancet 363:1139–1146, 2004

de la Torre JC: How do heart disease and stroke become risk factors for Alzheimer's disease? Neurol Res 28:637–644, 2006

Erkinjuntti T, Román G, Gauthier S: Treatment of vascular dementia: evidence from clinical trials with cholinesterase inhibitors. Neurol Res 26:603–605, 2004

Hébert R, Lindsay J, Verreault R, et al: Vascular dementia: incidence and risk factors in the Canadian Study of Health and Aging. Stroke 31:1487–1493, 2000

Kalaria RN: Vascular factors in Alzheimer's disease. Int Psychogeriatr 15 (suppl 1):47–52, 2003

Kramer JH, Reed BR, Mungas D, et al: Executive dysfunction in subcortical ischaemic vascular disease. J Neurol Neurosurg Psychiatry 72:217–220, 2002

Lojkowska W, Ryglewicz D, Jedrzejczak T, et al: SPECT as a diagnostic test in the investigation of dementia. J Neurol Sci 203–204:215–219, 2002

Naarding P, de Koning I, van Kooten F, et al: Post-stroke dementia and depression: frontosubcortical dysfunction as missing link? Int J Geriatr Psychiatry 22:1–8, 2007

8

Dementia With Lewy Bodies and Other Synucleinopathies

Rawan Tarawneh, M.D.

James E. Galvin, M.D., M.Sc.

The synucleinopathies are a group of neurodegenerative disorders that share the common pathology of fibrillar aggregates of α-synuclein protein in selective populations of neurons and glia. The most common of these disorders are dementia with Lewy bodies (DLB), Parkinson disease (PD), multiple system atrophy, and pure autonomic failure. The underlying pathological lesion in these disorders is the intracellular aggregation of α-synuclein. However, α-synuclein pathology is also present in many other neurodegenerative diseases, such as

This chapter was supported by grants from the National Institute on Aging (AG20764, AG03991, and AG05681) and by a generous gift from the Alan A. and Edith L. Wolff Charitable Trust.

Alzheimer disease (AD) and Down syndrome (Table 8–1). Synucleinopathies are characterized by variable degrees of progressive decline in cognitive, motor, behavioral, and autonomic function.

Aggregates of α-synuclein are present in neurons as Lewy bodies and dystrophic Lewy neurons, or as cytoplasmic inclusions in oligodendrocytes. The distribution of synuclein-related pathology is highly variable among these disorders. Lewy bodies predominate in the neocortex in diffuse Lewy body disease and the substantia nigra in PD. Cerebellar and brain stem tubulofilamentous inclusions are seen in multiple systems atrophy.

Dementia With Lewy Bodies

DLB is probably the second most common cause of neurodegenerative dementia after AD. Neocortical Lewy bodies were found, on autopsy, in up to 40% of elderly patients with dementia (Galasko et al. 1994).

Clinical Features and Diagnostic Criteria

The consensus criteria for diagnosing DLB require progressive cognitive decline severe enough to cause functional or occupational impairment (e.g., dementia). In addition to dementia, two of the following three core features are required for a diagnosis of probable DLB: fluctuating cognition, recurrent well-formed visual hallucinations, and spontaneous parkinsonism. At least one core feature is required for a diagnosis of possible DLB. In the absence of two core features, the diagnosis of probable DLB can be made if at least one core and one suggestive feature are present. Suggestive features include rapid eye movement (REM) sleep behavior disorder, severe neuroleptic sensitivity, and low dopamine transporter uptake in the basal ganglia demonstrated by single-photon emission computed tomography (SPECT) or positron emission tomography (PET). The diagnosis of probable DLB cannot be made on the basis of suggestive features alone (McKeith et al. 2005).

Supportive features for the diagnosis of DLB include repeated falls, syncope, transient loss of consciousness, severe autonomic dysfunction, depression, systematized delusions, and hallucinations in other modalities. Although these features may support the clinical diagnosis, they lack diagnostic specificity.

There are currently no radiological or biological markers that aid reliably in the diagnosis of DLB, and current therapies are limited to symptomatic ame-

Table 8–1.   Disorders with synuclein pathology

Dementia with Lewy bodies
Parkinson disease
  Sporadic
  Familial (with mutations other than the parkin gene)
Alzheimer disease
  Sporadic
  Familial forms (amyloid precursor protein, presenilin 1, and presenilin 2
    mutations)
Down syndrome
Multiple system atrophy
  Shy-Drager syndrome
  Olivopontocerebellar atrophy
  Striatonigral degeneration
Pure autonomic failure
Neurodegeneration with brain iron accumulation
  Type 1 (formerly Hallervorden-Spatz disease)
  Type 2 (neuroaxonal dystrophy)
Other disorders where synuclein inclusions have been described
  Amyotrophic lateral sclerosis
  Pick disease
  Creutzfeldt-Jakob disease
  Traumatic brain injury

lioration of cognitive and behavioral symptoms. Despite these limitations, early
detection is important. For example, these patients appear to have better responses to cholinesterase inhibitors than do patients with AD. Patients with
DLB are very sensitive to neuroleptics, even at very low dosages (McKeith et al.
1992). Early diagnosis will also allow families to enhance environmental safety
in response to the patients' tendency to fall.

Cognitive Profile

DLB is insidious in onset, with gradual progression. Whereas AD is characterized by a cortical pattern of deficits, DLB first involves frontal subcortical
structures. The frontal subcortical deficits mediate executive and visuospatial

functions in association with rapidly fluctuating attentional deficits, as well as memory loss (Salmon et al. 1996). Over time, symptoms occur that are related to temporoparietal cortical deficits, such as aphasia, apraxia, and spatial disorientation. In the following subsections, we describe the pattern of deficits in specific cognitive domains. In Table 8–2, we compare the patterns of cognitive impairment across various dementias.

Executive and Attentional Functions

Patients with DLB often have impaired judgment, organization, and planning. Attentional dysfunction is prominent. Executive demands seem to affect attentional variability, and greater performance variability is demonstrated in tasks that require more active recruitment of executive control processes.

Visuospatial Abilities

A consistent feature of DLB is impairment of visuospatial and visuoperceptual function. Patients with DLB often have difficulty navigating in their homes or even moving out of a bed or chair. Brief cognitive screening tests may miss visuospatial or constructive deficits at the very mildest stage, but visuospatial dysfunction can be readily detected by testing with the Block Design subtest of the Wechsler Adult Intelligence Scale, currently in its fourth edition (Wechsler 2008), or with figure copying.

Memory

Patients with pure Lewy body pathology have relative preservation of memory in the early stages compared to patients with AD. Memory impairment develops with disease progression, but the memory impairment in DLB predominantly reflects deficits in retrieval, whereas the primary substrate of memory impairment in AD is impaired encoding (Burn 2006).

Patients with DLB have poor initial learning and retrieval with mild deficits in delayed recall. Relative preservation of verbal skills is an important feature, and DLB patients show little or no impairment in verbal memory and confrontation naming (Johnson et al. 2005).

The performance of patients with combined Alzheimer and Lewy body pathology is similar to that of Alzheimer patients on the subsets of verbal memory, indicating that the additional Lewy body burden does not negatively affect verbal performance in patients with AD. This finding is in contrast to visuospatial

Table 8–2. Patterns of cognitive impairment between dementias

Disease	Learning and memory	Attention and concentration	Executive functioning	Language functioning	Visuospatial functioning
AD	+++	+ to +++	+ to +++	+ to +++	+ to +++
PD	0 to +	0 to ++	0 to ++	0	0
PDD	0 to +++	++ to +++	++ to +++	0 to ++	+ to +++
DLB	0 to +++	++ to +++	++ to ++	0 to ++	+ to +++

Note. 0 = no impairment; + = mild impairment; ++ = moderate impairment; +++ = severe impairment. AD = Alzheimer disease; DLB = dementia with Lewy bodies; PD = Parkinson disease; PDD = Parkinson disease with dementia.

dysfunction, on which the combined pathology has an additive effect (Johnson et al. 2005).

Language

Compared with AD patients, patients with DLB have more severe impairment in verbal fluency. In AD, category fluency is more severely impaired than letter fluency; however, both appear to be affected to the same degree in DLB. In addition, Lewy body patients may exhibit mild confrontation naming deficits.

Psychiatric Features

Visual hallucinations are frequently present early and occur intermittently throughout the course of DLB. They consist of fully formed, detailed, colored, three-dimensional images of objects, persons, or animals. The emotional response to hallucinations varies from indifference to excitement or fear, and the patient may have some insight into their unreality. Hallucinations occur in other modalities, including auditory, tactile, and olfactory, but auditory hallucinations rarely occur in the absence of visual hallucinations.

Visual hallucinations occur in 59%–85% of autopsy-confirmed Lewy body cases (Harding et al. 2002). The occurrence of visual hallucinations in the first 4 years after dementia onset has positive and negative predictive values for DLB of 81% and 79%, respectively (Ferman et al. 2003).

The hallucinations of DLB do not seem to correlate with the dose of L-dopa or the occurrence of motor fluctuations seen with dopaminergic therapy (Sanchez-Ramos et al. 1996). A strong association exists between visual hallucinations and cholinergic depletion in the temporal cortex and the basal fore-brain (Harding et al. 2002). Another suggested mechanism for visual hallucinations is dysregulation of REM sleep, with the intrusion of dreams into wakefulness (Boeve et al. 2003b).

Other psychiatric features in DLB include delusions. In contrast to the vague persecutory delusions often seen in AD, which are based mostly on confabulation and memory loss, delusions in DLB may be more fixed, be more complex, and represent recollections of hallucinations and perceptual disturbances (McKeith 2000).

Depression has been reported in 50% of persons with DLB (Klatka et al. 1996). Other psychiatric features include apathy, anxiety, illusions, Capgras syndrome, and reduplicative paramnesia.

Motor Features

Spontaneous parkinsonism is one of the core features of DLB (Table 8–3). The distinction between DLB and Parkinson disease with dementia (PDD) is based on the relationship of dementia onset to motor impairment. In DLB, cognitive impairment precedes motor impairment by more than 12 months; the reverse is true for PDD (McKeith et al. 1996). The onset and severity of parkinsonism in DLB are highly variable.

Many patients with DLB develop a symmetric akinetic-rigid syndrome. Tremor is less common than bradykinesia, facial masking, and rigidity, and tends to be maximal with posture/action rather than at rest. Myoclonus is seen in 18.5% of DLB patients and is rarely seen in PD patients who do not have dementia (Louis et al. 1997).

Postural instability and gait difficulty are more prominent features of DLB and PDD than of uncomplicated PD. Motor features in DLB patients are less responsive to dopaminergic treatment than are those in PD patients.

Cognitive Fluctuations

Fluctuations in cognition are seen in 15%–80% of DLB cases (Ballard et al. 2002). These involve waxing and waning of cognition, functional abilities, or arousal in the absence of a clear precipitant. They are often described as episodes of behavioral confusion, inattention, hypersomnolence, and incoherent speech, alternating with episodes of lucidity and capable task performance.

Table 8–3. Comparison of extrapyramidal features in dementias

Disease	Specific parkinsonian findings
Alzheimer disease	Parkinsonism tends to be later in course; rigidity, bradykinesia, and tremor (resting or postural) most obvious
Parkinson disease	Masked facies, stooped posture, and reduced arm swing; unilateral or asymmetric rigidity, bradykinesia, resting tremor, and postural instability; signs clearly are L-dopa responsive
Parkinson disease with dementia	Same as in Parkinson disease, but over time, bilateral involvement, marked postural instability, and loss of L-dopa responsiveness
Dementia with Lewy bodies	Masked facies, stooped posture, and reduced arm swing similar to Parkinson disease with or without dementia, but tremor is less asymmetric and more postural
Multiple system atrophy	Rigidity less asymmetric and minimally L-dopa responsive in the striatonigral variant; ataxia and spasticity prominent in the olivopontocerebellar atrophy variant; orthostatic hypotension prominent in the Shy-Drager syndrome variant

Patients may be described as staring into space or as dazed. These episodes can last minutes to days and can vary from alertness to stupor. Transient episodes of disturbed consciousness in which patients are found mute and unresponsive for a few minutes may represent an extreme form of fluctuations.

Excessive Daytime Drowsiness

Lewy body patients often experience daytime drowsiness or somnolence, but it is important to rule out secondary causes of daytime sleepiness, including medications and primary sleep disorders such as sleep apnea. Approximately three-quarters of patients have a significant number of arousals not accounted for by medication, periodic limb movements of sleep, or sleep apnea (Boeve et al. 2003b).

Rapid Eye Movement Sleep Behavior Disorder

REM sleep behavior disorder (RBD) is characterized by loss of normal muscle atonia during REM sleep, associated with excessive activity while dreaming. Increased muscle activity during REM sleep occurs along with dream content and can range from elevated muscle tone to complex behavioral sequences, such as acting out dreams.

RBD is associated with synucleinopathies, including DLB, PD, and multiple system atrophy, and may precede the synucleinopathy diagnosis by years, but it rarely occurs in tau-predominant conditions such as AD (Boeve et al. 2001). This relationship with synucleinopathies has been supported by neuropathological confirmation of Lewy bodies in patients with RBD and no clinical evidence of dementia or psychosis (Galvin et al. 2001).

Autonomic Dysfunction

Autonomic dysfunction is common and is a feature shared by most of the synucleinopathies (McKeith et al. 2000a). Autonomic dysfunction is not included in the criteria, but some of the supportive features, such as recurrent falls and transient loss of consciousness, might be explained by autonomic dysfunction. Although these autonomic features tend to occur late in the disease process, there have been cases with early and prominent involvement. There is also evidence of involvement of the peripheral nervous system, with numerous Lewy bodies in the sympathetic neurons and autonomic ganglia.

The most serious manifestation of autonomic dysfunction is orthostasis, which is symptomatic in approximately 15% of patients with DLB (McKeith et al. 2005). Other features include decreased sweating, sialorrhea, seborrhea, heat intolerance, urinary dysfunction, constipation or diarrhea, and erectile dysfunction.

Neuroleptic Sensitivity

Approximately 57% of patients with DLB, 39% of patients with PDD, and 27% of patients with PD develop severe neuroleptic sensitivity (Aarsland et al. 2005). It is not possible to predict the occurrence of these adverse motor reactions, but they are generally more common with the neuroleptics that are potent dopamine D_2 receptor antagonists.

Differential Diagnosis

Both baseline and longitudinal differences in cognitive, psychiatric, and functional deficits have been observed between DLB and AD. Men are more likely to have DLB; AD has a female predominance. Persons with Lewy bodies are also more likely to exhibit psychiatric symptoms and have greater functional impairment at the time of diagnosis. Furthermore, the diffuse cortical and subcortical Lewy body pathology produces cognitive impairment with predominant visuospatial and psychomotor deficits (Stern et al. 1993).

In general, memory and naming are less impaired in DLB than in AD. The performance of Lewy body patients on memory tests lies midway between that of patients with AD, who have more impairment (Helkala et al. 1988), and that of patients with other subcortical dementias such as progressive supranuclear palsy.

Lewy body patients have less impaired retention than do patients with AD, with more benefit from retrieval cues and less propensity to produce intrusion errors (Salmon et al. 1996). Recognition memory remains fairly stable in DLB and may be the only significant difference between cognitive performance in DLB and AD.

Parkinson Disease With Dementia

Up to 14% per year of patients with PD who are over age 70 will develop at least mild dementia (Galvin 2006). No operationalized criteria exist to characterize PDD or define the clinical boundaries between pure PD and PDD, which differ only in whether the cognitive impairment precedes or follows the motor signs by 12 months (McKeith et al. 2005).

Both DLB patients and PDD patients may have psychiatric symptoms, autonomic symptoms, RBD, cognitive fluctuations, and neuroleptic sensitivity. The neuropsychological profiles in PDD and DLB are similar, with prominent deficits in attention, executive dysfunction, visuospatial function, language function, memory retrieval, and behavior.

Risk Factors for Cognitive Decline in Parkinson Disease

Only a portion of patients with cognitive impairment develop dementia. Nonthreatening visual hallucinations, commonly reported in PD even prior to the use of L-dopa (Fénelon et al. 2006), are the strongest clinical predictor of dementia (Galvin et al. 2006). Age is another important risk factor. The cumulative risk of dementia by age 85 is over 65% (Martí et al. 2003). Advanced axial extrapyramidal involvement, such as bradykinesia, rigidity, or postural instability, also appears to increase the risk of dementia and the rate of cognitive decline once dementia develops. Among the motor predictors, bilateral onset of motor symptoms and declining response to L-dopa also appear to increase the risk of dementia (Padovani et al. 2006).

Cognitive Profile

The cognitive profile of PD is similar to that of DLB, with marked executive dysfunction and marked impairment in attention and visuospatial and constructional abilities (Lees and Smith 1983). Aside from verbal fluency, cortical functions such as language, limb praxis, and perceptual processing are relatively preserved in the early stages. Memory impairment is less prominent than in AD, and recall may be relatively preserved (Janvin et al. 2006).

Compared with PD patients who do not have dementia, PD patients with dementia are more likely to have visual or auditory hallucinations, delusions, and depression. They also tend to have a higher frequency of aphasia and impairment in visuoconstructional tasks such as clock drawing. Other distinctive clinical features of PDD include sensitivity to neuroleptic medications, fluctuations in cognition, myoclonus, and sleep disturbances.

Executive Function

Patients with PD have impaired ability to plan, organize, and regulate goal-directed behavior.

Visuospatial Abilities

Impairment in visuoperceptual and visuomotor abilities is seen in PD with and without dementia (Stern et al. 1983).

Memory

Patients with PD have impaired semantic and episodic memory with preserved recognition memory and benefit from cuing. The deficit in PD is mostly associated with impaired registration or retrieval of information during the early retention phase of short-term memory (Burn 2006).

Language

Language processing and comprehension are relatively well preserved in PDD compared with AD, but verbal fluency is more compromised in the former. Patients with PDD have also been reported to have naming deficits and difficulties with sentence comprehension. Decreased content of spontaneous speech is also seen but to a lesser degree than in AD. These patients exhibit motor speech abnormalities in the form of dysarthria, agraphia, decreased phrase length, and impaired speech melody.

Psychiatric Features

Approximately 61% of patients with PD exhibit neuropsychiatric disturbances. The most common are depression (38%), hallucinations (27%), delusions (6%), anxiety, sleep disturbances, and inappropriate sexual behavior. Visual hallucinations are aggravated by dopaminergic treatment.

Cognitive impairment is the main risk factor for hallucinations induced by L-dopa in PD patients (Fénelon et al. 2006). Other clinical correlates of psychosis in PD are old age, advanced disease, a history of depression, and coexistent sleep disorder, including altered dream phenomena and sleep fragmentation.

Depression is common in patients with PD and appears unrelated to the presence or absence of dementia or the severity of motor impairment (McKeith 2000). Anxiety co-occurs with depression in up to 40% of patients with PD (Menza et al. 1993), and apathy is common. It is important to recognize depression as a confounding factor in cognitive and motor impairment.

Fluctuations

PD patients usually have no cognitive fluctuations in the absence of dementia. On the other hand, PDD produces a pattern of impairment that is comparable to DLB (Ballard et al. 2002).

Autonomic Dysfunction

Autonomic dysfunction tends to occur in late PD, and features such as orthostatic hypotension appear to be related to disease severity and duration. About one-third of patients have clinical features of autonomic dysfunction. The most common autonomic features are decreased gastrointestinal mobility and bladder dysfunction. Constipation is very common, and serious complications such as intestinal pseudo-obstruction and toxic megacolon can occur. Other common features include bladder dysfunction with increased urgency, frequency, and incontinence, and sexual dysfunction such as decreased libido and erectile dysfunction. Almost 60% of patients with PD have orthostatic hypotension (a fall in systolic blood pressure by ≥20 mm Hg) by tilt table testing, with decreased cerebral perfusion, and approximately 20% of patients develop orthostatic symptoms related to reduced cerebral perfusion (Senard et al. 1997).

Preclinical Cognitive Impairment

Early cognitive deficits are usually in visuospatial and executive function and verbal memory (Mahieux et al. 1998). These deficits include decrements in planning, sequencing, concept formation, and working memory. A more rapid rate of cognitive decline has been associated with the severity of motor symptoms (Levy et al. 2002). In particular, motor symptoms believed to be mediated by nondopaminergic mechanisms, such as gait, speech, and postural control, have been associated with accelerated decline in cognition (Aarsland et al. 2004).

Neuropathology

Dementia With Lewy Bodies

Limbic and neocortical areas are preferentially involved in DLB, with a variable degree of Lewy body pathology in the brain stem (McKeith et al. 2005) (Figure 8–1). Over 70% of Lewy body patients have concurrent AD pathology. The neuritic plaques of AD include a dense core of amyloid-β peptide 40 ($A\beta_{40}$) with neuritic processes composed of tau protein, but plaques in Lewy body disease are typically diffuse and composed primarily of $A\beta_{42}$. So-called Lewy neurites are intracellular inclusions composed primarily of synuclein aggregated in the neural processes. They are found in brain regions rich in perikaryal Lewy bodies and preferentially affect limbic and temporal lobe structures. Striatal Lewy neurites in DLB may contribute to the extrapyramidal features. In addition to the involvement of the central autonomic nuclei, early involvement of the peripheral postganglionic autonomic neurons occurs in Lewy body disease (Tiraboschi et al. 2000).

Parkinson Disease With Dementia

The pathological substrates for PDD include cortical Lewy bodies, Alzheimer pathology, and restricted subcortical pathology (Galvin et al. 2006). Roughly one-third of PDD cases are associated with only neocortical Lewy bodies. Another one-third meet criteria for both PD and AD. The final one-third have only brain stem pathology comprising Lewy bodies (Braak et al. 2005).

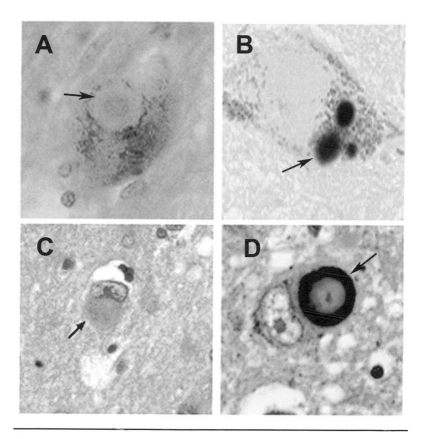

Figure 8–1. Brain stem Lewy bodies *(see color plate 9).*
Note. *(A)* A nigral Lewy body *(arrow)* after hematoxylin and eosin staining. *(B)* Multiple nigral Lewy bodies detected with antibodies against α-synuclein. *(C)* Cortical Lewy bodies, which tend to be eccentric and lack the defined core/halo appearance of nigral Lewy bodies with hematoxylin and eosin. *(D)* With the advent of immunohistochemistry, use of antibodies against α-synuclein makes it easier to detect cortical Lewy bodies.
Source. Reprinted from Tarawneh R, Galvin JE: "Dementia With Lewy Bodies and Other Synucleinopathies," in *The American Psychiatric Publishing Textbook of Alzheimer Disease and Other Dementias.* Edited by Weiner MF, Lipton AM. Washington, DC, American Psychiatric Publishing, 2009, pp. 195–217. Copyright 2009, American Psychiatric Publishing. Used with permission.

The neuropathological hallmark of PDD is the presence of Lewy bodies and neuronal loss in the substantia nigra. Cell loss is seen in the substantia nigra as well as in the dorsal motor nucleus of vagus, the nucleus basalis of Meynert, and the locus coeruleus.

DLB, whether in a pure form or in combination with AD, appears to begin rostrally and spread caudally, whereas the pathology of PDD appears to begin in the brain stem and spread rostrally (Braak et al. 2003).

Clinicopathological Correlates

The density of Lewy bodies in multiple brain regions correlates with the severity of cognitive impairment in Lewy body dementia. The total Lewy body burden seems to correlate with disease duration. Consistent correlations between the severity of neuropsychiatric symptoms and Lewy body load have not been established. Many investigations point to cholinergic depletion in the pathogenesis of fluctuations in DLB (Ballard et al. 2002). The response of these patients to cholinesterase inhibitors (McKeith et al. 2000b) and the worsening of delirium with the use of anticholinergic agents support this concept.

The presumed mechanism of RBD in DLB and PDD is damage to the descending pontine-medullary reticular formation or sublaterodorsal nucleus that leads to a loss of the normal REM sleep inhibition of the spinal alpha-motor neurons. In humans, polysomnographic evidence of REM sleep without atonia is considered the electrophysiological substrate of RBD and is found in patients with or without florid RBD (Lai and Siegel 2003).

Neurochemical Changes

Although loss of the nigrostriatal dopaminergic pathway is mostly responsible for the motor features of PD, the mesocorticolimbic dopaminergic system may have a more important role in cognitive dysfunction. The degree of striatal dopamine reduction is comparable between PDD and DLB (Piggott et al. 1999). The loss of striatal and putaminal D_2 receptors in DLB may contribute to neuroleptic sensitivity.

DLB and PDD are also associated with cholinergic dysfunction that occurs earlier and is more severe than in AD. Presynaptic depletion in the brain stem and basal forebrain structures results in more extensive cholinergic deficits and greater loss of postsynaptic mechanisms in Lewy body disease than in AD (Perry et al. 1994). Severe losses of basal forebrain acetylcholine can account for the hallucinations and fluctuations in arousal that characterize DLB. On the other hand, postsynaptic muscarinic receptors are better preserved and less functionally impaired in DLB than in AD. Given the greater cholinergic deficit and the potentially more reversible changes, patients with DLB might have greater benefit from the symptomatic and trophic effects of cholinergic stimulation than patients with AD.

Diagnostic Evaluation

Structural Imaging

Results from radiological investigations, along with other findings, may help in supporting clinical diagnosis (Table 8–4). Unlike in patients with AD, there is little difference in the size of the hippocampus between patients with DLB and normal control subjects (Barber et al. 1999). The degree of ventricular enlargement or white matter changes in DLB is comparable to that in AD (Barber et al. 2000).

Magnetic resonance imaging shows evidence of putaminal atrophy in DLB but not in AD (Cousins et al. 2003). Whole brain and caudate volumes are significantly reduced in subjects with AD compared with controls and subjects with PD, whereas both volumes are comparable between controls, subjects with PD, and subjects with PDD.

Functional Imaging

Functional brain imaging using ^{18}F-labeled fluorodeoxyglucose PET (FDG-PET) or ^{99m}Tc-hexamethylpropylene amine oxime (^{99m}Tc-HMPAO) SPECT shows only minor differences between DLB and AD (Table 8–4). However, FDG uptake studies show metabolic reduction in the visual association cortex in Lewy body disease that does not appear in AD (Higuchi et al. 2000).

In PET studies, frontal and temporoparietal hypometabolism can be seen in patients with PDD, superimposed on the milder global hypometabolism seen in nondemented subjects with PD. In a comparison of PDD patients to AD patients, the former had greater resting state hypometabolism in the visual cortex and relatively preserved medial temporal metabolism. This pattern of temporo-parieto-occipital hypometabolism with relative sparing of the medial temporal lobes may also be seen in patients with DLB (Vander Borght et al. 1997).

Functional brain imaging using ^{99m}Tc-HMPAO and N-isopropyl-p-[^{123}I] iodoamphetamine (IMP) SPECT in patients with PD shows reduced occipital perfusion as compared with other cortical areas (Matsui et al. 2005). Occipital hypoperfusion in SPECT can also be seen in DLB (Donnemiller et al. 1997). In fact, it has been suggested that reduced flow in the medial occipital lobe, including the cuneus and the lingual gyrus, can help discriminate DLB from AD (Shimizu et al. 2005).

Electrophysiological Studies

An electroencephalogram shows diffuse abnormalities in most cases of DLB, with early slowing of dominant rhythms, epoch-by-epoch fluctuation, and transient temporal slow wave activity (Briel et al. 1999).

Therapeutics

Cognitive Symptoms

Cholinesterase Inhibitors

Limbic and cortical cholinergic deficits are more severe in DLB than in AD; augmentation of cholinergic function by inhibition of acetylcholinesterase appears to provide symptomatic benefit. Attention, apathy, excessive somnolence, and hallucinations are most likely to benefit. In a double-blind, placebo-controlled, multicenter trial of patients with DLB, subjects treated with rivastigmine 12 mg/day for 20 weeks had better performance on tests of attention, working memory, and episodic secondary memory than the placebo group (McKeith et al. 2000b). A 24-week open-label study of galantamine showed improvement in visual hallucinations, nighttime behaviors, and fluctuating cognitive deficits. Patients also experienced a benefit in sleep abnormalities and RBD (Edwards et al. 2007).

Donepezil was evaluated in a randomized controlled trial involving patients with PD and dementia (Leroi et al. 2004). Results showed significant improvement in memory subscales and a trend toward improvement in psychomotor speed and attention. No differences were found between the treatment and placebo groups in psychiatric status, motor activity, or activities of daily living at baseline or at the endpoints. However, 25% of patients had side

Table 8–4. Neuroimaging findings (structural and functional imaging) between dementias

Disease	Pattern of atrophy on MRI	Pattern of hypoperfusion (SPECT) or hypometabolism (FDG-PET)
Alzheimer disease	Maximal in hippocampi, generalized cortical atrophy evolves over time	Maximal in temporoparietal cortex
Parkinson disease	Minimal to no significant cortical or hippocampal atrophy	Normal or minimally abnormal
Parkinson disease with dementia	Minimal to no significant cortical or hippocampal atrophy	Maximal in frontoparieto-occipital cortex
Dementia with Lewy bodies	Minimal to no significant cortical or hippocampal atrophy	Maximal in parieto-occipital cortex

Note. FDG-PET = ^{18}F-labeled fluorodeoxyglucose positron emission tomography; MRI = magnetic resonance imaging; SPECT = single-photon emission computed tomography.

effects requiring withdrawal of the medication; these included cholinergic side effects and worsening of parkinsonism. Nevertheless, the American Academy of Neurology suggests the use of acetylcholinesterase inhibitors for the treatment of PDD (Miyasaki et al. 2006).

Memantine

Controlled clinical trials suggest that memantine, which may diminish the toxic effects of glutamate, has a modest effect in DLB. In a small randomized study, patients with clinically diagnosed DLB or PDD who were taking memantine 20 mg/day had significantly better scores after 24 weeks on the Clinical Global Impression—Change (CGI-C) scale than those patients taking placebo (Aarsland et al. 2009). In a larger 24-week trial of memantine 20 mg/day versus placebo in patients with DLB or PDD, the DLB group had a mean 0.6-point improved score on the CGI-C, but no difference was seen in the PDD group's score (Emre et al. 2010).

Motor Symptoms

L-Dopa is the standard treatment for extrapyramidal symptoms in PD. However, its use in DLB has been limited because of adverse effects on cognitive and behavioral features and worsening of psychosis. There have been reports of increased adverse events with the combined use of L-dopa and cholinesterase inhibitors in patients with PD (Okereke et al. 2004).

Although some reports suggest that dopaminergic treatment increases impulsivity or decreases performance, neither of these side effects has been confirmed. In fact, L-dopa replacement improves working memory, particularly visuospatial and object tasks, in patients with PD (Costa et al. 2003), and dopamine withdrawal may "unmask" dysfunction in executive functions, spatial working memory, and thinking time and accuracy.

Dopamine agonists have been less effective and less well tolerated than L-dopa. Therefore, a trial of L-dopa is recommended in patients with DLB, with slow titration of the dose to symptomatic benefit.

Other PD medications such as amantadine, catechol O-methyltransferase (COMT) inhibitors, monoamine oxidase inhibitors, and anticholinergics tend to exacerbate cognitive impairment, whereas cholinesterase inhibitors can worsen parkinsonism (McKeith et al. 2000b).

Behavioral Pathology

Anxiety and depression are common in patients with DLB and PDD, and both groups respond to selective serotonin reuptake inhibitors and anxiolytics. Benzodiazepines are better avoided given their risk of sedation, paradoxical agitation, and falls.

Nonpharmacological Approaches

Education of caregivers is an essential part of managing behavioral pathology. Often, patients' behaviors are reactions to external stimuli that can be identified and reduced or eliminated. Hallucinations and delusions should not be confronted and argued about. Validation of the patients' feelings and reassurance that their concerns are taken seriously can often be calming. Although education can provide caregivers with better understanding of the nature of the condition and improve their skills in managing difficult situations, caregivers should also be made aware of available support systems (see listing of resources in appendix at end of book).

Acetylcholinesterase Inhibitors

A meta-analysis of large acetylcholinesterase inhibitor trials in patients with AD showed that the medications had a small but significant benefit in treating neuropsychiatric symptoms (Trinh et al. 2003). Psychosis, agitation, wandering, and anxiety are the most consistently responsive symptoms, whereas depression, apathy, and eating behaviors are less responsive.

Antipsychotics

Visual hallucinations occur in up to 80% of patients with DLB and have been suggested as predictors of a good response to cholinesterase inhibitors (McKeith et al. 2004). The management of psychosis in DLB has been mostly based on trials in AD. In addition, some recommendations for the use of antipsychotics in DLB are based on studies in PD, because of its similar pathology. Treatment of psychosis can be very challenging given the sensitivity of patients with DLB to antipsychotics, as well as these patients' complex neurochemical and pathological deficits and wide phenotypic variations.

The first approach is to attempt reduction of dopaminergic agents. Dopaminergic agents are likely only to exacerbate factors in patients with predisposition to psychosis. The dose, duration, or number of dopaminergic agents does not seem to relate to the risk of psychosis in patients with PD (Aarsland et al. 1999).

Typical neuroleptics such as haloperidol and atypical neuroleptics with D_2 receptor antagonism (e.g., olanzapine and risperidone) should be avoided because of the risk of neuroleptic malignant syndrome, parkinsonism, somnolence, and orthostatic hypotension. Experience with atypical antipsychotics in Lewy body disease has been mixed. Risperidone and olanzapine have been shown to reduce psychosis and agitation in AD in randomized trials. Although low doses of risperidone (0.5 mg) and olanzapine (2.5 mg) are usually well tolerated, they may aggravate extrapyramidal symptoms (Walker et al. 1999), especially in advanced cases. Quetiapine, which has little D_2 activity, is used frequently for psychosis in DLB. Efficacy and tolerability have been documented in both PD and DLB (Fernandez et al. 2002).

Sleep Disorders

Clonazepam is the usual therapy for RBD, at 0.25–0.5 mg/night, but doses above 1 mg/night are necessary in some patients. Melatonin may also offer some benefit as monotherapy or in conjunction with clonazepam. There are reports of persistent efficacy beyond 1 year with melatonin (Boeve et al. 2003a). Other drugs reported to improve RBD include pramipexole, donepezil, L-dopa, carbamazepine, triazolam, clozapine, and quetiapine.

Treatment for insomnia can be attempted with low dosages of benzodiazepines (e.g., zolpidem) or with trazodone. For excessive daytime sleepiness, treatment options include bupropion, modafinil, and psychostimulants.

Autonomic Dysfunction

Management of orthostatic hypotension includes measures such as leg elevation, elastic stockings, increasing salt and fluid intake, and avoiding medications that exacerbate orthostasis. If these measures fail, midodrine or fludrocortisone can be used.

Supine hypertension is a common manifestation of autonomic dysfunction and can lead to serious complications. Treatment of supine hypertension is difficult, and multiple trials of different medications may be required. Simple measures include avoiding the supine position in the daytime and using a tilt-up position at night, which will decrease nocturnal natriuresis and may also improve morning orthostatic hypotension.

Bladder dysfunction in Lewy body and Parkinson diseases is often associated with nocturia, urgency with or without urge incontinence, and detrusor hyperreflexia. Decreasing fluid intake in the evening can often improve nocturia. Medications with anticholinergic activity can be used to treat urinary urgency, frequency, and urge incontinence, but they can exacerbate cognitive problems. Other risks include precipitating orthostatic hypotension if these drugs are used early in the day. Although these medications are effective for detrusor hyperreflexia, they may worsen urine retention in patients with detrusor hyporeflexia or flaccid bladder. Another precaution concerns men who have concomitant prostate hypertrophy or bladder outlet obstruction. Anticholinergics should be avoided in this group, and urine retention should be prevented by intermittent catheterization.

Constipation can usually be treated by exercise and dietary modifications with at least two high-fiber meals each day. Laxatives such as lactulose at dosages of 10–20 g/day can be helpful. Cholinergic stimulation by acetylcholinesterase inhibitors used for cognitive treatment might improve constipation in some patients.

Although autonomic dysfunction plays a major role in impotence, there is often contribution from depression and nocturnal akinesia. Treatment often necessitates specialized care with urological consultation.

Conclusion

Dementia with Lewy bodies and Parkinson disease with dementia are common causes of cognitive, behavioral, affective, movement, and autonomic dysfunction in older adults. They are associated with the accumulation of Lewy bodies in subcortical, limbic, and neocortical regions and characterized clinically by progressive dementia, parkinsonism, cognitive fluctuations, and visual hallucinations. There is essentially no difference in the clinical phenotype between the two clinical entities. The presence of neocortical Lewy bodies imparts a distinctive clinical phenotype that is well captured by published criteria regardless of the temporal relationship of motor to cognitive symptoms. An important goal is to widen the spectrum of understanding of neurodegenerative diseases and change concepts of Lewy body disease from a movement disorder to a disorder associated with wider neuropsychiatric disturbances, impaired cognition, episodic confusion, and the development of dementia. As the ability to refine clinical and cognitive profiles of PDD and DLB increases, the development of pharmacotherapeutic agents that may be more selective or potentially specific for these syndromes becomes more possible.

Key Clinical Points

- The synucleinopathies are characterized by α-synuclein-containing intraneuronal inclusion bodies called Lewy bodies.
- The diseases associated with Lewy bodies are the second largest group of dementing illnesses; their clinical manifestation depends on the distribution of Lewy bodies in the central and autonomic nervous system.
- The most common Lewy body diseases are Parkinson disease, Parkinson disease with dementia (PDD), dementia with Lewy bodies (DLB), and multiple system atrophy.

- These diseases have in common a degree of cognitive impairment, extrapyramidal symptoms, neuroleptic sensitivity, sleep disorders, and dysautonomia.

- DLB is probably the second most common cause of dementia; however, it remains an underdiagnosed cause of dementia.

- The cognitive profiles of DLB and PDD are very similar; the main differentiation is the temporal sequence of dementia and motor involvement.

- DLB and PDD have prominent involvement of executive function, attention, and visuospatial skills.

- Cholinesterase inhibitors are used to treat the cognitive and behavioral pathology of DLB.

- Neuroleptic sensitivity is a serious, unpredictable, and potentially fatal side effect in this group of patients.

- If L-dopa is used to treat the motor symptoms of DLB, the dosage should be titrated gradually to avoid the risk of worsening psychosis.

References

Aarsland D, Larsen JP, Cummings JL, et al: Prevalence and clinical correlates of psychotic symptoms in Parkinson disease: a community-based study. Arch Neurol 56:595–601, 1999

Aarsland D, Andersen K, Larsen JP, et al: The rate of cognitive decline in Parkinson disease. Arch Neurol 61:1906–1911, 2004

Aarsland D, Perry R, Larsen JP, et al: Neuroleptic sensitivity in Parkinson's disease and parkinsonian dementias. J Clin Psychiatry 66:633–637, 2005

Aarsland D, Ballard C, Walker Z, et al: Memantine in patients with Parkinson's disease dementia or dementia with Lewy bodies: a double-blind, placebo-controlled multicentre trial. Lancet Neurol 8:613–618, 2009

Ballard CG, Aarsland D, McKeith I, et al: Fluctuations in attention: PD dementia vs. DLB with parkinsonism. Neurology 59:1714–1720, 2002

Barber R, Gholkar A, Scheltens P, et al: Medial temporal lobe atrophy on MRI in dementia with Lewy bodies. Neurology 52:1153–1158, 1999

Barber R, Ballard C, McKeith IG, et al: MRI volumetric study of dementia with Lewy bodies: a comparison with AD and vascular dementia. Neurology 54:1304–1309, 2000

Boeve BF, Silber MH, Ferman TJ, et al: Association of REM sleep behavior disorder and neurodegenerative disease may reflect an underlying synucleinopathy. Mov Disord 16:622–630, 2001

Boeve BF, Silber MH, Ferman TJ: Melatonin for treatment of REM sleep behavior disorder in neurologic disorders: results in 14 patients. Sleep Med 4:281–284, 2003a

Boeve BF, Silber MH, Parisi JE, et al: Synucleinopathy pathology and REM sleep behavior disorder plus dementia or parkinsonism. Neurology 61:40–45, 2003b

Braak H, Del Tredici K, Rub U, et al: Staging of brain pathology related to sporadic Parkinson's disease. Neurobiol Aging 24:197–211, 2003

Braak H, Rub U, Jansen Steur EN, et al: Cognitive status correlates with neuropatho-logic stage in Parkinson disease. Neurology 64:1404–1410, 2005

Briel RC, McKeith IG, Barker WA, et al: EEG findings in dementia with Lewy bodies and Alzheimer's disease. J Neurol Neurosurg Psychiatry 66:401–403, 1999

Burn DJ: Cortical Lewy body disease and Parkinson's disease dementia. Curr Opin Neurol 19:572–579, 2006

Costa A, Peppe A, Dell'Agnello G, et al: Dopaminergic modulation of visual-spatial working memory in Parkinson's disease. Dement Geriatr Cogn Disord 15:55–66, 2003

Cousins DA, Burton EJ, Burn D, et al: Atrophy of the putamen in dementia with Lewy bodies but not Alzheimer's disease: an MRI study. Neurology 61:1191–1195, 2003

Donnemiller E, Heilmann J, Wenning GK, et al: Brain perfusion scintigraphy with 99mTc-HMPAO or 99mTc-ECD and 123I-beta-CIT single-photon emission tomography in dementia of the Alzheimer-type and diffuse Lewy body disease. Eur J Nucl Med 24:320–325, 1997

Edwards K, Royall D, Hershey L, et al: Efficacy and safety of galantamine in patients with dementia with Lewy bodies: a 24-week open-label study. Dement Geriatr Cogn Disord 23:401–405, 2007

Emre M, Tsolaki M, Bonucelli U, et al: Memantine for patients with Parkinson's disease dementia or dementia with Lewy bodies: a randomised, double-blind, placebo-controlled trial. Lancet Neurol 10:967–977, 2010

Fénelon G, Goetz CG, Karenberg A: Hallucinations in Parkinson disease in the prelevodopa era. Neurology 66:93–98, 2006

Ferman TJ, Dickson DW, Graff-Radford N, et al: Early onset of visual hallucinations in dementia distinguishes pathologically confirmed Lewy body disease from AD (abstract). Neurology 60 (suppl 5):264, 2003

Fernandez HH, Trieschmann ME, Burke MA, et al: Quetiapine for psychosis in Parkinson's disease versus dementia with Lewy bodies. J Clin Psychiatry 63:513–515, 2002

Galasko D, Hansen LA, Katzman R, et al: Clinical-neuropathological correlations in Alzheimer's disease and related dementias. Arch Neurol 51:888–895, 1994

Galvin JE: Cognitive change in Parkinson disease. Alzheimer Dis Assoc Disord 20:302–310, 2006

Galvin JE, Lee VM, Trojanowski JQ: Synucleinopathies: clinical and pathological implications. Arch Neurol 58:186–190, 2001

Galvin JE, Pollack J, Morris JC: Clinical phenotype of Parkinson disease dementia. Neurology 67:1605–1611, 2006

Harding AJ, Broe GA, Halliday GM: Visual hallucinations in Lewy body disease relate to Lewy bodies in the temporal lobe. Brain 125:391–403, 2002

Helkala EL, Laulumaa V, Soininen H, et al: Recall and recognition memory in patients with Alzheimer's and Parkinson's diseases. Ann Neurol 24:214–217, 1988

Higuchi M, Tashiro M, Arai H, et al: Glucose hypometabolism and neuropathological correlates in brains of dementia with Lewy bodies. Exp Neurol 162:247–256, 2000

Janvin CC, Larsen JP, Salmon DP, et al: Cognitive profiles of individual patients with Parkinson's disease and dementia: comparison with dementia with Lewy bodies and Alzheimer's disease. Mov Disord 21:337–342, 2006

Johnson DK, Morris JC, Galvin JE: Verbal and visuospatial deficits in dementia with Lewy bodies. Neurology 65:1232–1238, 2005

Klatka LA, Louis ED, Schiffer RB: Psychiatric features in diffuse Lewy body disease: a clinicopathologic study using Alzheimer's disease and Parkinson's disease comparison groups. Neurology 47:1148–1152, 1996

Lai YY, Siegel JM: Physiological and anatomical link between Parkinson-like disease and REM sleep behavior disorder. Mol Neurobiol 27:137–152, 2003

Lees AJ, Smith E: Cognitive deficits in the early stages of Parkinson's disease. Brain 106:257–270, 1983

Leroi I, Brandt J, Reich SG, et al: Randomized placebo-controlled trial of donepezil in cognitive impairment in Parkinson's disease. Int J Geriatr Psychiatry 19:1–8, 2004

Levy G, Schupf N, Tang MX, et al: Combined effect of age and severity on the risk of dementia in Parkinson's disease. Ann Neurol 51:722–729, 2002

Louis ED, Klatka LA, Liu Y, et al: Comparison of extrapyramidal features in 31 pathologically confirmed cases of diffuse Lewy body disease and 34 pathologically confirmed cases of Parkinson's disease. Neurology 48:376–380, 1997

Mahieux F, Fénelon G, Flahault A, et al: Neuropsychological prediction of dementia in Parkinson's disease. J Neurol Neurosurg Psychiatry 64:178–183, 1998

Martí MJ, Tolosa E, Campdelacreu J: Clinical overview of the synucleinopathies. Mov Disord 18 (suppl 6):S21–S27, 2003

Matsui H, Udaka F, Miyoshi T, et al: N-Isopropyl-p-123I iodoamphetamine single photon emission computed tomography study of Parkinson's disease with dementia. Intern Med 44:1046–1050, 2005

McKeith IG: Spectrum of Parkinson's disease, Parkinson's dementia, and Lewy body dementia. Neurol Clin 18:865–902, 2000

McKeith IG, Fairbairn A, Perry R, et al: Neuroleptic sensitivity in patients with senile dementia of Lewy body type. BMJ 305:673–678, 1992

McKeith IG, Galasko D, Kosaka K, et al: Consensus guidelines for the clinical and pathologic diagnosis of dementia with Lewy bodies (DLB): report of the Consortium on DLB international workshop. Neurology 47:1113–1124, 1996

McKeith IG, Ballard CG, Perry RH, et al: Prospective validation of consensus criteria for the diagnosis of dementia with Lewy bodies. Neurology 54:1050–1058, 2000a

McKeith I, Del Ser T, Spano P, et al: Efficacy of rivastigmine in dementia with Lewy bodies: a randomised, double-blind, placebo-controlled international study. Lancet 356:2031–2036, 2000b

McKeith IG, Wesnes KA, Perry E, et al: Hallucinations predict attentional improvements with rivastigmine in dementia with Lewy bodies. Dement Geriatr Cogn Disord 18:94–100, 2004

McKeith IG, Dickson DW, Lowe J, et al: Diagnosis and management of dementia with Lewy bodies: third report of the DLB Consortium. Neurology 65:1863–1872, 2005

Menza MA, Robertson-Hoffman DE, Bonapace AS: Parkinson's disease and anxiety: comorbidity with depression. Biol Psychiatry 34:465–470, 1993

Miyasaki JM, Shannon K, Voon V, et al: Practice parameter: evaluation and treatment of depression, psychosis, and dementia in Parkinson disease (an evidence-based review). Report of the Quality Standards Subcommittee of the American Academy of Neurology. Neurology 66:996–1002, 2006

Okereke CS, Kirby L, Kumar D, et al: Concurrent administration of donepezil HCl and levodopa/carbidopa in patients with Parkinson's disease: assessment of pharmacokinetic changes and safety following multiple oral doses. Br J Clin Pharmacol 58:41–49, 2004

Padovani A, Costanzi C, Gilberti N, et al: Parkinson's disease and dementia. Neurol Sci 27 (suppl 1):S40–S43, 2006

Perry EK, Haroutunian V, Davis KL, et al: Neocortical cholinergic activities differentiate Lewy body dementia from classical Alzheimer's disease. Neuroreport 5:747–749, 1994

Piggott MA, Marshall EF, Thomas N, et al: Striatal dopaminergic markers in dementia with Lewy bodies, Alzheimer's and Parkinson's diseases: rostrocaudal distribution. Brain 122:1449–1468, 1999

Salmon DP, Galasko D, Hansen LA, et al: Neuropsychological deficits associated with diffuse Lewy body disease. Brain Cogn 31:148–165, 1996

Sanchez-Ramos JR, Ortoll R, Paulson GW: Visual hallucinations associated with Parkinson disease. Arch Neurol 53:1265–1268, 1996

Senard JM, Rai S, Lapeyre-Mestre M, et al: Prevalence of orthostatic hypotension in Parkinson's disease. J Neurol Neurosurg Psychiatry 63:584–589, 1997

Shimizu S, Hanyu H, Kanetaka H, et al: Differentiation of dementia with Lewy bodies from Alzheimer's disease using brain SPECT. Dement Geriatr Cogn Disord 20:25–30, 2005

Stern Y, Mayeux R, Rosen J, et al: Perceptual motor dysfunction in Parkinson's disease: a deficit in sequential and predictive voluntary movement. J Neurol Neurosurg Psychiatry 46:145–151, 1983

Stern Y, Richards M, Sano M, et al: Comparison of cognitive changes in patients with Alzheimer's and Parkinson's disease. Arch Neurol 50:1040–1045, 1993

Tiraboschi P, Hansen LA, Alford M, et al: Cholinergic dysfunction in diseases with Lewy bodies. Neurology 54:407–411, 2000

Trinh NH, Hoblyn J, Mohanty S, et al: Efficacy of cholinesterase inhibitors in the treatment of neuropsychiatric symptoms and functional impairment in Alzheimer disease: a meta-analysis. JAMA 289:210–216, 2003

Vander Borght T, Minoshoma S, Giordani B, et al: Cerebral metabolic differences in Parkinson's and Alzheimer diseases matched for dementia severity. J Nucl Med 38:797–802, 1997

Walker Z, Grace J, Overshot R, et al: Olanzapine in dementia with Lewy bodies: a clinical study. Int J Geriatr Psychiatry 14:459–466, 1999

Wechsler DA: Wechsler Adult Intelligence Scale, 4th Edition. San Antonio, TX, Pearson, 2008

Further Reading

Galpern WR, Lang AE: Interface between tauopathies and synucleinopathies: a tale of two proteins. Ann Neurol 59:449–458, 2006

Jellinger KA: Neuropathological spectrum of synucleinopathies. Mov Disord 18 (suppl 6):S2–S12, 2003

Lee VM, Trojanowski JQ: Mechanisms of Parkinson's disease linked to pathological alpha-synuclein: new targets for drug discovery. Neuron 52:33–38, 2006

Tarawneh R, Galvin JE: Distinguishing Lewy body dementias from Alzheimer's disease. Expert Rev Neurother 7:1499–1516, 2007

Frontotemporal Dementia and Other Tauopathies

Anne M. Lipton, M.D., Ph.D.

Adam Boxer, M.D., Ph.D.

In its broadest sense, the term *frontotemporal dementia* (FTD) refers to a number of neurodegenerative diseases that vary in clinical presentation and pathological findings. FTD is also known as *frontotemporal lobar degeneration* (FTLD) (Neary et al. 1998). The clinical and research nosology for this disease continue to evolve and sometimes create controversy or confusion. *Frontal-variant FTD* (fvFTD) refers to the specific FTD clinical subtype characterized by executive dysfunction and apathy. Although the clinical syndromes vary, they characteristically involve problems with language, behavior, and/or motor findings, such

Preparation of portions of this chapter was supported by National Institutes of Health Grant K23NS048855 and the John Douglas French Foundation.

as parkinsonism. Research in FTD, including genetic discoveries and the application of modern neuroimaging techniques, has led to remarkable advances.

History

The archetypal FTD is Pick disease, first clinically delineated by Arnold Pick (1892), who described language impairments and behavioral disturbances in the setting of focal brain atrophy. Alois Alzheimer (1911) provided the first histopathological description of Pick disease with argyrophilic inclusions (later called Pick bodies) and swollen, achromatic cells (later called Pick cells). The Lund-Manchester criteria (Lund and Manchester Groups 1994) delineated the clinical features of FTD; these criteria were later refined by a consensus panel that used the term *frontotemporal lobar degeneration* (Neary et al. 1998). Additional clinical consensus criteria for FTD have been published (McKhann et al. 2001).

FTD occurs, on average, in individuals in their 50s and may be the most common cause of dementia in this age group (Knopman et al. 2004). Onset before age 65 years is one of the clinical diagnostic criteria for FTD (Neary et al. 1998).

Clinical Subtypes of FTD

Patients with FTD present with the insidious onset of a behavioral syndrome or a language variant. FTD progresses gradually, but survival is generally shorter than for Alzheimer disease. Hodges et al. (2003) reported that median survival from symptom onset and from diagnosis was about 6 years for fvFTD and about 3 years for FTD associated with motor neuron disease.

Frontal Variant FTD

The frontal or behavioral variant of FTD is an FTD subtype characterized by executive dysfunction and problems with social conduct and interpersonal skills associated with abnormalities of the right frontotemporal lobe on neuroimaging (Mychack et al. 2001). Lack of insight is a hallmark of the fvFTD subtype. Patients are often impulsive and oblivious to societal or other limitations on their actions. Compulsions, hoarding, and decline in hygiene frequently occur.

An individual with fvFTD may display disinhibition, apathy, or both. Patients with orbitofrontal dysfunction are more "disagreeable" and less modest and altruistic (Rankin et al. 2004). Damage in the ventromedial frontal lobes is associated with disinhibited, impulsive, antisocial, and compulsive behaviors (Rosen et al. 2002a). Patients with fvFTD may have some aspects of a Klüver-Bucy syndrome, including eating (or drinking) to excess, with an emphasis on carbohydrate-laden junk food.

Primary Progressive Aphasia

Patients with a language variant of FTD—either progressive nonfluent aphasia or semantic dementia—frequently have one or more extensive evaluations for stroke due to their aphasia. The aphasia worsens, and they may become mute. Some also develop behaviors similar to those seen in fvFTD or in motor dysfunctions such as amyotrophic lateral sclerosis (ALS) or parkinsonism.

Artistic abilities often manifest in patients with a language variant of FTD, but they may emerge in patients with nonlanguage presentations of FTD as well (Miller et al. 1998). These talents may manifest de novo or as a modification of a skill previously evident in an individual.

Progressive Nonfluent Aphasia

Progressive nonfluent aphasia involves expressive aphasia with word finding difficulty, agrammatism, and phonemic paraphasias. Unlike patients with the other forms of FTD, patients with progressive nonfluent aphasia usually have little functional or behavioral impairment until late in their disease.

Semantic Dementia

Semantic dementia, also called the *temporal lobe variant of FTD,* is caused by a progressive loss of information about the world and is associated with degeneration of the anterior temporal lobes. It usually manifests as a fluent dysphasia with impairment of semantic verbal memory (severe difficulty in naming and in understanding the meaning of words) and an associative agnosia (e.g., difficulty in stating or demonstrating the function of an object, such as a tool or utensil) in individuals with more left temporal lobe involvement. Prosopagnosia (inability to recognize faces) may rarely occur and is associated with right temporal lobe damage. More commonly, behavioral problems similar to those in fvFTD occur in individuals with more right lobar dysfunction.

Overlap of FTD Clinical Syndromes

Because the three FTD clinical syndromes often overlap (as can be seen in some of the above examples), and because they may also overlap with motor syndromes such as motor neuron disease/ALS and parkinsonism (including corticobasal syndrome and progressive supranuclear palsy [PSP]), some authors suggest the term *Pick complex* to encompass all of these syndromes.

The current consensus clinical criteria for FTD are useful but still lack precision. New guidelines are in development. The current clinical criteria fail to account for many neurogenetic and neuroimaging aspects of the diagnosis of FTD. Rosen et al. (2002b) found that the Neary et al. (1998) clinical consensus criteria efficiently separated 30 autopsy-proven cases of Alzheimer disease and 30 autopsy-proven cases of FTLD. They found that the following five clinical features best distinguished FTLD from Alzheimer disease: presence of social conduct disorders, hyperorality, akinesia, and absence of amnesia and perceptual disorder.

Clinical Syndromes Associated With FTD

A number of diseases overlap clinically and pathologically with FTD, including motor neuron disease/ALS, corticobasal syndrome, and PSP.

Motor Neuron Disease/Amyotrophic Lateral Sclerosis

Of 100 ALS patients studied prospectively with extensive neuropsychological assessment, about one-third met criteria for FTLD (Lomen-Hoerth et al. 2003). Many patients clinically diagnosed with FTLD have motor neuron–type inclusions on histopathology, either with or without clinical motor neuron disease (Bigio et al. 2003). Moreover, both chronic traumatic encephalopathy and FTLD may include TAR-DNA binding protein 43 (TDP-43)–positive inclusions in the brain. These inclusions have been shown in the spinal cord in a few cases of chronic traumatic encephalopathy associated with motor neuron disease (McKee et al. 2010).

Corticobasal Syndrome

Corticobasal syndrome is the current nomenclature used to describe the unifying clinical and pathological characteristics of FTD and corticobasal degeneration, also known as corticobasal ganglionic degeneration (CBGD). CBGD is a Parkinson-plus syndrome (classically manifested as unilateral rigidity, apraxia, the alien hand syndrome, reflex myoclonus, and/or cortical sensory loss) that tends to progress more rapidly than Parkinson disease and is usually less amenable to treatment.

Progressive Supranuclear Palsy

PSP is another Parkinson-plus syndrome possessing clinical and pathological overlap with FTD. Both FTD and PSP are tauopathies (pathologically classified as abnormalities of the cytoskeletal protein tau) with clinical onset in late life. PSP is characterized by balance difficulty, falls, visual disturbances, slurred speech, dysphagia, and personality change (Richardson et al. 1963). The dementia of PSP is consistent with FTD. A characteristic triad of ophthalmoplegia, pseudobulbar palsy, and axial dystonia develops. First, downward gaze is impaired, then upward gaze, then voluntary gaze in all directions. If the eyes are fixed on a target and the head is turned, full eye movement occurs (doll's eye phenomenon), indicating that the motor nerves are intact.

The etiology of PSP is unknown. Pathological findings include loss of neurons; gliosis; and the presence of neurofibrillary tangles in the surviving neurons in the midbrain, cerebellar peduncles, and subthalamic nucleus. Functional impairment proceeds to anarthria and total immobility, usually within a few years.

Neuropathology

FTD is pathologically distinct from Alzheimer disease. Historically, the FTD disorders have been divided into Pick disease and non-Pick lobar atrophy (Dickson 1998). Both have grossly appreciable frontal and temporal atrophy. Pick bodies are seen only in Pick disease.

Tau and ubiquitin immunohistochemistries are important in classifying pathological FTD subtypes. Motor neuron–type, ubiquitin-positive inclusions are the most common histopathological type of FTLD (Lipton et al. 2004). The chief protein associated with ubiquitinated inclusions is now recognized to be TDP-43 (Neumann et al. 2006). Frontotemporal degeneration with neuronal loss and spongiosis has no tau or ubiquitin inclusions, but some of these cases are classifiable as FTLD–motor neuron disease (Lipton et al. 2004). Corticobasal degeneration has tau-positive neuronal inclusions and glial plaques, along with ballooned neurons, in cortex, basal ganglia, brain stem, and cerebellum. Despite the shared pathology in patients with FTD, there may be a variety of pathological findings within the same clinical FTD subtype. Familial multiple system tauopathy is one of the many cases of familial FTD and parkinsonism linked to chromosome 17 (FTDP-17). These families have a variety of clinical presentations, including disinhibition-dementia-parkinsonism-amyotrophy complex, and neuropathological findings always associated with tau deposition. In contrast, individuals with progranulin mutations, an even more common form of autosomal dominant FTD, are found to have ubiquitin pathology at autopsy. Validity of the FTLD diagnostic consensus criteria has been verified histopathologically (Knopman et al. 2005).

Diagnostic Evaluation

Clinical evaluation, including history from a reliable collateral source, such as a close family member, is crucial in the diagnosis of FTD. Family history of neurological disease and psychiatric illness is important, because FTD is hereditary in some cases and is often not diagnosed as FTD per se, but rather may manifest as motor neuron disease or parkinsonism, go undiagnosed, or be misdiagnosed (as depression, bipolar disorder, another form of dementia, etc.). Neurological evaluation may elicit abnormalities, such as motor weakness, parkinsonism, or frontal reflexes, that may provide additional diagnostic certainty. Patients with FTD, particularly the FTD clinical profile, will often display echopraxia (imitating the examiner), perseveration, and motor impersistence. Patients can also be tested for frontal release signs, such as suck, snout, rooting, palmomental, and Babinski reflexes.

Neuropsychological Testing

A comprehensive neuropsychological evaluation is often helpful in diagnostic differentiation (see Chapter 3, "Neuropsychological Assessment"), if the patient can comprehend and cooperate with such testing. Usual clinical tests, such as the Mini-Mental State Examination (MMSE; Folstein et al. 1975), do not directly assess executive functioning and may be relatively normal in patients with FTD (due to relative sparing of memory) or may show profound impairment in patients with the language variants of FTD. However, MMSE scores do decline at a greater rate in FTD than in Alzheimer disease (Chow et al. 2006). Neuropsychological evaluation may reveal executive dysfunction on commonly performed assessments, including the Stroop Test, the Trail Making Test, tests of verbal and design fluency, and the Wisconsin Card Sorting Test (Hodges and Graham 2001).

Tests reported to be sensitive to FTD include the Frontal Behavioral Inventory (Kertesz et al. 1997) and the Frontal Assessment Battery (FAB; Dubois et al. 2000). The FAB has been shown to distinguish healthy control subjects from patients with mild Parkinson disease, multiple system atrophy, corticobasal degeneration, and PSP. Total FAB scores did not differentiate FTLD from Alzheimer disease, but some subscores (of mental flexibility and environmental autonomy) did (Lipton et al. 2005), and patients with Alzheimer disease and FTLD patients actually performed comparably on the Luria maneuver (Weiner et al. 2011).

Speech-Language Cognitive Evaluation

A speech-language cognitive evaluation is often helpful, especially in diagnosing specific language variants (see also Chapter 1, "Neuropsychiatric Assessment and Diagnosis"). Some patients may also benefit from further therapy to assist in maintaining communication.

Neuroimaging

Prominent frontal lobe atrophy on structural magnetic resonance imaging is a common feature of FTD, particularly in individuals without motor neuron disease (Figure 9–1). Neuroimaging with ^{18}F-labeled fluorodeoxyglucose positron emission tomography (FDG-PET) is sometimes helpful in the differential diagnosis of FTD (Foster et al. 2007) and has been approved by Medicare for this purpose in the context of a comprehensive clinical evaluation (see also Chapter 4, "Neuroimaging"). The amyloid imaging agent Pittsburgh compound B, or PIB, may be even more valuable for ruling out atypical forms of Alzheimer disease that mimic FTD (Rabinovici et al. 2007).

Electroencephalography

Electroencephalography (EEG) is not generally helpful for diagnosis. EEG has been shown to be normal in many cases. One study showed that electroencephalographic abnormalities correlated with severity of FTD but that this correlation was not helpful in differentiating FTD from Alzheimer disease (Chan et al. 2004).

Genetics

Genetic tests are not available commercially but are a major area of research interest. Multiple genetic loci (on chromosomes 3p, 9p, 9q, 17q21, and 17q24) and five genes (those for microtubule-associated protein tau, progranulin, valosin-containing protein, and charged multivesicular body protein 2B [CHMP2B]) have been associated with inherited FTD (Mackenzie and Rademakers 2007; Rademakers and Hutton 2007). FTD with parkinsonism (FTDP-17) has been linked to mutations in the gene coding for the microtubule-associated protein tau (Hutton et al. 1998). FTD with ubiquitin-positive inclusions (FTDU-17) is caused by loss-of-function mutations in the TAR-DNA binding protein gene coding for progranulin (PGRN), a growth factor involved in neuronal survival (Baker et al. 2006).

Treatment

No treatment for FTD has been approved by the U.S. Food and Drug Administration, but antidepressants, including selective serotonin reuptake inhibitors, are useful in treating many of the behavioral symptoms (Huey et al. 2006). Trazodone is the only medication for FTD behavioral symptoms studied in a double-blind, randomized controlled trial (Lebert et al. 2004). Trazodone is beneficial for a number of behavioral problems in FTD, including irritability, agitation, depressive symptoms, and eating disorders.

FTD does not entail a cholinergic deficit, and the use of cholinesterase inhibitors is controversial. In an open-label study, rivastigmine ameliorated behavioral problems in FTD (Moretti et al. 2004), but donepezil worsened behavioral symptoms (Mendez et al. 2007). Other symptomatic treatments that have been tried are dopaminergic therapies for parkinsonism and language problems. A prospective 26-week open-label trial of memantine 20 mg/day in FTD showed that patients with progressive nonfluent aphasia maintained relative cognitive stability over the 26 weeks, whereas the subjects with semantic aphasia had a decline in cognitive ability (Boxer et al. 2009). In a double-blind study of memantine 20 mg/day in 18 human subjects with primary progres-

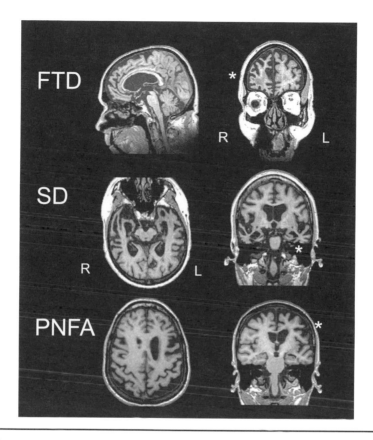

Figure 9–1.   Magnetic resonance imaging (MRI) findings in frontotemporal dementia (FTD).

FTD: parasagittal and coronal images from T_1-weighted MRI. Note asymmetric right frontal atrophy on coronal image (*), and lack of significant atrophy posterior to frontal lobe on sagittal image.

Semantic dementia (SD): axial and coronal images; atrophy is most severe anteriorly and involves both medial and lateral temporal lobe structures (*).

Progressive nonfluent aphasia (PNFA): axial and coronal images show asymmetric left frontal atrophy with minimal temporal lobe involvement (*).

Source.   Reprinted from Lipton AM, Boxer A: "Frontotemporal Dementia," in *The American Psychiatric Publishing Textbook of Alzheimer Disease and Other Dementias.* Edited by Weiner MF, Lipton AM. Washington, DC, American Psychiatric Publishing, 2009, pp. 219–227. Copyright 2009, American Psychiatric Publishing. Used with permission.

sive aphasia, the treated group showed less decline on the Western Aphasia Battery than did the placebo group (Johnson et al. 2010).

Key Clinical Points

- Frontotemporal dementia (FTD) may be the most common cause of dementia for adults under age 65.

- Gradual personality change with impaired judgment in the fifth or sixth decade of life should elicit suspicion for the frontal/ behavioral variant of FTD.

- FTD may manifest as a disorder of language expression or comprehension.

- FTD overlaps clinically and pathologically with a number of neurological syndromes, including amyotrophic lateral sclerosis, corticobasal syndrome, and progressive supranuclear palsy.

References

Alzheimer A: Über eigenartige Krankheitsfälle des späteren Alters. Zeitschrift für die gesamte Neurologie und Psychiatrie 4:356–385, 1911

Baker M, Mackenzie IR, Pickering-Brown SM, et al: Mutations in progranulin cause tau-negative frontotemporal dementia linked to chromosome 17. Nature 24:916–919, 2006

Bigio EH, Lipton AM, White CL III, et al: Frontotemporal and motor neuron degeneration with neurofilament inclusion bodies: additional evidence for overlap between FTD and ALS. Neuropathol Appl Neurobiol 29:239–253, 2003

Boxer AL, Lipton AM, Womack K, et al: An open-label study of memantine treatment in 3 types of frontotemporal lobar degeneration. Alzheimer Dis Assoc Disord 23:211–217, 2009

Chan D, Walters RJ, Sampson EL, et al: EEG abnormalities in frontotemporal lobar degeneration. Neurology 62:1628–1630, 2004

Chow TW, Hynan LS, Lipton AM: MMSE scores decline at a greater rate in frontotemporal degeneration than in AD. Dement Geriatr Cogn Disord 22:194–199, 2006

Dickson DW: Pick's disease: a modern approach. Brain Pathol 8:339–354, 1998

Dubois B, Slachevsky A, Litvan I, et al: The FAB: a frontal assessment battery at bedside. Neurology 55:1622–1625, 2000

Folstein MF, Folstein SE, McHugh PR: "Mini-mental state": a practical method for grading the cognitive state of patients for the clinician. J Psychiatr Res 12:189–198, 1975

Foster NL, Heidebrink JL, Clark CM, et al: FDG-PET improves accuracy in distinguishing frontotemporal dementia and Alzheimer's disease. Brain 130:2616–2635, 2007

Hodges JR, Graham KS: Episodic memory: insights from semantic dementia. Philos Trans R Soc Lond B Biol Sci 356:1423–1434, 2001

Hodges JR, Davies R, Xuereb J, et al: Survival in frontotemporal dementia. Neurology 61:349–354, 2003

Huey ED, Putnam KT, Grafman J: A systematic review of neurotransmitter deficits and treatments in frontotemporal dementia. Neurology 66:17–22, 2006

Hutton M, Lendon CL, Rizzu P: Association of missense and 5'-splice-site mutations in tau with the inherited dementia FTDP-17. Nature 393:702–705, 1998

Johnson NA, Rademaker A, Weintraub S, et al: Pilot trial of memantine in primary progressive aphasia (letter). Alzheimer Dis Assoc Disord 24:308, 2010

Kertesz A, Davidson W, Fox H: Frontal Behavioral Inventory: diagnostic criteria for frontal lobe dementia. Can J Neurol Sci 24:9–36, 1997

Knopman DS, Petersen RC, Edland SD, et al: The incidence of frontotemporal lobar degeneration in Rochester, Minnesota, 1990 through 1994. Neurology 62:506–508, 2004

Knopman DS, Boeve BF, Parisi JE, et al: Antemortem diagnosis of frontotemporal lobar degeneration. Ann Neurol 57:480–488, 2005

Lebert F, Stekke W, Hasenbroekx C: Frontotemporal dementia: a randomised, controlled trial with trazodone. Dement Geriatr Cogn Disord 17:355–359, 2004

Lipton AM, White CL III, Bigio EH: Frontotemporal lobar degeneration with motor neuron disease–type inclusions predominates in 76 cases of frontotemporal degeneration. Acta Neuropathol 108:379–385, 2004

Lipton AM, Ohman KA, Womack KB, et al: Subscores of the FAB differentiate frontotemporal lobar degeneration from AD. Neurology 65:726–731, 2005

Lomen-Hoerth C, Murphy J, Langmore S, et al: Are amyotrophic lateral sclerosis patients cognitively normal? Neurology 60:1094–1097, 2003

Lund and Manchester Groups: Clinical and neuropathological criteria for frontotemporal dementia. J Neurol Neurosurg Psychiatry 57:416–418, 1994

Mackenzie IR, Rademakers R: The molecular genetics and neuropathology of frontotemporal lobar degeneration: recent developments. Neurogenetics 8:237–248, 2007

McKee AC, Gavett BE, Stern RA, et al: TDP-43 proteinopathy and motor neuron disease in chronic traumatic encephalopathy. J Neuropathol Exp Neurol 69:918–929, 2010

McKhann GM, Albert MS, Grossman M, et al: Clinical and pathological diagnosis of frontotemporal dementia. Arch Neurol 58:1803–1809, 2001

Mendez MF, Shapira JS, McMurtray A, et al: Preliminary findings: behavioral worsening on donepezil in patients with frontotemporal dementia. Am J Geriatr Psychiatry 15:84–87, 2007

Miller BL, Cummings J, Mishkin F, et al: Emergence of artistic talent in frontotemporal dementia. Neurology 51:978–982, 1998

Moretti R, Torre P, Antonello RM, et al: Rivastigmine in frontotemporal dementia: an open-label study. Drugs Aging 21:931–937, 2004

Mychack P, Kramer JH, Boone KB, et al: The influence of right frontotemporal dysfunction on social behavior in frontotemporal dementia. Neurology 56 (suppl 4):S11–S15, 2001

Neary D, Snowden JS, Gustafson L, et al: Frontotemporal lobar degeneration: a consensus on clinical diagnostic criteria. Neurology 51:1546–1554, 1998

Neumann M, Sampathu DM, Kwong LK, et al: Ubiquitinated TDP-43 in frontotemporal lobar degeneration and amyotrophic lateral sclerosis. Science 314:130–133, 2006

Pick A: Über die Beziehungen der senilen Hirnatrophie zur Aphasie. Prager medizinische Wochenschrift 17:165–167, 1892

Rabinovici GD, Furst AJ, O'Neil JP, et al: 11C-PIB PET imaging in Alzheimer disease and frontotemporal lobar degeneration. Neurology 68:1205–1212, 2007

Rademakers R, Hutton M: The genetics of frontotemporal lobar degeneration. Curr Neurol Neurosci Rep 7:434–442, 2007

Rankin KP, Rosen HJ, Kramer JH, et al: Right and left medial orbitofrontal volumes show an opposite relationship to agreeableness in FTD. Dement Geriatr Cogn Disord 17:328–332, 2004

Richardson JC, Steele J, Olszewski J: Supranuclear ophthalmoplegia, pseudobulbar palsy, nuchal dystonia and dementia. Trans Am Neurol Assoc 88:25–29, 1963

Rosen HJ, Hartikainen KM, Jagust W, et al: Utility of clinical criteria in differentiating frontotemporal lobar degeneration from Alzheimer's disease. Neurology 58:1608–1615, 2002a

Rosen HJ, Perry RJ, Murphy J, et al. Emotion comprehension in the temporal variant of frontotemporal dementia. Brain 125:2286–2295, 2002b

Weiner MF, Hynan LS, Rossetti H, et al: Luria's three-step test: what is it and what does it tell us? Int Psychogeriatr May 4, 2011 (Epub ahead of print)

Further Reading

Brun A: Identification and characterization of frontal lobe degeneration: historical perspective on the development of FTD. Alzheimer Dis Assoc Disord 21:3–4, 2007

Caselli R, Yaari R: Medical management of frontotemporal dementia. Am J Alzheimers Dis Other Demen 22:489–498, 2007

Hallam BJ, Silverberg ND, Lamarre AK, et al: Clinical presentation of prodromal frontotemporal dementia. Am J Alzheimers Dis Other Demen 22:456–457, 2007

Levy JA, Chelune GJ: Cognitive-behavioral profiles of neurodegenerative dementias: beyond Alzheimer's disease. J Geriatr Psychiatry Neurol 20:227–238, 2007

10

Traumatic Brain Injury

Erin D. Bigler, Ph.D.

More than 80,000 individuals become disabled from traumatic brain injuries (TBIs) each year (Thurman 2007). Thus, TBI represents a substantial source of neuropsychiatric morbidity and disability. From a cognitive perspective, the three likely proximal outcomes of a TBI are complete recovery after a period of recuperation, mild to moderate residual cognitive impairment, and dementia. However, even in those who appear to fully recover from the proximal effects of TBI, the brain injury may become a vulnerability factor that during aging interacts with other environmental, constitutional, and genetic factors to produce later cognitive decline and earlier onset of frank dementia

The technical expertise and manuscript assistance of Tracy Abildskov, Craig Vickers, and Jo Ann Petrie are gratefully acknowledged. Much of the research reported on in this chapter was supported by a grant from the Ira Fulton Foundation.

in late life (Gavett et al. 2010; van den Heuvel et al. 2007). Acute TBI induces several histopathological changes that also occur in age-related degenerative diseases such as Alzheimer disease (AD) (DeKosky et al. 2010). Indeed, much has been written about TBI as a substantial risk factor for dementia and other neuropsychiatric problems later in life (Rao and Lyketsos 2002; Starkstein and Jorge 2005), although much needs to be discovered and scientifically established about the distant effects of TBI (Blennow et al. 2006).

By the standards of DSM-IV-TR (American Psychiatric Association 2000), dementia due to head trauma is diagnosed when the dementia is judged to be a direct pathophysiological consequence of head trauma (see Table 10–1). Head trauma is a common cause of acquired dementia (Kim et al. 2011). By definition, when head injury is the *proximal* cause of a dementia syndrome, the person never recovers sufficiently to overcome or compensate for the substantial cognitive and behavioral residuals of the brain injury. However, the majority of TBIs are in the mild to moderate range, and although cognitive impairments are commonplace, most TBIs at this level of severity do not cause dementia. A more common diagnosis attributable to TBI is cognitive disorder not otherwise specified (NOS).

Head injury can be a *remote* contributor to the later development of dementia even if the individual experienced an apparent complete recovery from the original brain injury (Bigler 2007). These remote effects of TBI are discussed later in this chapter after a discussion of proximal effects.

Proximal Effects of TBI: Dementia Due to Head Trauma

Dementia due to head trauma usually results from a moderate to severe brain injury. As indicated in Table 1–2 of Chapter 1, DSM-IV-TR criteria for dementia require multiple cognitive deficits, including memory impairment and at least one of the following cognitive disturbances: aphasia, apraxia, agnosia, or a disturbance in executive functioning. The deficits that make up dementia are diagnosed clinically. The deficits must be sufficient to cause functional impairment in home or work life and must represent a decline from previous functioning. Because a distinct antecedent event is known in TBI-associated cognitive disorders, little doubt exists about the causal relationship of the head injury in dementia due to head trauma.

Table 10–1. Dementia due to head trauma

The essential feature of dementia due to head trauma is the presence of a dementia that is judged to be the direct pathophysiological consequence of head trauma. The degree and type of cognitive impairments or behavioral disturbances depend on the location and extent of the brain injury. Posttraumatic amnesia is frequently present, along with persisting memory impairment. A variety of other behavioral symptoms may be evident, with or without the presence of motor or sensory deficits. These symptoms include aphasia, attentional problems, irritability, anxiety, depression or affective lability, apathy, increased aggression, or other changes in personality. Alcohol or other substance intoxication is often present in individuals with acute head injuries, and concurrent substance abuse or dependence may be present. Head injury occurs most often in young males and has been associated with risk-taking behaviors. When it occurs in the context of a single injury, dementia due to head trauma is usually nonprogressive, but repeated head injury (e.g., from boxing) may lead to a progressive dementia (so-called dementia pugilistica). A single head trauma that is followed by a progressive decline in cognitive function should raise the possibility of another superimposed process such as hydrocephalus or a major depressive episode.

Source.   Reprinted from American Psychiatric Association: *Diagnostic and Statistical Manual of Mental Disorders,* 4th Edition, Text Revision. Washington, DC, American Psychiatric Association, 2000, p. 164. Copyright 2000, American Psychiatric Association. Used with permission.

In the most severe cases, TBI-related cognitive impairment can be detected during standard mental status examination, using screening psychometric tests such as the Mini-Mental State Examination (MMSE; Lorentz et al. 2002). In some cases, more detailed neuropsychological testing may be necessary. The drawing presented in Figure 10–1 is by a patient with dementia due to head injury. He had sustained a severe TBI as an adolescent, and despite extensive inpatient and outpatient treatment and although physically intact, he never recovered enough cognitive and praxic functions to live independently. When the patient was tested postinjury as a young adult, his Full Scale IQ score was 78 and his MMSE score was 17. Preinjury school records reflected average academic performance with no history of learning or developmental disorder, and he had never been diagnosed prior to injury with a neuropsychiatric condition. He had striking impairment in short-term memory and severe constructional apraxia, as evidenced in the drawing shown in Figure 10–1. Over a 5-year span of monitoring, he never changed significantly. Unlike dementias associated with progressive degenerative diseases such as AD, dementia associated with head trauma is static.

Neuroimaging for Estimating Severity of Brain Injury in TBI

Significant advancements in detecting TBI abnormalities have come from contemporary high-field magnetic resonance imaging (MRI) and functional neuroimaging techniques (Metting et al. 2007; Taber and Hurley 2007). Using neuroimaging findings to visualize the degree and extent of structural and functional damage greatly assists clinicians in understanding the effects of TBI (Bigler 2011). Computed tomography (CT) studies have demonstrated that the extent of TBI-induced structural brain damage is linearly related to the severity of brain injury and that both are coarsely related to the degree of cognitive impairment (Cullum and Bigler 1986). Wilde et al. (2006) examined the association between posttraumatic amnesia (PTA) and the development of MRI-identified cerebral atrophy in patients with TBI. PTA is often used as a marker of initial injury severity: PTA<1 hour is consistent with mild TBI, PTA=1–24 hours indicates moderate TBI, and PTA>24 hours indicates severe injury (Lezak et al. 2004). Wilde et al. (2006) calculated that the odds of developing generalized cerebral atrophy on quantitative MRI increases by 6% with each day of PTA. In addition to greater amounts of cerebral atrophy, longer PTA is associated with worse functional outcome. The combination of longer PTA and greater amounts of cerebral atrophy is associated in turn with the poorest TBI outcome (Bigler et al. 2006). Thus, for the clinician making predictions about clinical outcome, markers of brain injury severity, including PTA, or severity of coma, as indicated by the Glasgow Coma Scale (GCS), and their duration directly relate to the likelihood of developing dementia following TBI.

MRI studies of the brain readily demonstrate clinically relevant TBI-related atrophy, when present. The MRI findings of the patient whose apraxia was evident from the drawing in Figure 10–1 are shown in Figure 10–2; they demonstrate extensive structural damage to the entire brain, particularly in frontotemporal regions, readily appreciated by viewing the reconstructed brain in three-dimensional views. The scan, in conjunction with the patient's neuropsychological test performance, initial GCS score of 3 (GCS scores range from 3 [deep coma] to 15 [alert, oriented, and following commands]), and history of weeks of coma and months of PTA, points to the greater likelihood of a residual dementia due to head trauma.

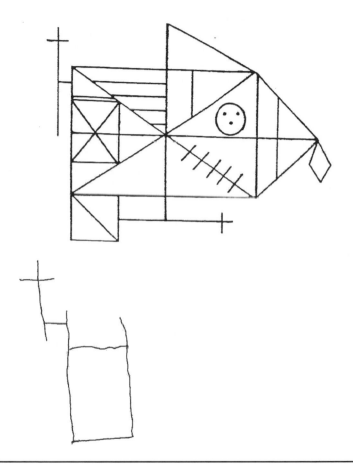

Figure 10–1.   Drawing by patient with dementia due to head injury *(lower portion)* in response to model *(upper portion)*.

At the time of neuropsychological assessment and neuroimaging, this patient was 22 years old and 2 years post–traumatic brain injury. He had severe constructional apraxia, as demonstrated by his inability to copy the Rey-Osterrieth Complex Figure (Lezak et al. 2004). He performed below the first percentile on all measures of short-term memory and was unable to perform any standardized executive function tasks.

As shown in Figure 10–2, because of the particular vulnerability for focal damage in TBI to occur in the frontal and temporal lobe regions of the brain, frontal and temporal lobe atrophy is often observed to develop after injury (Bigler 2011). Injury significant enough to produce focal damage typically occurs amid a backdrop of diffuse injury. TBI-induced damage to frontotemporal systems increases the likelihood of cognitive impairment and disability (Wilde et al. 2005), in part because of the disruption of cholinergic systems subserved by these regions and the critical role that cholinergic neurons play in cognition (Salmond et al. 2005). Damage to these regions represents another common connection between TBI and the development of a dementing illness such as AD later in life.

Progression of Atrophy From Day of Injury Until Stabilization

Viewing the progression of cerebral damage from acute to chronic stage helps to demonstrate how TBI alters brain structure that is pertinent to developing dementia. This progression can be straightforwardly observed in sequential neuroimaging, as shown in Figure 10–3. The day-of-injury (DOI) scan demonstrates multiple hemorrhagic lesions, intraventricular hemorrhage, and generalized edema in a brain with no identifiable preinjury abnormalities. Although the acute scan demonstrates prominent neuropathological changes, the otherwise intact features help the clinician establish baseline information for future comparison. Subsequent neuroimaging shows over time how hydrocephalus ex vacuo emerges as a reflection of brain parenchyma volume loss. In a postmortem study of patients who would likely have met criteria for dementia due to head trauma, Adams et al. (2011) found that the majority of individuals with severe to moderate disability from TBI who subsequently died had cortical contusions, diffuse traumatic axonal injury (TAI), and ventricular dilation as a reflection of cerebral atrophy; specific to level of disability, the extensiveness of TAI, presence of thalamic lesions, and increased ventricular dilation were particularly prognostic for worse outcome. Viewing the scans in Figure 10–3 serially, one can see that the brain injury has resulted in extensive cerebral atrophy that stabilizes a few months posttrauma. Given the severity of his TBI (GCS= 3), the extensive nature of the cerebral damage documented by the emergence of cerebral atrophy, his impaired cognition on examination and MMSE score of < 10, and his unchanging status for several years postinjury, this patient also

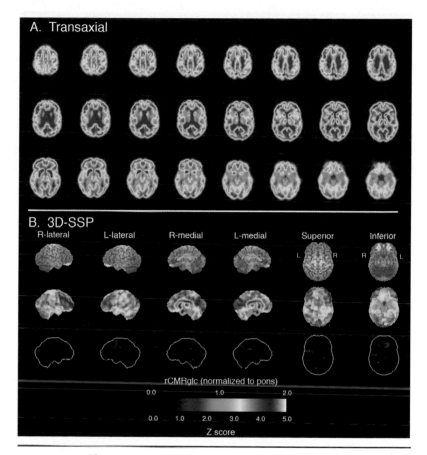

PLATE 1. [¹⁸F]Fluorodeoxyglucose positron emission tomography images from a cognitively normal elderly individual displayed as transaxial *(A)* and three-dimensional stereotactic surface projection (3D SSP) *(B)* metabolic and statistical maps.

FDG-PET scans produce up to 128 transaxial images, here truncated to the most relevant brain slices for easier display. Relative rates of glucose metabolism, in this case relative to pons, are displayed using a color scale shown below the images, with hotter colors representing higher rates of glucose metabolism. Scan data were summarized and displayed in uniform space by 3D SSP, an analysis software program.

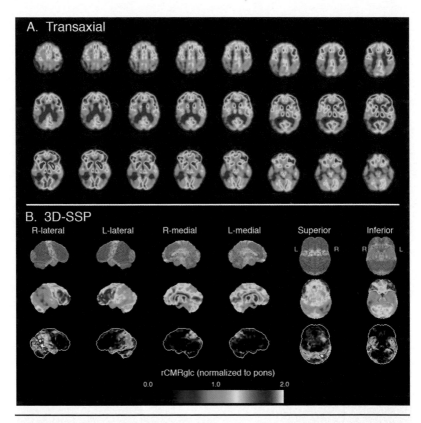

PLATE 2. [^{18}F]Fluorodeoxyglucose positron emission tomography images from a patient with Alzheimer disease displayed as transaxial *(A)* and three-dimensional stereotactic surface projection (3D-SSP) *(B)* metabolic and statistical maps.

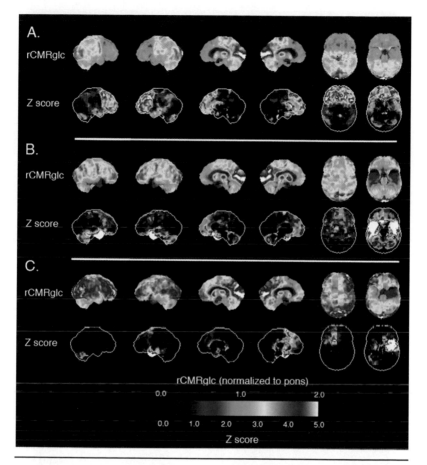

PLATE 3. [^{18}F]Fluorodeoxyglucose positron emission tomography images from three patients with frontotemporal dementia displayed as three-dimensional stereotactic surface projection metabolic and statistical maps, two with bifrontal hypometabolism *(A, B)* and the third with asymmetric predominantly temporal hypometabolism *(C)*.

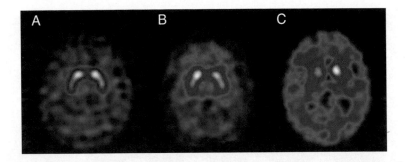

PLATE 4. Single-photon emission computed tomography scans showing binding to dopamine uptake sites in the striatum from a cognitively normal individual *(A)*, an 83-year-old patient with Alzheimer disease *(B)*, and an 81-year-old patient with probable DLB *(C)*.

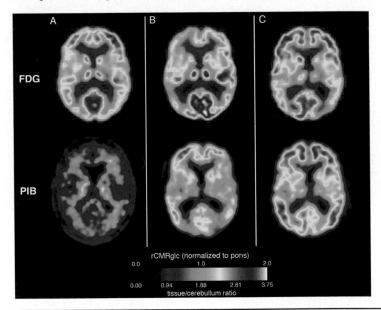

PLATE 5. Transaxial [^{18}F]fluorodeoxyglucose positron emission tomography (FDG-PET) *(top row)* and Pittsburgh compound B (PIB)–PET *(bottom row)* images from a cognitively normal elderly individual *(A)* and two patients with Alzheimer disease *(B, C)*.

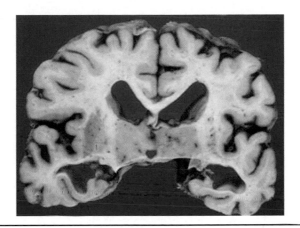

PLATE 6. Coronal pathological section of a patient with confirmed Alzheimer disease with hippocampal complex atrophy and dilatation of the temporal horn of the lateral ventricle.

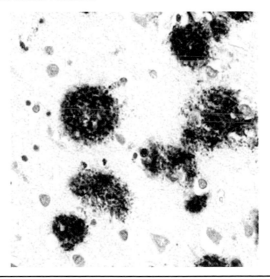

PLATE 7. Photomicrograph of plaques in the cerebral cortex of a patient with Alzheimer disease.

The section is immunostained for amyloid-β, which appears as dark extracellular granular material. The plaques are large compared with surrounding cellular nuclei.

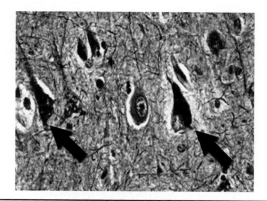

PLATE 8. High-power photomicrograph of Bielschowsky-stained neuro-fibrillary tangles *(see arrows)* in the cerebral cortex of a patient with Alzheimer disease.

Tangles are intraneuronal and consist of collapsed cytoskeletal elements, including characteristic paired helical filaments. Tangle development interferes with normal neuronal function through loss of axonal transport and other vital homeostatic mechanisms.

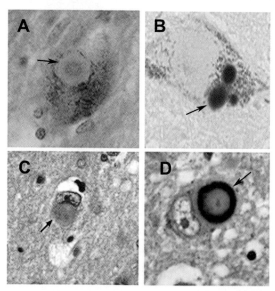

PLATE 9. Brain stem Lewy bodies. *(A)* A nigral Lewy body *(arrow)*. *(B)* Multiple nigral Lewy bodies detected with antibodies against α-synuclein. *(C)* Cortical Lewy bodies. *(D)* Easier detection of cortical Lewy bodies with advent of immunohistochemistry.

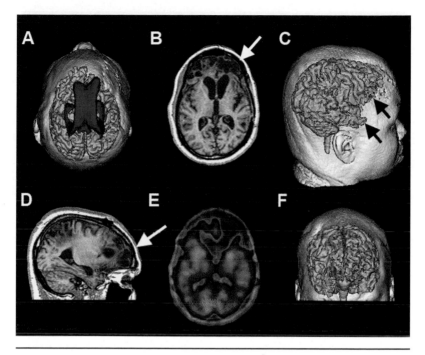

PLATE 10. Neuroimaging studies for the patient with dementia due to head injury whose drawing is shown in Figure 10–1 *(see text)*.
B is an axial T_1-weighted magnetic resonance image showing extensive frontal damage (white arrow) as a result of the severe traumatic brain injury. D is a sagittal T_1-weighted image showing the extensive frontal pathology present in this patient *(white arrow)*. A, C, and F are three-dimensional magnetic resonance image reconstructions visualizing the ventricles *(shown in blue)* in the dorsal view in A, the extensive frontotemporal wasting *(black arrows)* in C, and the bifrontal atrophy, particularly in the inferior frontal region in F. E—a view of single-photon emission computed tomography findings at the same axial level depicted in B—shows extensive loss of frontal perfusion. There is generalized ventricular dilation *(see Plate 11 [Figure 10–4H in text] for a normal dorsal view)*. These imaging findings demonstrate diffuse brain damage and generalized loss of total brain volume.

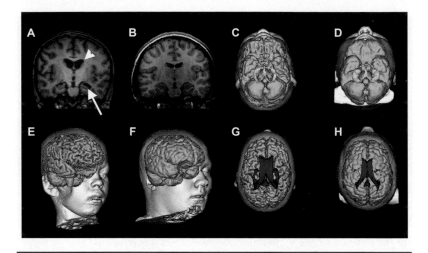

PLATE 11. Neuroimaging studies for an adolescent patient who sustained a severe traumatic brain injury (TBI) in a motor vehicle accident, contrasted with those of an age-matched control.

The coronal T_1-weighted magnetic resonance image shown in *A* shows pronounced hippocampal atrophy *(arrow)*, along with dilated anterior horns of the lateral ventricular system *(arrowhead)* and prominence of cortical sulci, all indicating generalized cerebral volume loss due to TBI as compared with an age-matched control *(B)*. The three-dimensional (3D) reconstructions of the TBI patient *(E)* and an age-matched control subject *(F)* show the frontotemporal atrophy present in the TBI case patient *(E)*, defined by more prominent sulci than in the age-matched control. The TBI patient has profound hippocampal volume loss that can be readily appreciated in the 3D reconstruction *(C, ventral view)* of the hippocampal formation and fornix as shown in *yellow,* compared with the normal appearance of the hippocampus in the control subject *(D)*. A 3D dorsal view reconstruction of the surface anatomy shows generalized atrophy with prominent sulcal widening in the TBI patient *(G)* compared with the control subject *(H)*, along with a dilated ventricular system.

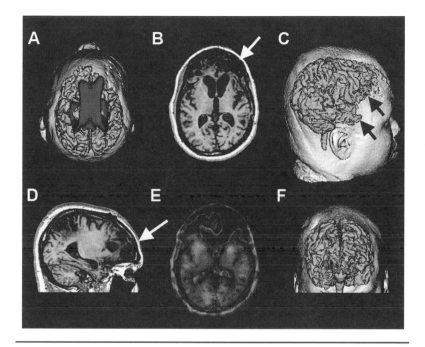

Figure 10–2. Neuroimaging studies for the patient with dementia due to head injury whose drawing is shown in Figure 10–1 *(see color plate 10)*.

B is an axial T_1 weighted magnetic resonance image showing extensive frontal damage *(white arrow)* as a result of the severe traumatic brain injury. *D* is a sagittal T_1-weighted image showing the extensive frontal pathology present in this patient *(white arrow)*. *A, C,* and *F* are three-dimensional magnetic resonance image reconstructions visualizing the ventricles *(shown in blue in Plate 10; shown here in gray)* in the dorsal view in *A,* the extensive frontotemporal wasting *(black arrows)* in *C,* and the bifrontal atrophy, particularly in the inferior frontal region in *F. E*—a view of single-photon emission computed tomography findings at the same axial level depicted in *B*—shows extensive loss of frontal perfusion. There is generalized ventricular dilation *(see Figure 10–4H for a normal dorsal view)*. These imaging findings demonstrate diffuse brain damage and generalized loss of total brain volume.

Source. Reprinted from Bigler ED: "Traumatic Brain Injury," in *The American Psychiatric Publishing Textbook of Alzheimer Disease and Other Dementias.* Edited by Weiner MF, Lipton AM. Washington, DC, American Psychiatric Publishing, 2009, pp. 229–246. Copyright 2009, American Psychiatric Publishing. Used with permission.

meets the criteria for dementia due to head trauma. Therefore, starting with the DOI scan, the degree of resultant cerebral atrophy can be documented over time and typically stabilized within 6 months postinjury, with level of atrophy coarsely associated with degree of cognitive impairment. Such neuroimaging findings in association with the mental status findings reflective of cognitive impairment are the type most likely to be associated with dementia due to head trauma.

Additional Factors That Contribute to Severity of Functional Injury

Damage to Critical Limbic System Structures

Both animal models and human studies have demonstrated the vulnerability of the hippocampus to TBI (Bigler et al. 2010). In humans, this vulnerability of the medial temporal lobe and hippocampus is due in part to their location in the middle cranial fossa and also to excitotoxic reactions that occur in traumatically injured hippocampal neurons (Geddes et al. 2003); diaschisis plays a role as well because hippocampal neurons have diverse afferent and efferent cortical connections throughout the brain (Wilde et al. 2007). Because the medial temporal cortex (and in particular the hippocampus) is so critical to all cognitive functions, damage to this region has a high likelihood for disrupting cognition; however, even with extensive damage, the patient may not meet criteria for dementia.

Figure 10–4 shows scans from an adolescent patient who sustained a severe TBI in a motor vehicle accident (GCS score=3). The scan demonstrates medial temporal lobe atrophy with prominent hippocampal atrophy. Positron emission tomography imaging confirmed reduced radiotracer uptake throughout the medial temporal lobes bilaterally, yet neuropsychological studies demonstrated only mild memory impairment and related cognitive impairments. The patient's MMSE score was 26. Thus, despite these rather dramatic imaging findings and the presence of some cognitive sequelae from the TBI that certainly met criteria for cognitive disorder NOS, the level of cognitive impairment did not warrant a diagnosis of dementia.

Wilde et al. (2007) have also shown that in comparison to all other brain structures, the hippocampus exhibits the greatest atrophic changes in response to TBI. From this and other research, one can conclude that hippocampal injury is found in most cases of moderate to severe TBI. Additionally, it should

DOI	8 days	4 months	9 months	17 months

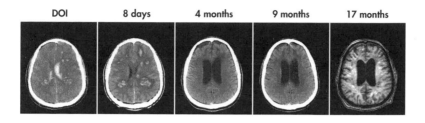

Figure 10–3.   Progression of cerebral damage from acute to chronic stage of traumatic brain injury (TBI).

This patient sustained a severe TBI (Glasgow Coma Scale score = 3) with months of coma and persistent posttraumatic amnesia. Since the patient regained consciousness, his MMSE score has been consistently below 10. The sequential imaging shows brain changes over time. The day-of-injury (DOI) computed tomography scan shows multiple intraparenchymal and intraventricular hemorrhagic lesions scattered throughout the brain, some of which "'blossom" 8 days postinjury. However, by 4 and 9 months postinjury, ventricular dilation, as a sign of generalized brain volume loss, has peaked and shows little change thereafter.

Source.   Reprinted from Bigler ED: "Traumatic Brain Injury," in *The American Psychiatric Publishing Textbook of Alzheimer Disease and Other Dementias.* Edited by Weiner MF, Lipton AM. Washington, DC, American Psychiatric Publishing, 2009, pp. 229–246. Copyright 2009, American Psychiatric Publishing. Used with permission.

be noted that the hippocampus, which also plays a role in emotional control, is potentially injured by stress-related hormones that are part of both the physical and emotional reaction to injury (Wolkowitz et al. 2007). The high incidence of neuropsychiatric sequelae, including depression, in individuals with TBI (Holsinger et al. 2002), as well as the potential part that damage to limbic structures such as the hippocampus may play in mood disorders following TBI (Jorge et al. 2007), underscores the role that hippocampal damage may play in the emotional and cognitive aftermath of TBI. There is even evidence that injury may disrupt hippocampal neurogenesis and that the presence of amyloid may reduce the rate of neurogenesis (Morgan 2007). Because neuropsychiatric disorders may also be a vulnerability factor for later expression of dementia (Starkstein and Jorge 2005), anything that increases the likelihood of neuropsychiatric disorder over the life span may have adverse consequences on the aging process.

Speed-of-Processing Deficits

A nearly universal consequence of TBI, directly related to the severity of injury and persistence of neurobehavioral symptoms, is reduced speed of cognitive processing (Ben-David et al. 2011). Two main neuropathological consequences of TBI impair processing speed. Because recovery from focal pathology is probably due to alternate, redundant, or adaptive pathways taking over function, this less direct way of processing increases response time. The other main factor is the selective vulnerability of white matter to TBI (Vannorsdall et al. 2010). Diminished white matter integrity results in less efficient neural transmission. In normal aging, the extent of white matter pathology directly relates to speed of processing, and both are related to the clinical presentation of age-related mild cognitive impairment (MCI) and dementia (Burns et al. 2005). Because diminished speed of processing is a natural consequence of aging that impacts executive function, and alterations in processing speed mirror normal changes in white matter integrity with aging, the older the individual is at the time of sustaining a TBI, the less resilient the brain is to injury.

Genetics

Many studies have demonstrated that presence of the apolipoprotein E4 allele *(APOE4)* may adversely affect the outcome of any type of acquired brain injury (Mayeux et al. 1995; Verghese et al. 2011). The role of *APOE4* or any other genetic factor in recovery from TBI is beyond the scope of this review, and there are negative reports or findings of minimal association (Han et al. 2007). Nonetheless, genetic factors likely affect recovery from TBI.

Associated Vascular Effects

TAI is associated with microvascular damage in addition to direct damage to the axon, and damage to the underlying cerebral microvasculature can, by itself, cause dementia (Holsinger et al. 2007). The combination of TAI and microvascular damage can lead to widespread changes in cerebral integrity (Petrov and Rafols 2001). Ueda et al. (2006) reported changes in the vascular reactivity and local autoregulation of cerebrovasculature following a TBI, suggesting that localized cerebral perfusion may be disrupted, affecting the energy needs of neurons. In this scenario, neurons may not be specifically damaged but are nonetheless rendered functionally impaired because of diminished autoregulatory factors resulting from vascular rather than neuronal injury.

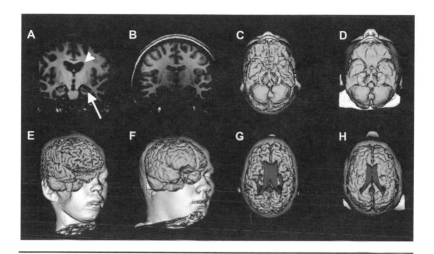

Figure 10–4. Neuroimaging studies for an adolescent patient who sustained a severe traumatic brain injury (TBI) in a motor vehicle accident, contrasted with those of an age-matched control *(see color plate 11)*.

The coronal T_1-weighted magnetic resonance image shown in *A* shows pronounced hippocampal atrophy *(arrow)*, along with dilated anterior horns of the lateral ventricular system *(arrowhead)* and prominence of cortical sulci, all indicating generalized cerebral volume loss due to TBI as compared with an age-matched control *(B)*. The three-dimensional (3D) reconstructions of the TBI patient *(E)* and an age-matched control subject *(F)* show the frontotemporal atrophy present in the TBI case patient *(E)*, defined by more prominent sulci than in the age-matched control. The TBI patient has profound hippocampal volume loss that can be readily appreciated in the 3D reconstruction *(C, ventral view)* of the hippocampal formation and fornix as shown in *yellow (see color plate 11)*, compared with the normal appearance of the hippocampus in the control subject *(D)*. A 3D dorsal view reconstruction of the surface anatomy shows generalized atrophy with prominent sulcal widening in the TBI patient *(G)* compared with the control subject *(H)*, along with a dilated ventricular system.

Source. Reprinted from Bigler ED: "Traumatic Brain Injury," in *The American Psychiatric Publishing Textbook of Alzheimer Disease and Other Dementias.* Edited by Weiner MF, Lipton AM. Washington, DC, American Psychiatric Publishing, 2009, pp. 229–246. Copyright 2009, American Psychiatric Publishing. Used with permission.

Inflammatory Effects of Injury

Inflammatory reactions in the brain are associated with injury, aging, disease, and dementia vulnerability (Loane and Byrnes 2010). At the moment of first injury, the biomechanics of damage include stretching and shear-tensile forces on neural structures that physically damage the cell, inducing immediate changes in the form of increased membrane permeability to ions and other molecules that in turn may stimulate various inflammatory reactions (Laplaca et al. 2007). These changes are widespread and extend into the subacute and chronic phases of recovery (Pineda et al. 2007) and, in turn, may be very important in aging and the age-mediated effects of an injury. The restoration that follows a TBI is through active neuron–glial cell repair mechanisms, in which the control of localized inflammatory reactions is key to maximum recovery (Floyd and Lyeth 2007). Complex environment-stress responses to psychosocial factors may also be at play, and these stress-mediated responses may also be influenced by local and global inflammatory reactions that, if sustained, may be adverse to optimum recovery. Increases in psychosocial stress response during recovery or adaptation to a TBI may have long-term adverse effects on cognition (Lee et al. 2007). TBI is itself a psychosocial stressor, and potential environmental influences must also be considered when discussing inflammatory reactions.

Stability of Dementia Due to Head Trauma: Living With Brain Injury and Aging

In longitudinal surveys of patients followed for decades postinjury, cognitive and neuropsychiatric symptoms suggest that when injury occurs in childhood or early adulthood, the patients generally are stable through midlife (Brown et al. 2011). Because the greatest occurrence of TBI is between ages 15 and 30 years, the majority of those who develop dementia due to head trauma will survive for many years. The assumption has been that the dementia acquired early in life due to head trauma will remain relatively stable at least through the fifth decade of life. However, no study has prospectively followed a group of patients with dementia due to head trauma for the remainder of their lives. Himanen et al. (2006) examined 61 individuals who had sustained a TBI (mild, moderate, or severe) earlier in life and followed them for 30 years, but the authors did not specifically focus on those patients meeting criteria for dementia. Nonetheless, in the patients as a group, cognitive impairments were present, as expected, at baseline and at the end of 30 years, and the authors described the cognitive decline with age during this time interval as being only "mild." As discussed in the following section, there may indeed be more accelerated neurodegeneration in late life because of a prior head injury. Hinkebein et al. (2003) proposed that neurocognitive deficits associated with TBI become more influential with age in altering the patient's cognitive status. For patients with dementia due to head trauma, especially those injured earlier in life, there may be a few decades of stable cognition, but ultimately aging will adversely interact with the effects of the TBI, and the combination will have a greater effect than aging or the prior injury alone.

Remote Effects of TBI: Relation to Late-Life Neurodegenerative Changes

The majority of persons with moderate to severe TBI have potential for good cognitive recovery (Wood and Rutterford 2006). Most TBI patients in the mild to moderate range recover sufficiently to resume some level of normal personal, vocational, and psychosocial functioning (Brown et al. 2011). However, neuropathological residuals are probably present in *all* individuals who have sustained a significant head injury. Their injury-related effects will be expressed only later in life and only with the co-occurrence of yet unknown vulnerability factors or age itself. Additional candidate risk factors are other chronic illnesses such as diabetes and cerebrovascular disease, genetic predisposition (e.g., *APOE4*), additional head injuries, and other environmental factors, including drug and alcohol abuse. Mild TBI has been shown to be comorbid with the development of posttraumatic stress disorder (PTSD), and a very large U.S. Department of Veterans Affairs investigation found a nearly twofold higher risk of developing dementia in those veterans with a prior diagnosis of PTSD (Yaffe et al. 2010).

TBI as Risk Factor for Alzheimer Disease and Frontotemporal Dementia

Epidemiological studies have suggested that TBI is a risk factor for AD later in life (van den Heuvel et al. 2007). Other studies have reported no or limited association of prior head injury with AD (see review by Starkstein and Jorge [2005]).

Rao et al. (2010), in their population-based sample, did not observe higher rates of dementia in participants with predementia history of self-reported head injury, but those in the group with prior head injury were more likely to exhibit disinhibition.

A problem with research on this topic has been reliance on self-report of head injury. For that reason, Plassman et al. (2000) examined medical records of a cohort of military veterans to independently establish presence of head injury. The authors gauged head injury severity as follows: 1) mild injury=loss of consciousness (LOC) or PTA <30 minutes; 2) moderate injury=LOC or PTA >30 minutes but <24 hours and/or a skull fracture; and 3) severe injury=LOC or PTA >24 hours. There was a clear relationship to injury severity and later diagnosis of dementia, including AD.

Rosso et al. (2003), in a retrospective case-control study, observed that patients with sporadic frontotemporal dementia were more likely (odds ratio=3.3) than control subjects to have a history of head trauma.

Pathophysiological Link of TBI to Subsequent Dementia

Dementia pugilistica (punch-drunk syndrome) was the first clinical syndrome linking repetitive head trauma to development of dementia (Jordan 1992). Postmortem histopathological analysis of the brains of boxers showed neurofibrillary tangles and diffuse plaques of amyloid-β (Aβ) similar to lesions observed in AD (Tokuda et al. 1991), and neuroimaging studies have demonstrated widespread cerebral atrophy (Handratta et al. 2010). Graham et al. (1995) subsequently demonstrated that a single brain trauma from an automobile accident resulted in widespread deposition of Aβ, a metabolite of amyloid precursor protein (APP). APP is a membrane glycoprotein produced in the cytoplasm of all cells and in brain may play a role in cell adhesion and neuroprotection (LeBlanc et al. 1992). Accumulation of the APP metabolite Aβ in the neuritic plaques of AD is one of the potential links between prior TBI and subsequent development of AD (Lee et al. 2007; Nakagawa et al. 1999). Additionally, Aβ burden relates to integrity of memory function in normal and pathological states (Morgan 2005).

Diffuse axonal injury, a subset of TAI, is widespread but particularly evident in the corpus callosum, the central white matter of the cerebral hemispheres, and the pons (Xu et al. 2007), as well as the thalamus (Lifshitz et al. 2007). TAI occurs from primary axotomy associated with direct injury to the axon from shear-strain forces at the time of initial impact and from secondary injury effects, including ischemia, disrupted cytoarchitecture, associated metabolic injury, and wallerian degeneration. Thus, not only is the overall Aβ burden in the brain elevated following TBI, but the white matter structural damage from diffuse axonal injury can be widespread and nonspecific (Bigler et al. 2010), thereby disrupting the general connectivity of the brain. The loss of white matter connectivity probably has disruptive influences on cognitive reserve during the aging process, increasing the likelihood of dementia later in life for those who have experienced a significant TBI.

Alzheimer Pathology in Surgically Excised TBI Tissue

Increased levels of Aβ can be detected very shortly after brain injury, and Aβ deposition—along with a host of other acute neuropathological effects—induces inflammatory cytokine infiltrations with microglial activation and oxidative stress that relate to the ultimate effects of an acquired brain injury. These same factors are also considered important neuropathological antecedents in the development of AD (Butterfield et al. 2007). In an important histological study, Ikonomovic et al. (2004) examined excised tissue from persons who underwent neurosurgical intervention for treatment of severe TBI. They observed that extracellular Aβ deposits and other related degenerative changes occurred in the temporal lobe within 2 hours after injury. This association with AD-like degenerative changes that occur early in response to TBI gives considerable credence to a link between prior head injury and development of dementia later in life. Furthermore, Swartz et al. (2006) examined temporal lobe tissue specimens from 21 patients treated for posttraumatic epilepsy by partial temporal lobectomy and found that 94% of the specimens exhibited hippocampal neuronal loss. This finding underscores the vulnerability of the hippocampus and the likelihood that in the majority of patients with moderate to severe TBI, there will be some loss of hippocampal neurons.

Time Course of Atrophy in TBI

Progressive parenchymal volume loss in brain has been associated with normal aging (Blatter et al. 1995). In degenerative disorders, there is greater than expected atrophy for age. In such cases, degree of hippocampal and total brain volume (TBV) loss predicts crossing over to dementia (Ridha et al. 2007). More than a decade ago, Blatter et al. (1997) demonstrated that in TBI, normal age-related progression does not return to equilibrium until about 3 years postinjury and that there is, on average, a 50- to 100-cc TBV loss from moderate to severe TBI. However, 60%–90% of total volume changes in TBV occur within 6 months of injury. Blatter et al. assumed that this volume loss occurred because of TAI, apoptosis, reduced synaptic complexity, and so forth, during this recovery cycle. This conjecture has now been supported by animal studies of TBI, where progressive changes appear to represent the brain's attempts at neural repair and reintegration after injury. Animal studies have shown that active neuropathological changes can be detected during the postinjury year and even longer (Chen et al. 2004). If the TBI is complicated by hypoxic-ischemic injury, often related to compromised pulmonary/airway dysfunction or shock, then the progressive changes may be more severe than with TBI alone (Truettner et al. 2007).

As indicated above, moderate to severe TBI results in significant reduction in TBV, so an interesting heuristic can be developed, as shown in Figure 10–5. Absolute TBV values are not strongly predictive of TBI outcome because TBV relates to body, head size, and sex differences. To overcome this variability in using TBV as a metric of brain health, a ventricle-to-brain ratio (VBR) is used. VBR, as a metric of generalized cerebral atrophy, remains relatively stable until the sixth decade of life, when age-related changes begin to be detected. VBR has been extensively studied in the aging process as well as in TBI. The patient in Figure 10–4 had a severe TBI with marked generalized atrophic changes but did not meet clinical criteria for dementia; nonetheless, by superimposing the patient's VBR value and comparing it to normative values, it is obvious that the patient's VBR crosses the mean age-related VBR values for MCI and AD years before normally expected. Similar findings have been reported for hippocampal volume (Bigler 2007). In fact, whole brain and hippocampal volumetrics over time can be used to predict progression from asymptomatic, to symptomatic, to age-related MCI, and to clinical AD (Devanand et al. 2007). Also, Olesen et al. (2011) showed that greater amounts of cerebral atrophy at age 85, even in individuals who did not meet the criteria for dementia, were associated with decreased survival.

Repetitive Head Injuries

Animal models of repetitive head injury suggest that once the brain is injured, it becomes more susceptible to repeated injury and that repeated injuries have

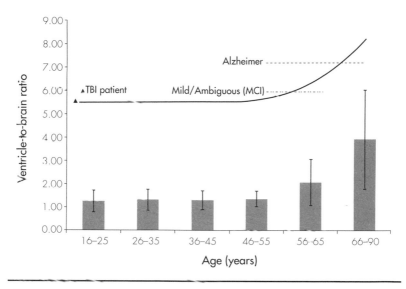

Figure 10–5.   Normative ventricle-to-brain ratio (VBR) values from ages 16 to 90.

VBR is stable over the first five decades of life but then increases with normal aging. Moderate to severe traumatic brain injury (TBI) results in significant elevations of VBR. The TBI patient presented in Figure 10–4 had a VBR of approximately 5.55, markedly above the normative value for his age *(see triangle on graph)*. The graph reflects the slope of VBR changes over age, with the starting point *(triangle)* being the patient's elevated VBR at age 15 when the imaging was performed. The horizontal lines reflect the VBR values for subjects with mild cognitive impairment (MCI) and Alzheimer disease in a large population-based study that calculated VBR in subjects age 65 or older (see Plassman et al. 2000). Using this simplistic heuristic, this young patient is already very near the degree of generalized cerebral atrophy found in patients with MCI and Alzheimer disease much later in life.

Source.   Adapted from Bigler 2007.

Reprinted from Bigler ED: "Traumatic Brain Injury," in *The American Psychiatric Publishing Textbook of Alzheimer Disease and Other Dementias.* Edited by Weiner MF, Lipton AM. Washington, DC, American Psychiatric Publishing, 2009, pp. 229–246. Copyright 2009, American Psychiatric Publishing. Used with permission.

a cumulative effect (Weber 2007). Postmortem studies of professional athletes with repetitive head injuries indicate a relationship between earlier injury, neuropsychiatric disorder, and dementia (Omalu et al. 2006), which is now termed *chronic traumatic encephalopathy* (Omalu et al. 2011). Similarly, high-field MRI studies demonstrate microstructural abnormalities that clearly indicate that subtle neuropathological changes occur in the brains of boxers, even those who do not meet clinical criteria for concussion (Zhang et al. 2006). Likewise, cerebrospinal fluid markers of neuronal injury are seen in boxers (Zetterberg et al. 2006).

Although no large-scale epidemiological studies have been reported at this time, considerable anecdotal information implicates head injury, including repetitive head injuries, as a trigger initiating a cascade of changes that ultimately lead to dementia (Leung et al. 2006). In the short term, however, repeated sports concussions may not always have a detectable cumulative effect. A study by De Beaumont et al. (2007) is most interesting in this regard. They examined college athletes with histories of single or multiple concussions using a visual evoked-response paradigm (oddball visual search), specifically measuring the third positive wave component (P3), and found that those who had sustained multiple concussions had significant amplitude suppression. What is particularly important about this observation is that the multiply concussed and singly concussed athletes did *not* differ on neuropsychological measures. This study supports the notion that repeated concussive head injury, even in those who are asymptomatic, may nonetheless alter neural functioning in the athlete.

Conclusion

Moderate to severe TBI can result in dementia, but the more common result of TBI is cognitive disorder NOS, with residual cognitive impairments that place an individual at increased risk for accelerated cognitive decline. Additionally, TBI has pathological features in common with those associated with aging and degenerative disease, creating a circumstance in which aging, genetics, environmental factors, and other health-related factors may interact with head injury to increase the risk of dementia later in life. These latter effects may even occur in those who appeared to fully recover from a brain injury.

Key Clinical Points

- Moderate to severe traumatic brain injury (TBI) can cause a dementia syndrome.

- Dementia due to head trauma earlier in life is typically nonprogressive but may progress in late life because of interaction with normal aging and other factors.

- The proximal cause of dementia due to head trauma is a combination of diffuse injury and more specific pathological changes in frontotemporal and limbic structures.

- There is neuropathological overlap, including presence of amyloid-β, associated with TBI and age-related degenerative disorders.

- Head injury is a risk factor for dementia later in life that is dependent on the expression of other vulnerability factors.

References

Adams JH, Jennett B, Murray LS, et al: Neuropathological findings in disabled survivors of a head injury. J Neurotrauma 28:701–709, 2011 [Epub ahead of print]

American Psychiatric Association: Diagnostic and Statistical Manual of Mental Disorders, 4th Edition, Text Revision. Washington, DC, American Psychiatric Association, 2000

Ben-David BM, Nguyen LL, van Lieshout PH, et al: Stroop effects in persons with traumatic brain injury: selective attention, speed of processing, or color-naming? A meta-analysis. J Int Neuropsychol Soc 17:354–363, 2011

Bigler ED: Traumatic brain injury and cognitive reserve, in Cognitive Reserve: Theory and Applications. Edited by Stern Y. New York, Taylor & Francis Group, 2007, pp 85–116

Bigler ED: Structural imaging, in Textbook of Traumatic Brain Injury, 2nd Edition. Edited by Silver JM, Yudofsky SC, McAllister TW. Washington, DC, American Psychiatric Publishing, 2011, pp 73–90

Bigler ED, Ryser DK, Gandhi P, et al: Day-of-injury computerized tomography, rehabilitation status, and development of cerebral atrophy in persons with traumatic brain injury. Am J Phys Med Rehabil 85:793–806, 2006

Bigler ED, Abildskov TJ, Wilde EA, et al: Diffuse damage in pediatric traumatic brain injury: a comparison of automated versus operator-controlled quantification methods. Neuroimage 50:1017–1026, 2010

Blatter DD, Bigler ED, Gale SD, et al: Quantitative volumetric analysis of brain MR: normative database spanning 5 decades of life. AJNR Am J Neuroradiol 16:241–251, 1995

Blatter DD, Bigler ED, Gale SD, et al: MR-based brain and cerebrospinal fluid measurement after traumatic brain injury: correlation with neuropsychological outcome. AJNR Am J Neuroradiol 18:1–10, 1997

Blennow K, de Leon MJ, Zetterberg H: Alzheimer's disease. Lancet 368:387–403, 2006

Brown AW, Moessner AM, Mandreker JN, et al: A survey of very-long-term outcomes after traumatic brain injury among members of a population-based incident cohort. J Neurotrauma 28:167–176, 2011

Burns JM, Church JA, Johnson DK, et al: White matter lesions are prevalent but differentially related with cognition in aging and early Alzheimer disease. Arch Neurol 62:1870–1876, 2005

Butterfield DA, Reed T, Newman SF, et al: Roles of amyloid beta-peptide–associated oxidative stress and brain protein modifications in the pathogenesis of Alzheimer's disease and mild cognitive impairment. Free Radic Biol Med 43:658–677, 2007

Chen XH, Siman R, Iwata A, et al: Long-term accumulation of amyloid-beta, beta-secretase, presenilin-1, and caspase-3 in damaged axons following brain trauma. Am J Pathol 165:357–371, 2004

Cullum CM, Bigler ED: Ventricle size, cortical atrophy and the relationship with neuropsychological status in closed head injury: a quantitative analysis. J Clin Exp Neuropsychol 8:437–452, 1986

De Beaumont L, Brisson B, Lassonde M, et al: Long-term electrophysiological changes in athletes with a history of multiple concussions. Brain Inj 21:631–644, 2007

DeKosky ST, Ikonomovic MD, Gandy S: Traumatic brain injury: football, warfare, and long-term effects. N Engl J Med 363:1293–1296, 2010

Devanand DP, Pradhaban G, Liu X, et al: Hippocampal and entorhinal atrophy in mild cognitive impairment: prediction of Alzheimer disease. Neurology 68:828–836, 2007

Floyd CL, Lyeth BG: Astroglia: important mediators of traumatic brain injury. Prog Brain Res 161:61–79, 2007

Gavett BE, Stern RA, Cantu RC, et al: Mild traumatic brain injury: a risk factor for neurodegeneration (editorial). Alzheimers Res Ther 2:18, 2010

Geddes DM, LaPlaca MC, Cargill RS Jr: Susceptibility of hippocampal neurons to mechanically induced injury. Exp Neurol 184:420–427, 2003

Graham DI, Gentleman SM, Lynch A, et al: Distribution of beta-amyloid protein in the brain following severe head injury. Neuropathol Appl Neurobiol 21:27–34, 1995

Han SD, Drake AI, Cessante LM, et al: APOE and TBI in a military population: evidence of a neuropsychological compensatory mechanism? J Neurol Neurosurg Psychiatry 78:1103–1108, 2007

Handratta V, Hsu E, Vento J, et al: Neuroimaging findings and brain-behavioral correlates in a former boxer with chronic traumatic brain injury. Neurocase 16:125–134, 2010

Himanen L, Portin R, Isoniemi H, et al: Longitudinal cognitive changes in traumatic brain injury: a 30-year follow-up study. Neurology 66:187–192, 2006

Hinkebein JH, Martin TA, Callahan CD, et al: Traumatic brain injury and Alzheimer's: deficit profile similarities and the impact of normal ageing. Brain Inj 17:1035–1042, 2003

Holsinger T, Steffens DC, Phillips C, et al: Head injury in early adulthood and the lifetime risk of depression. Arch Gen Psychiatry 59:17–22, 2002

Holsinger T, Deveau J, Boustani M, et al: Does this patient have dementia? JAMA 297:2391–2404, 2007

Ikonomovic MD, Uryu K, Abrahamson EE, et al: Alzheimer's pathology in human temporal cortex surgically excised after severe brain injury. Exp Neurol 190:192–203, 2004

Jordan B: Medical Aspects of Boxing. Boca Raton, FL, CRC Press, 1992

Jorge RE, Acion L, Starkstein SE, et al: Hippocampal volume and mood disorders after traumatic brain injury. Biol Psychiatry 62:332–338, 2007

Kim KW, Park JH, Kim MH, et al: A nationwide survey on the prevalence of dementia and mild cognitive impairment in South Korea. J Alzheimers Dis 23:281–291, 2011

Laplaca MC, Simon CM, Prado GR, et al: CNS injury biomechanics and experimental models. Prog Brain Res 161:13–26, 2007

LeBlanc AC, Kovacs DM, Chen HY, et al: Role of amyloid precursor protein (APP): study with antisense transfection of human neuroblastoma cells. J Neurosci Res 31:635–645, 1992

Lee BK, Glass TA, McAtee MJ, et al: Associations of salivary cortisol with cognitive function in the Baltimore memory study. Arch Gen Psychiatry 64:810–818, 2007

Leung FH, Thompson K, Weaver DF, et al: Evaluating spousal abuse as a potential risk factor for Alzheimer's disease: rationale, needs and challenges. Neuroepidemiology 27:13–16, 2006

Lezak MD, Howieson DB, Loring DW: Neuropsychological Assessment. New York, Oxford University Press, 2004

Lifshitz J, Kelley BJ, Povlishock JT, et al: Perisomatic thalamic axotomy after diffuse traumatic brain injury is associated with atrophy rather than cell death. J Neuropathol Exp Neurol 66:218–229, 2007

Loane DJ, Byrnes KR: Role of microglia in neurotrauma. Neurotherapeutics 7:366–377, 2010

Lorentz WJ, Scanlan JM, Borson S, et al: Brief screening tests for dementia. Can J Psychiatry 47:723–733, 2002

Mayeux R, Ottman R, Maestre G, et al: Synergistic effects of traumatic head injury and apolipoprotein-epsilon 4 in patients with Alzheimer's disease. Neurology 45:555–557, 1995

Metting Z, Rödiger LA, De Keyser J, et al: Structural and functional neuroimaging in mild-to-moderate head injury. Lancet Neurol 6:699–710, 2007

Morgan D: Mechanisms of A beta plaque clearance following passive A beta immunization. Neurodegener Dis 2:261–266, 2005

Morgan D: Amyloid, memory and neurogenesis. Exp Neurol 205:330–335, 2007

Nakagawa Y, Nakamura M, McIntosh TK, et al: Traumatic brain injury in young, amyloid-beta peptide overexpressing transgenic mice induces marked ipsilateral hippocampal atrophy and diminished Abeta deposition during aging. J Comp Neurol 411:390–398, 1999

Olesen PJ, Guo X, Gustafson D, et al: A population-based study on the influence of brain atrophy on 20-year survival after age 85. Neurology 76:879–886, 2011

Omalu BI, DeKosky ST, Hamilton RL, et al: Chronic traumatic encephalopathy in a National Football League player, part II. Neurosurgery 59:1086–1092; discussion 1092–1093, 2006

Omalu B, Bailes J, Hamilton RL, et al: Emerging histomorphologic phenotypes of chronic traumatic encephalopathy in American athletes. Neurosurgery 69:173–183, 2011 [Epub ahead of print]

Petrov T, Rafols JA: Acute alterations of endothelin-1 and iNOS expression and control of the brain microcirculation after head trauma. Neurol Res 23:139–143, 2001

Pineda JA, Lewis SB, Valadka AB, et al: Clinical significance of alphaII-spectrin breakdown products in cerebrospinal fluid after severe traumatic brain injury. J Neurotrauma 24:354–366, 2007

Plassman BL, Havlik RJ, Steffens DC, et al: Documented head injury in early adulthood and risk of Alzheimer's disease and other dementias. Neurology 55:1158–1166, 2000

Rao V, Lyketsos CG: Psychiatric aspects of traumatic brain injury. Psychiatr Clin North Am 25:43–69, 2002

Rao V, Rosenberg P, Miles QS, et al: Neuropsychiatric symptoms in dementia patients with and without a history of traumatic brain injury. J Neuropsychiatry Clin Neurosci 22:166–172, 2010

Ridha BH, Barnes J, van de Pol LA, et al: Application of Automated Medial Temporal Lobe Atrophy Scale to Alzheimer disease. Arch Neurol 64:849–854, 2007

Rosso SM, Landweer EJ, Houterman M, et al: Medical and environmental risk factors for sporadic frontotemporal dementia: a retrospective case-control study. J Neurol Neurosurg Psychiatry 74:1574–1576, 2003

Salmond CH, Chatfield DA, Menon DK, et al: Cognitive sequelae of head injury: involvement of basal forebrain and associated structures. Brain 128:189–200, 2005

Starkstein SE, Jorge R: Dementia after traumatic brain injury. Int Psychogeriatr 17 (suppl 1): S93–S107, 2005

Swartz BE, Houser CR, Tomiyasu U, et al: Hippocampal cell loss in posttraumatic human epilepsy. Epilepsia 47:1373–1382, 2006

Taber KH, Hurley RA: Traumatic axonal injury: atlas of major pathways. J Neuropsychiatry Clin Neurosci 19:iv–104, 2007

Thurman DJ, Coronado V, Selassie A: The epidemiology of TBI: implications for public health, in Brain Injury Medicine. Edited by Zasler ND, Katz DI, Zafonte RD. New York, Demos Medical, 2007, pp 45–55

Tokuda T, Ikeda S, Yanagisawa N, et al: Re-examination of ex-boxers' brains using immunohistochemistry with antibodies to amyloid beta-protein and tau protein. Acta Neuropathol 82:280–285, 1991

Truettner JS, Hu B, Alonso OF, et al: Subcellular stress response after traumatic brain injury. J Neurotrauma 24:599–612, 2007

Ueda Y, Walker SA, Povlishock JT, et al: Perivascular nerve damage in the cerebral circulation following traumatic brain injury. Acta Neuropathol 112:85–94, 2006

van den Heuvel C, Thornton E, Vink R: Traumatic brain injury and Alzheimer's disease: a review. Prog Brain Res 161:303–316, 2007

Vannorsdall TD, Cascella NG, Rao V, et al: A morphometric analysis of neuroanatomic abnormalities in traumatic brain injury. J Neuropsychiatry Clin Neurosci 22:173–181, 2010

Verghese PB, Castellano JM, Holtzman DM: Apolipoprotein E in Alzheimer's disease and other neurological disorders. Lancet Neurol 10:241–252, 2011

Weber JT: Experimental models of repetitive brain injuries. Prog Brain Res 161:253–261, 2007

Wilde EA, Hunter JV, Newsome MR, et al: Frontal and temporal morphometric findings on MRI in children after moderate to severe traumatic brain injury. J Neurotrauma 22:333–344, 2005

Wilde EA, Bigler ED, Pedroza C, et al: Post-traumatic amnesia predicts long-term cerebral atrophy in traumatic brain injury. Brain Inj 20:695–699, 2006

Wilde EA, Bigler ED, Hunter JV, et al: Hippocampus, amygdala, and basal ganglia morphometrics in children after moderate-to-severe traumatic brain injury. Dev Med Child Neurol 49:294–299, 2007

Wolkowitz OM, Lupien SJ, Bigler ED: The "steroid dementia syndrome": a possible model of human glucocorticoid neurotoxicity. Neurocase 13:189–200, 2007

Wood RL, Rutterford NA: Long-term effect of head trauma on intellectual abilities: a 16-year outcome study. J Neurol Neurosurg Psychiatry 77:1180–1184, 2006

Xu J, Rasmussen IA, Lagopoulos J, et al: Diffuse axonal injury in severe traumatic brain injury visualized using high-resolution diffusion tensor imaging. J Neurotrauma 24:753–765, 2007

Yaffe K, Vittinghoff E, Lindquist K, et al: Posttraumatic stress disorder and risk of dementia among U.S. veterans. Arch Gen Psychiatry 67:608–613, 2010

Zetterberg H, Hietala MA, Jonsson M, et al: Neurochemical aftermath of amateur boxing. Arch Neurol 63:1277–1280, 2006

Zhang L, Heier LA, Zimmerman RD, et al: Diffusion anisotropy changes in the brains of professional boxers. AJNR Am J Neuroradiol 27:2000–2004, 2006

Further Reading

Arciniegas DB, Vanderploeg R, Zasler ND, et al: Management of Traumatic Brain Injury. Washington, DC, American Psychiatric Publishing, 2013

Ashley MJ (ed): Traumatic Brain Injury: Rehabilitation, Treatment, and Case Management, 3rd Edition. Boca Raton, FL, CRC Press, 2010

Silver JM, McAllister TW, Yudofsky SC: Textbook of Traumatic Brain Injury, 2nd Edition. Washington, DC, American Psychiatric Publishing, 2011

11

Other Causes of Dementia

Edward Y. Zamrini, M.D.

Mary Quiceno, M.D.

The focus of this chapter is uncommon causes of dementia. The most common causes of dementia—Alzheimer disease, stroke, synucleinopathies, tauopathies, and traumatic brain injury—have been described in preceding chapters. Other dementias, as they are referred to here, account for less than 15% of cases (Larson et al. 1984). They can be divided into four categories: 1) diseases primarily affecting the central nervous system (CNS), 2) diseases primarily affecting organs outside the CNS, 3) diseases caused by exposure to substances (toxins), and 4) diseases due to deficiency of essential substances (e.g., vitamins). Many of these conditions are arrestable or at least partly reversible, particularly if detected and managed early. Although the other dementias are subdivided into distinct etiologies here, many patients have more than one cause of cognitive impairment.

Diseases Primarily Affecting the Central Nervous System

Autoimmune Disorder: Multiple Sclerosis

Multiple sclerosis (MS) can cause both physical and mental disability. The triggers are unknown, but there may be a genetic predisposition. At least half of persons afflicted by MS will become cognitively impaired (Bobholz and Rao 2003).

Cognitive profiles and the severity of cognitive deficits vary depending on the subtype of MS. Huijbregts et al. (2004) found that the most severe cognitive deficits occurred in subjects with secondary progressive MS and the least severe in people with relapsing-remitting MS. Cognitive impairment may occur within 24 months of diagnosis (Schulz et al. 2006) and may herald a poor prognosis (Deloire et al. 2010).

The most common cognitive impairments in MS are slowed information processing and impaired visual learning and memory. Problems with attention, executive functioning, and long-term memory also occur, but language typically is preserved.

Memory impairment is found in up to 60% of patients with MS (Brassington and Marsh 1998). Compared with control subjects, patients with MS tend to need more time to learn a set of given information and are more susceptible to interference (Chiaravalloti and DeLuca 2008). Recognition is usually intact. Executive dysfunction may be seen in one-third of patients, and visuospatial difficulties of some form, such as facial recognition or visual organization problems, may be experienced by up to one-fifth of patients (Feinstein 2007).

Assessments must be done for depression, fatigue, and sedating medications, any of which can contribute to cognitive impairment. Cognitive screening at least annually should be considered. Screening instruments include the Multiple Sclerosis Neuropsychological Screening Questionnaire, a short, sensitive, specific, and self-administered instrument (Benedict et al. 2004), and the Minimal Assessment of Cognitive Function in Multiple Sclerosis, a battery of seven tests that takes approximately 90 minutes (Benedict et al. 2002).

Direct correlations between MS plaque location, lesion burden, and cognitive deficits are difficult to make. Sperling et al. (2001) found a relationship between frontoparietal white matter lesion load and cognitive performance on attentional tasks. They also confirmed an association between total lesion burden and cognitive performance, but the strongest associations were seen with regional lesion burden in the frontal and parietal lobes (Figure 11–1). Central atrophy, as estimated by third ventricle size, and corpus callosum atrophy are associated with neuropsychological deficits (Filippi et al. 2010).

Amato et al. (2006) summarized the results from trials of interferon beta-1b, interferon beta-1a, and glatiramer acetate on cognitive decline. In two small trials of interferon beta-1b, cognitive improvement was demonstrated. Patients from the original cohort in the interferon beta-1a trial were followed over 2 years, and the treatment group did better on all measures of cognition tested. None of the subjects in either the treated or the control group in the Phase III trial of glatiramer acetate showed cognitive decline after 2 years. Natalizumab may reduce the risk of cognitive worsening, but long-term studies are needed. It is not known if agents for fatigue, such as amantadine, 4-aminopyridine, and modafinil, improve cognition. Donepezil has been studied in a number of trials, but a recent large trial failed to show a benefit (Krupp et al. 2010). Memantine is not helpful and may worsen fatigue and neuropsychiatric symptoms (Lovera 2010).

Genetic Disorders

Huntington Disease

Huntington disease is a progressive autosomal dominant neurodegenerative disease characterized by a hyperkinetic movement disorder and changes involving cognition and personality. Prevalence of the disease is 4–8 cases per 100,000 population, but five times as many individuals are at 50:50 risk of having inherited the genetic predisposition (Harper 1992). Most patients present in their fourth or fifth decades, although the range of onset can vary from juvenile to over age 65.

Huntington disease is due to the expansion of a trinucleotide repeat mutation of cytosine-adenine-guanine $(CAG)_n$ in the IT-15 gene on chromosome 4p16.3 encoding the protein huntingtin (Huntington's Disease Collaborative Research Group 1993). The length of the CAG trinucleotide repeat mutation is inversely related to age at disease onset, accounting for at least 50% of the variance in onset age, but can be modified by genetic factors in addition to the huntingtin gene (Duyao et al. 1993; Wexler et al. 2004).

Usually, a patient with Huntington disease has an affected parent, although spontaneous mutations may occur. In addition to choreic, hyperkinetic movements, dystonia and apraxia may be present. Walking may elicit the chorea in more subtle cases. Later, gait may become ataxic or dancelike. Orolingual apraxia is common. Parkinsonian features include decreased arm swing, bradykinesia, and dystonia. In the Westphal variant, more frequent in juvenile-onset disease, patients are hypokinetic and rigid. Cognitive and personality changes may precede the movement disorder; these may include obsessive and compulsive symptoms.

Patients and at-risk individuals can be tested for the triple CAG polymorphism. A polymorphism number greater than 39 is definitive evidence of the disease. The disease may occur late or may not occur if there are 36–39 repeats. About 1% of patients suspected to have Huntington disease do not have $(CAG)_n$ expansion but have phenocopy syndromes (chorea, psychiatric and cognitive decline). These patients may have spinocerebellar atrophy type 17, Huntington disease–like syndrome 2, familial prion disease, or Friedreich ataxia, among others. Computed tomography (CT) or magnetic resonance imaging (MRI) may show caudate atrophy, whereas ^{18}F-labeled fluorodeoxyglucose positron emission tomography (FDG-PET) scanning can demonstrate striatal hypometabolism early on.

Treatment of Huntington disease is symptomatic and palliative. In-depth information on management is provided in a physician's guide available through the Huntington's Disease Society of America (Nance et al. 2011). It is important to attend to weight, because these patients may use up to 5,000 kcal per day and weight is inversely related to the amount of dyskinesias. Weighted wristbands can reduce the amplitude of dyskinesias. Speech therapy can improve communication and reduce risk of aspiration. Exercises and special equipment can improve mobility and comfort. Dopamine antagonists are the mainstay of drug treatment for the dyskinesias. Common side effects include drowsiness, parkinsonism (an age-associated effect), depression, and akathisia. Potentially neuroprotective therapies include the antibiotic minocycline, which is well tolerated at 100 mg bid. Other potentially neuroprotective therapies are glutamate release inhibitors (riluzole), glutamate receptor blockers (amantadine, memantine, lamotrigine), tetrabenazine, ubiquinone, creatine, ethyl eicosapentaenoic acid, and phenylbutyrate (Reynolds 2007). Genetic counseling and presymptomatic testing of at-risk relatives should be considered part of the management. Affected

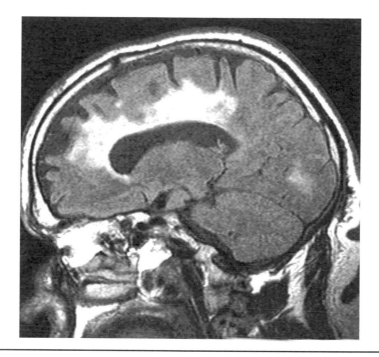

Figure 11–1.   Sagittal fluid-attenuated inversion recovery (FLAIR) magnetic resonance image demonstrating significant periventricular white matter hyperintensity oriented perpendicular to the long axis of the lateral ventricle and extending through the deep white matter into subcortical areas. There is also greater than expected sulcal widening consistent with mild atrophy.
Source.   Reprinted from Zamrini E, Quiceno M: "Other Causes of Dementia," in *The American Psychiatric Publishing Textbook of Alzheimer Disease and Other Dementias.* Edited by Weiner MF, Lipton AM. Washington, DC, American Psychiatric Publishing, 2009, pp. 247–262. Copyright 2009, American Psychiatric Publishing. Used with permission.

individuals are at high risk for suicide. Death occurs 10–20 years after onset from swallowing or breathing difficulties and their consequences.

Wilson Disease

Wilson disease (hepatolenticular degeneration) is an autosomal recessive disorder of copper metabolism. The disease may manifest between ages 6 and 60 years but affects most individuals in the first two decades of life. Excess copper deposition results from the dysfunction of a copper-transporting adenosine-triphosphatase (ATPase) encoded on chromosome 13. The process of copper transport into ceruloplasmin and subsequent excretion into bile is disrupted. Copper accumulates in and damages the liver, the basal ganglia of the brain, the kidneys, the cornea, and other tissues by inducing free-radical reactions and lipid peroxidation. More than 200 mutations of the Wilson disease gene have been detected.

Family history is often negative because carriers do not manifest the disease. The disease may have different presentations even in the same family. Positive family history is noted in 47% and consanguinity in 54% of cases (Taly et al. 2007). Presentations can include dystonia and the characteristic risus sardonicus, a facial dystonia mimicking a sardonic smile, which result from striatal deposition of copper. Vertical eye movements, in particular vertical pursuits, are impaired. Electro-oculographic abnormalities can be found in patients who do not yet exhibit lesions on MRI (Ingster-Moati et al. 2007). Other presentations include encephalopathy secondary to metabolic problems, steatosis, cirrhosis, jaundice, and occasionally fulminant liver failure, kidney failure, or hemolytic anemia. Characteristic Kayser-Fleischer rings around the cornea are present in 100% of neurological patients, 86% of hepatic patients, and 59% of presymptomatic patients. In one series, predominant neurological features were as follows: parkinsonism, 62.3%; dystonia, 35.4%; cerebellar abnormalities, 28%; pyramidal signs, 16%; chorea, 9%; athetosis, 2.2%; myoclonus, 3.4%; and behavioral abnormalities, 16% (Taly et al. 2007). Behavioral manifestations include disorders of mood, behavior, and personality, and may include psychosis. Psychiatric symptoms occur during the early phase in approximately 50% of patients (Wichowicz et al. 2006). High levels of copper are found in blood, urine, and the liver; serum ceruloplasmin is low. Because of the high number of mutations, genetic testing is not practical. CT or MRI shows diffuse cerebral atrophy. The most common initial MRI abnormality among patients with Wilson disease is high T_1 signal intensity in the globus pallidus, putamen, and mesencephalon in association with hepatic dysfunction or high T_2 signal intensity in the striatum among patients with neurological symptoms. Treatment involves the use of metal chelators such as *d*-penicillamine or zinc sulfate.

Choreoacanthocytosis

Choreoacanthocytosis is a rare autosomal recessive disorder that is due to a frameshift mutation on chromosome 9q21 encoding chorein (Ueno et al. 2001). It is manifested by chorea, dystonia and tics, psychiatric symptoms, and cognitive decline.

Clinical features that distinguish it from Huntington disease are orofacial dystonia with tongue protrusion and biting of the tongue and lips. Additional features include seizures, distal amyotrophy, and neuropathy. Laboratory findings include characteristic red cell acanthocytes on peripheral blood smears and elevated serum creatine kinase.

Porphyria

The porphyrias are a group of inherited or acquired disorders of metabolism of the heme biosynthesis pathway. Each of the eight reactions in this pathway is catalyzed by a specific enzyme. The two major subtypes are hepatic and erythropoietic, depending on whether the metabolic step occurs in the liver or the bone marrow. The principal cause of CNS abnormalities is intermittent acute porphyria, which is often asymptomatic but may result in motor peripheral neuropathy, optic nerve atrophy, seizures, delirium, and coma. Porphyrias can cause a posterior leukoencephalopathy syndrome and cortical blindness. Porphyric encephalopathy is typically acute and intermittent. Neuroimaging may reveal multiple large contrast-enhancing subcortical white matter lesions, which regress with glucose and hematin infusions. Diagnostic tests depend on the suspected subtype of porphyria. Plasma fluorescence scanning can detect porphyrins in blood. Quantitative chromatography can detect and measure porphyrins in urine, stool, or serum. Enzyme assay of the heme synthetic pathway is particularly useful in acute intermittent porphyria. There is no consensus on treatment of the porphyrias, but many drugs are unsafe in persons with porphyria; these include hormonal contraceptives, local and general anesthetics, and anticonvulsants.

Neurodegeneration With Accumulation

Formerly known as Hallervorden-Spatz syndrome, neurodegeneration with brain iron accumulation is actually a heterogeneous group of disorders with different treatments. Common clinical manifestations are motor symptoms such as dystonia or parkinsonism, mental deterioration, retinitis pigmentosa, and iron accumulation in the brain. The differential diagnosis includes pantothenate kinase–associated neurodegeneration, an autosomal recessive disorder involving mutations in the pantothenate kinase 2 gene on chromosome 20p13, corticobasal degeneration, progressive supranuclear palsy, Parkinson disease, multiple system atrophy, giant axonal neuropathy, neuroaxonal dystrophy, Guam dementia, and HARP (hypoprebetalipoproteinemia, acanthocytosis, retinitis pigmentosa, and pallidal degeneration) syndrome (Zhou et al. 2001). Neuroimaging with MRI shows prominent T_1 signal hyperintensity in addition to the "eye of the tiger" sign on T_2 in the globus pallidus bilaterally. Susceptibility-weighted imaging, fast low-angle shot, and BOLD (blood oxygen level–dependent) MRI techniques demonstrate mineral deposition in the globi pallidi better than conventional imaging does.

Idiopathic Basal Ganglia Calcification

Idiopathic basal ganglia calcification is a rare autosomal dominant neurodegenerative disease. Clinical features include parkinsonism, cognitive decline, and psychosis (Le Ber et al. 2007).

Mitochondrial Multisystem Disorders

A large number of mitochondrial disorders can produce neurological symptoms (muscle-specific symptoms, vision problems, or hearing deficits) and cognitive symptoms. Cerebral autosomal dominant arteriopathy with subcortical infarcts and leukoencephalopathy (CADASIL) can produce multiple small cerebral infarcts resulting in dementia (see Figure 4–11 in Chapter 4, "Neuroimaging"). MRI reveals diffuse white matter disease (leukoaraiosis) and lacunar infarcts in nonhypertensive patients. Neuropsychological testing can reveal frontal-subcortical dysfunction. CADASIL can be challenging to diagnose because of the wide range of mutations that can cause disease, but an immunohistochemical technique using a skin biopsy appears to be highly sensitive and specific. Granular osmophilic material within the basement membrane of vascular smooth muscle cells demonstrated on electron microscopy is pathognomonic (Ishiko et al. 2005).

In a landmark Icelandic study, linkage was established between stroke and a locus on chromosome 5q12 designated STRK1 (Meschia and Worrall 2004). The pathology is believed to be secondary to gradual destruction of vascular smooth muscle cells of arterioles, leading to progressive wall thickening and fibrosis and luminal narrowing. Resultant lacunar infarcts have a predilection for the basal ganglia and frontotemporal white matter.

Mitochondrial encephalomyopathy, lactic acidosis, and strokelike episodes (MELAS) can produce similar symptoms, absent infarcts.

Neuronal Ceroid-Lipofuscinosis

Neuronal ceroid-lipofuscinosis is an autosomal recessive lysosomal storage disorder that can affect people at different ages. Clinical characteristics include seizures, progressive loss of vision, and loss of cognitive and motor functions, leading to premature demise. The juvenile form (often called Batten disease or Spielmeyer-Vogt-Sjögren-Batten disease) is caused by mutations of the ceroid-lipofuscinosis, neuronal 3 gene *(CLN3),* which encodes a hydrophobic transmembrane protein (Rakheja et al. 2007).

Leukodystrophies

Leukodystrophies are a group of degenerative diseases that primarily involve disturbances in the synthesis or catabolism of myelin. Metachromatic leukodystrophy results from a disorder of catabolism of sulfatides, Krabbe disease results from a disorder of catabolism of galactocerebrosides, and Pelizaeus-Merzbacher disease results from abnormal synthesis of proteolipid protein. In Canavan disease, there is accumulation of *N*-acetylaspartic acid. Common clinical features include neurological deterioration following a period of normal development; predominant involvement of motor function, at least initially; and absence of convulsions or myoclonus. MRI shows changes in density or signal from central white matter (Aicardi 1993). Treatment is symptomatic.

X-linked adrenoleukodystrophy is an X-linked peroxisomal disease associated with accumulation of very long chain fatty acids in different tissues. Many carriers are asymptomatic. Clinical manifestations in symptomatic patients include signs of progressive brain and peripheral demyelination and adrenal cortical insufficiency (Sutovsky et al. 2007).

Disorder With Unknown Etiology: Normal-Pressure Hydrocephalus

The prevalence of normal-pressure hydrocephalus (NPH) is unknown, but NPH is rare at best. The classical clinical diagnostic triad involves gait disturbance, incontinence, and cognitive impairment in temporal sequence. Unfortunately, this triad is seen in a number of neurodegenerative disorders, including some presentations of frontotemporal dementia, multiple system atrophy, Parkinson disease, and dementia with Lewy bodies. These diseases may also share ventricular enlargement disproportionate to the level of cortical atrophy or sulcal enlargement noted on neuroimaging. Other contributing MRI findings include periventricular hyperintensity consistent with transependymal flow of cerebrospinal fluid (CSF), prominent flow void in the aqueduct and third ventricle (jet sign), rounding of the frontal horns, and elevation of the corpus callosum. Significant improvement in gait immediately after high volume (30-cc) lumbar puncture is strongly suggestive. The best method for diagnosis is intraventricular pressure monitoring.

NPH has two major categories: idiopathic NPH and secondary NPH. The latest guidelines recommend that idiopathic NPH be classified into probable, possible, and unlikely categories based on history, imaging, and clinical criteria (Relkin et al. 2005). Treatment involves implantation of a ventricular shunt to the peritoneum or the atrium, but shunt complications occur in up to 40% of cases. In cases of cognitive impairment or with concomitant cerebrovascular disease, prognosis for cognitive recovery after shunting is poor.

Infections of the Central Nervous System

Encephalitis

Most cases of encephalitis do not have an identifiable etiology. Only 16% of 1,570 cases studied between 1998 and 2005 had identifiable causes: viral (in 69% of these cases), bacterial (20%), prion (7%), parasitic (3%), and fungal (1%). An additional 13% of cases had a suspected etiology, 8% were noninfectious, and the remaining 63% were unidentified (Glaser et al. 2006).

The herpes zoster virus rarely produces encephalitis. Herpes simplex virus encephalitis causes acute fever and altered behavior. Because this infection may produce lasting neurocognitive deficits, early recognition and management are very important. The virus has a predilection for the limbic system. Neuropsychiatric manifestations include anterograde amnesia, retrograde amnesia (Damasio et al. 1985), and various kinds of aphasia. MRI reveals increased T_2/fluid-attenuated inversion recovery (FLAIR) signal in the limbic areas (Figure 11–2). Diagnosis is by detection of virus in CSF. For patients with untreated herpetic encephalitis, morbidity and mortality are high. Therapy is acyclovir 30 mg/kg per day.

Subacute sclerosing panencephalitis is a delayed manifestation of measles. It typically occurs 7–10 years after infection. Patients present with cognitive decline, behavioral changes, headache, myoclonic jerks, and possibly seizures. CSF has inflammatory features and a high immunoglobulin G (IgG) level. There is no definitive treatment, but intrathecal interferon alpha-2 with or without an antiviral immunomodulatory agent has been used.

Prion diseases are fatal neurodegenerative disorders responsible for transmissible spongiform encephalopathies in animals and humans. The normal cellular form of encoded prion protein (PrP^C) undergoes a conformational change to an abnormal isoform, PrP^{Sc}. In humans, this conversion can result in Creutzfeldt-Jakob disease (CJD), Gerstmann-Sträussler-Scheinker disease, fatal or sporadic familial insomnia, or kuru. Most cases are sporadic, although about 15% are inherited and associated with mutations in the PrP gene, and a minority of cases are acquired through exposure to infected material. The latter group includes iatrogenic CJD, kuru, and variant CJD in humans.

Prion diseases occur at a rate of about 1 per million per year, with predilection for ages 55–65 years. Variant CJD tends to affect young individuals, averaging age 27 years. Incubation periods are long (years), but survival from first symptom is brief: 6 months for sporadic CJD and 15 months for variant CJD. Most cases occur in homozygotes at codon 129 of the PRNP (prion protein) gene, where either methionine or valine may be encoded. They include a large number of mutations and a wide spectrum of clinical and histopathological phenotypes. Dementia, ataxia, and psychiatric symptoms are present in all cases, and extrapyramidal symptoms are evident in 88% of patients. Increased T_2-weighted MRI signal is seen in the basal ganglia in 90% and in the thalamus in 88% of cases. CSF tau protein is elevated in 83%, and 14-3-3 protein is positive in 76%. Diagnosis can be difficult and requires brain tissue for definite confirmation. The typical picture is one of rapidly progressive cognitive decline and behavioral change, often accompanied with gait disturbance and myoclonic jerks. However, up to two-thirds of patients may present with atypical features such as fatigue and wasting; focal neurological symptoms suggesting stroke; wasting and fasciculations suggesting amyotrophic lateral sclerosis; or features that mimic other neurological syndromes. Clinical variants include occipital, ataxic, extrapyramidal, amyotrophic, frontopyramidal, and panencephalopathic. The characteristic electroencephalographic (EEG) biphasic or triphasic synchronized sharp wave complexes are not often present. Presence of 14-3-3 protein, neuron-specific enolase, and S100 calcium-binding protein B in the CSF is highly suggestive but not specific. MRI may show multifocal areas of reduced diffusion involving the basal ganglia and the cerebral cortex on T_2-weighted and diffusion-weighted images. Combining CSF total tau protein and MRI can identify 98% of early cases (Zeidler and Green 2004). Treatment is symptomatic and supportive.

HIV/AIDS

HIV/AIDS is currently the most common cause of dementia in persons under age 40 years. Over 33 million persons are infected with HIV worldwide (UN-AIDS 2007). HIV causes immunosuppression by infecting $CD4^+$ T lymphocytes. Disease stage is associated with reduction in $CD4^+$ cells: >500 cells/mL= asymptomatic, 201–500 cells/mL=constitutional symptoms, ≤200 cells/mL= full-blown AIDS (Centers for Disease Control and Prevention 1992).

Mild cognitive disturbances associated with HIV may occur without frank dementia in up to 35% of otherwise asymptomatic individuals (Selnes and Miller 1992). Symptoms include forgetfulness, decreased attention/concentration, slowed thinking, and mild tremor. Patients complain that they cannot retain information or remember recent events. On neuropsychological testing, reduction in psychomotor speed is a prominent feature. Treatment of HIV with antiretroviral therapy can control the disease for many years and eliminate the occurrence of HIV-associated dementia.

Dementia or cognitive impairment secondary to complications of HIV may be due to opportunistic infections or malignancies, such as CNS lymphoma. Potential secondary infections include viral, fungal, parasitic, and bacterial infections. These can usually be ascertained by neuroimaging and CSF analysis for cells and titers.

Hepatitis C

Hepatitis C virus (HCV) infection is common, affecting up to 2% of the world's population. The rate of comorbid infection with HCV in patients with HIV is high (30%) and even higher in intravenous drug users (60%–90%). Up to 20% of chronically HCV-infected patients may develop cirrhosis over 20 years and possibly cirrhosis-associated encephalopathy; however, up to one-third of people with chronic HCV infection experience cognitive impairment

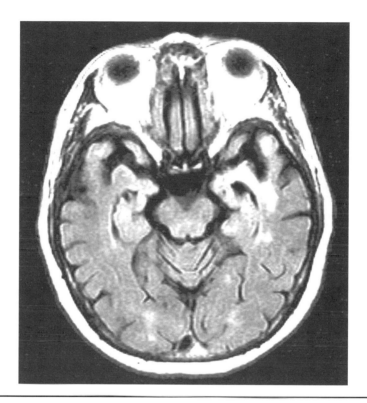

Figure 11–2.   Fluid-attenuated inversion recovery (FLAIR) magnetic resonance image showing increased signal in the anterior left temporal lobe, demonstrating secondary gliosis in a patient previously treated for herpetic encephalitis.

Source.   Reprinted from Zamrini E, Quiceno M: "Other Causes of Dementia," in *The American Psychiatric Publishing Textbook of Alzheimer Disease and Other Dementias.* Edited by Weiner MF, Lipton AM. Washington, DC, American Psychiatric Publishing, 2009, pp. 247–262. Copyright 2009, American Psychiatric Publishing. Used with permission.

in the absence of cirrhosis (Perry et al. 2008). Early symptoms include fatigue, malaise, weakness, anorexia, and occasionally jaundice. Some persons complain of problems with attending to and recalling everyday information. This is most consistent with frontal-subcortical dysfunction and similar to attention and memory problems reported by patients with HIV. Interferon-alpha is the primary antiviral therapy.

West Nile Virus

West Nile virus is transmitted by mosquitoes from birds to humans. The incubation period is between 3 and 14 days. About 1 in 150 infected persons will develop severe illness. Clinical manifestations of infection can mimic many neurological syndromes. Symptoms can include high fever, headache, neck stiffness, stupor, disorientation, coma, tremors, convulsions, muscle weakness, vision loss, numbness, and paralysis. These symptoms may last several weeks, and neurological effects may be permanent (Centers for Disease Control and Prevention 2006). EEG findings are nonspecific. Moderate to severe generalized slowing is present, and triphasic waves may appear. Treatment is supportive. Efforts at controlling the disease involve eliminating mosquito breeding sites and limiting exposure to mosquitoes.

Syphilis

Syphilis has become rare in settings outside of HIV. Infection with *Treponema pallidum* passes through three clinical stages. In primary syphilis, a chancre develops at the site of contact. Secondary syphilis occurs 6–8 weeks later, manifested by constitutional symptoms, a generalized lymphadenitis, and a mucocutaneous rash over the palms, soles, face, or scalp. After an asymptomatic latent stage that may last many years, one-third of patients may develop tertiary syphilis (neurosyphilis). This typically occurs in the fourth and fifth decades of life. It may present as any combination of delirium, dementia, other neuropsychiatric conditions, stroke, spinal cord disease, and/or seizures. Syphilitic myelopathy (tabes dorsalis) has become uncommon. In patients with neurosyphilis, CSF may show elevated protein and cell count. The CSF-VDRL (Venereal Disease Research Laboratory) test is positive, with titers greater than 1:8 in about 77% of cases. When neurosyphilis is suspected, CSF fluorescent treponemal antibody absorption can be performed. Neuroimaging shows cerebral atrophy. MRI may show meningeal enhancement. Treatment is with 20 million units/day of penicillin G for 14 days. The rate of residual symptoms can be high.

Lyme Disease

Lyme disease is caused by infection with *Borrelia burgdorferi,* transmitted by the bite of ixodid ticks. It may have a wide variety of clinical manifestations. Typically, an expanding bull's-eye rash appears at the site of the bite. This may be followed some months later by cardiac and neurological symptoms, typically radiculitis or neuropathy, particularly involving the facial nerve. A minority of patients may develop arthritic or dermatological symptoms years later. Rarely, encephalomyelitis and encephalopathy occur. Potential neuropsychiatric manifestations include virtually every psychiatric syndrome (Fallon and Nields 1994). Diagnosis is with a positive CSF polymerase chain reaction test. Various antibiotic regimens have been tried, but treatment of late manifestations with antibiotics may lead to only a partial response. Prolonged (14–30 days) parenteral cephalosporin treatment is preferred.

Fungal Meningoencephalitis

Fungal meningoencephalitis occurs mostly in HIV-positive and other immunocompromised patients. The more common culprits are *Cryptococcus neoformans,* coccidioidomycosis, histoplasmosis, blastomycosis, and species of *Aspergillus* and *Candida.*

Diseases Primarily Affecting an Organ Outside the Central Nervous System

Systemic Lupus Erythematosus

Systemic lupus erythematosus (SLE) is an autoimmune disease that affects multiple organ systems, including the CNS. Many studies have reported that 50% or more of persons with SLE will experience neuropsychiatric symptoms at some point during their illness (Berlit 2007; Emori et al. 2005).

The neuropsychiatric syndromes defined by the American College of Rheumatology (1999a) include cognitive dysfunction. In people with SLE, higher cortical functions could be influenced by many factors, such as medications, metabolic derangements, underlying psychiatric disorders, and cerebrovascular disease (Ad Hoc Committee on Lupus Response Criteria 2007). Reports of the presence of cognitive dysfunction range from 12% to 87% (Ad Hoc Committee 2007; Berlit 2007); it may be the most prevalent SLE-related disease manifestation (McLaurin et al. 2005). The pattern of cognitive impairment is diverse, but the impairment appears to involve a subcortical process (Harrison and Ravdin 2002).

A meta-analysis of 25 studies found that most cognitive deficits were in the domains of attention, with lesser involvement of visual memory, verbal memory, and psychomotor speed. Testing demonstrated that language, visuospatial processing, and concept formation were generally intact. Persons with a prior history of American College of Rheumatology–defined neuropsychiatric syndromes in SLE were more likely to experience cognitive dysfunction (Monastero et al. 2001) and more likely to have severe cognitive impairment. The American College of Rheumatology (1999b) recommends a battery of neuropsychological tests to assess cognition in people with SLE; this battery takes about 1 hour and is valid and reliable (Kozora et al. 2004).

McLaurin et al. (2005) reported on 123 patients with SLE who were followed for at least 3 years for cognitive dysfunction. Most participants were women; their mean age was 41 years. Regular use of prednisone and consistently positive antiphospholipid antibodies were predictive of cognitive dysfunction, as was the presence of diabetes mellitus, depression, and lower levels of education. Regular aspirin use was associated with improved cognition, even if prednisone was being concurrently taken; all ages seemed to benefit, but the effect was strongest in the group over age 48 years.

It is unknown if any particular treatment for SLE will prevent cognitive impairment. The relationship between steroid use and the development of cognitive dysfunction is not truly known in SLE (McLaurin et al. 2005).

Autoantibodies have been investigated as potential mediators of neuropsychiatric syndromes in SLE. Zandman-Goddard et al. (2007) suggested that cognitive dysfunction is associated with seven different antibody types. The antibodies were found in serum and/or CSF, and none was specific for cognitive dysfunction. The antibodies most commonly associated with SLE-associated cognitive dysfunction were anticardiolipin antibodies. Menon et al. (1999) found that persistently elevated anticardiolipin antibodies over a 2- to 3-year period were associated with dysfunction in word fluency, concentration, attention, and reaction time. A 5-year prospective study found that persistently elevated IgG anticardiolipin antibody levels were associated with decreased psychomotor speed, problems with conceptual reasoning, and executive dysfunction (Hanly et al. 1999).

Hashimoto's Encephalopathy

Hashimoto's encephalopathy, also known as steroid-responsive encephalopathy associated with autoimmune thyroiditis, may present with atypical psychosis, myoclonus, seizures, dementia, and disturbances of consciousness. Median age at onset is 56 years. In a series of 20 patients, the most frequent clinical features were tremor in 16 (80%), transient aphasia in 16 (80%), myoclonus in 13 (65%), gait ataxia in 13 (65%), seizures in 12 (60%), and sleep abnormalities in 11 (55%) (Castillo et al. 2006). The presentation can often be mistaken for viral encephalitis, CJD, or a degenerative dementia. Liver enzymes may be elevated, and thyroid hormone levels may remain normal. MRI is often normal or shows nonspecific white matter changes on T_2/FLAIR images (Figure 11–3). EEG findings may be nonspecific. Antithyroid antibodies are present. Treatment with high-dose prednisolone (1 g/day for 5 days) can result in significant or full recovery.

Inflammatory/Paraneoplastic Diseases

Limbic Encephalitis

Another autoimmune disease, limbic encephalitis, may be viral or nonviral in etiology. Nonviral limbic encephalitis can result from antibodies to proteins of the CNS. Broadly, two categories of antigens have been identified: 1) intracellular or classical paraneoplastic antigens and 2) cell membrane antigens expressed in hippocampal neuropil and cerebellum (Tüzün and Dalmau 2007). Limbic encephalitis is characterized by short-term memory impairment, complex partial seizures, and psychiatric symptoms. Signal abnormalities in the mesial temporal lobes without contrast enhancement are the typical MRI findings (Vernino et al. 2007) (Figure 11–4). Assays may not be positive for anti-Ma antibodies, anti-Ta 1 and 2 antibodies, anti-CV2 autoantibody, antineuronal nuclear and anti–Purkinje cell antibodies, anti-RI antibodies, and paraneoplastic opsoclonus-myoclonus antibody. Treatment of limbic encephalitis includes removal of the underlying tumor, if present, and treatments to remove pathogenic antibodies (plasma exchange) or modulate the immune response (steroids or immunosuppressants).

Morvan Syndrome

Morvan syndrome is an autoimmune disorder affecting both the peripheral and central nervous systems. It presents with behavioral changes, hallucina-

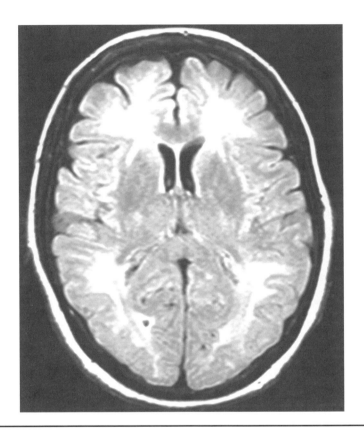

Figure 11–3.   Fluid-attenuated inversion recovery (FLAIR) magnetic resonance image demonstrating white matter hyperintensities involving the subcortical U fibers.

Source.   Reprinted from Zamrini E, Quiceno M: "Other Causes of Dementia," in *The American Psychiatric Publishing Textbook of Alzheimer Disease and Other Dementias.* Edited by Weiner MF, Lipton AM. Washington, DC, American Psychiatric Publishing, 2009, pp. 247–262. Copyright 2009, American Psychiatric Publishing. Used with permission.

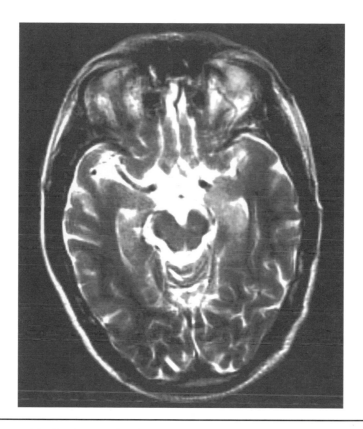

Figure 11–4. T$_2$-weighted magnetic resonance image demonstrating increased signal in mesial temporal lobes.

Source. Reprinted from Zamrini E, Quiceno M: "Other Causes of Dementia," in *The American Psychiatric Publishing Textbook of Alzheimer Disease and Other Dementias.* Edited by Weiner MF, Lipton AM. Washington, DC, American Psychiatric Publishing, 2009, pp. 247–262. Copyright 2009, American Psychiatric Publishing. Used with permission.

tions, severe insomnia, autonomic hyperactivity, and neuromyotonia (spontaneous muscle activity). It may be associated with high levels of voltage-gated potassium channel antibodies (Josephs et al. 2004).

Lymphomatosis Cerebri

Lymphomatosis cerebri is a rare variant of primary CNS lymphoma that may manifest with a rapidly progressive dementia and unsteady gait. MRI findings may show an isolated lesion or diffuse leukoencephalopathy without contrast enhancement or may be nonspecific, and CSF may have elevated 14-3-3 protein. Diagnosis is often made only after brain biopsy.

Diseases Caused by Exposure to Toxic Substances

Ethyl Alcohol

Alcohol can cause acute and chronic complications. Acute alcohol intoxication causes temporary disinhibition, followed by sedation and an unsteady gait. Heavy alcohol consumption can result in amnesia of Korsakoff syndrome, alcoholic cognitive impairment, and Marchiafava-Bignami disease. Indirectly, alcoholism may result in hepatic encephalopathy by causing hepatic cirrhosis. Other side effects include the Wernicke triad of ataxia, nystagmus, and ophthalmoplegia; however, this triad is often not present in its entirety. Neurological complications include myopathy, cardiomyopathy, and peripheral polyneuropathy, with predominantly sensory and autonomic deficits and often with a loss of deep tendon reflexes. Alcohol consumption can also adversely affect vestibular function.

The Wernicke-Korsakoff syndrome is a consequence of thiamine deficiency due to poor nutrition. It is accompanied by anterograde and retrograde amnesia. Patients have difficulty forming new memories, and old memories are less distinct. Patients confabulate. They may mix up information from different time points or make up new stories, usually with some element of factual information. When one patient was asked who the person next to him was, he pointed to his wife and stated, "They say she's my wife."

On neuroimaging of patients with chronic alcohol consumption, one may see atrophy of the brain in general and, more specifically, of the cerebellum; areas

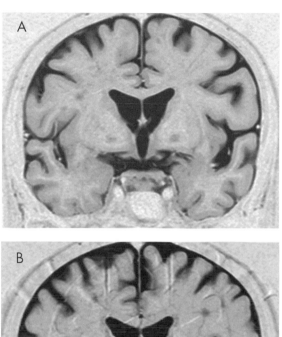

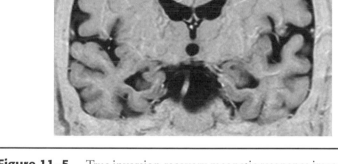

Figure 11–5.   True inversion recovery magnetic resonance images demonstrating atrophy of the mamillary bodies *(A)* and atrophy of the fornices and hippocampi *(B)*.

Source.   Reprinted from Zamrini E, Quiceno M: "Other Causes of Dementia," in *The American Psychiatric Publishing Textbook of Alzheimer Disease and Other Dementias.* Edited by Weiner MF, Lipton AM. Washington, DC, American Psychiatric Publishing, 2009, pp. 247–262. Copyright 2009, American Psychiatric Publishing. Used with permission.

of increased T_2/FLAIR signal in midline periventricular structures; and atrophy of the anterior diencephalon and mamillary bodies (Figure 11–5).

Marchiafava-Bignami disease is a dissociation disorder from acute demyelination of the corpus callosum classically associated with chronic alcoholism. Patients have attentional deficits, language difficulty, personality changes, and signs of interhemispheric disconnection (apraxia, agraphia, and left hand anomia) (Berek et al. 1994).

Radiation Therapy

Ionizing radiation for the treatment of brain tumors can damage double-stranded DNA, RNA, proteins, lipids, and cellular membranes. Radiotherapy-induced cerebral injury can generally be classified by its time of onset as acute encephalopathy, early-delayed, delayed, and late-delayed forms. Delayed forms are typically not reversible. Late-delayed cerebral injury can occur months to years after treatment if the brain was included in the radiation portal. Cognitive consequences are dose related and range from short-term memory impairment to dementia. The following is a case that was evaluated by one of the authors (see also Figure 11–6).

> A man in his 70s developed progressive memory loss and language deficits four decades after irradiation for an unspecified intracranial tumor. He had disproportionate atrophy of the left temporal lobe corresponding to the radiation therapy window indicated by permanent tattoos over the left side of his head. Although lobar atrophy secondary to Alzheimer disease or frontotemporal dementia could not be completely excluded, the clinical localization of his symptoms, neuroimaging, and radiation window tattoo made late-delayed radiation a more likely diagnosis.

Heavy Metals

Multiple metals, including lead, mercury, arsenic, manganese, and bismuth, have been associated with cognitive impairment. Lead may produce anemia, abdominal pain, aminoaciduria, bone changes, and peripheral and CNS damage. Lead encephalopathy results in impaired attention, concentration, and memory. Emotional lability and psychosis may also occur. Inorganic mercury poisoning causes stomatitis, irritability, tremor, and peripheral neuropathy. Organic mercury causes paresthesias, ataxia, and visual problems. Arsenic can cause myelopathy, peripheral neuropathy, optic neuropathy, somnolence, disorientation, and impaired memory. Manganese toxicity can cause parkinsonism

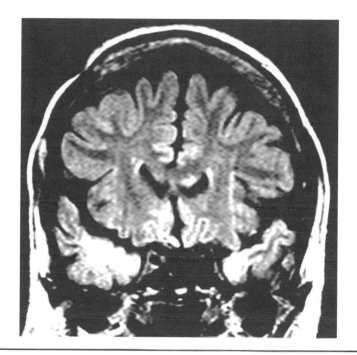

Figure 11–6.   Fluid-attenuated inversion recovery (FLAIR) magnetic resonance image, coronal section, demonstrating white matter hyperintensities in bilateral temporal lobes.

The right side, which received the greatest amount of radiation, is significantly more affected than the left side.

Source.   Reprinted from Zamrini E, Quiceno M: "Other Causes of Dementia," in *The American Psychiatric Publishing Textbook of Alzheimer Disease and Other Dementias.* Edited by Weiner MF, Lipton AM. Washington, DC, American Psychiatric Publishing, 2009, pp. 247–262. Copyright 2009, American Psychiatric Publishing. Used with permission.

with gait disturbance, tremor, increased muscle tone, memory problems, aggressiveness, and hallucinations. Bismuth toxicity can result in depression, anxiety, hallucinations, and delusions.

Cancer Chemotherapy

Cyclosporine may produce leukoencephalopathy. Other chemotherapeutic agents can produce multifocal inflammatory leukoencephalopathies. Symptoms include subacute confusion, seizures, and focal neurological symptoms and may last long after the medications have been stopped. Steroids may help reduce the symptoms.

Diseases Due to Deficiency of an Essential Substance

Certain vitamin and mineral deficiencies can cause dementia. Beriberi is caused by thiamine (vitamin B_1) deficiency. This may result from poor diet such as high consumption of milled rice, severe gastrointestinal disease, alcoholism, HIV infection, gastric bypass surgery, and even hyperemesis gravidarum. Clinical manifestations include apathy, fatigue, irritability, depression, and poor concentration. Dry beriberi symptoms include peripheral neuropathy, paresthesias, weakness, pallor, wasting, and hepatomegaly. Wet beriberi is associated with cardiac symptoms, including edema, tachycardia, and cardiomegaly.

Pellagra is a systemic disease resulting from severe niacin deficiency. Causes include conditions resulting in severe malnutrition, including alcoholism and anorexia nervosa. Clinical manifestations include dermatitis resembling sunburn, diarrhea, and dementia. Features of pellagra encephalopathy include confusion, clouding of consciousness, and myoclonus. Symptoms respond to treatment with nicotinic acid.

Cyanocobalamin (vitamin B_{12}) is an essential cofactor in the conversion of homocysteine to methionine. Vitamin B_{12} deficiency results in macrocytic anemia and subacute combined degeneration, a disorder of the posterior and lateral columns of the spinal cord resulting in loss of vibratory and position sense, ataxia, weakness, and loss of sphincter control. Optic neuropathy, memory dysfunction, and encephalopathy may ensue. Psychotic symptoms may also occur, with or without anemia or spinal cord symptoms. Outright dementia is rare. Vitamin B_{12} deficiency may result from poor nutrition, loss of intrinsic factor, or gastric bypass surgery. Exposure to nitrous oxide anesthesia may precipitate symptoms in otherwise asymptomatic patients with low vitamin B_{12} values. Copper deficiency may also result in subacute combined degeneration.

Folate modulates the transmethylation and transsulfuration pathways of homocysteine elimination. Several studies have found an association between low levels of folate and cognitive impairment in the elderly (Hassing et al. 1999). Folic acid deficiency is unlikely in the United States today because since January

1998, the U.S. Food and Drug Administration has required folic acid fortification of grain products (140 μg of folic acid per 100 g), with the goal of reducing neural tube defects.

Severe vitamin E deficiency can result in spinocerebellar degeneration, with gait unsteadiness, ataxia, hyporeflexia, loss of both vibratory and joint-position sensations, limitations in upward gaze, strabismus, long-tract defects, profound muscle weakness, and visual field constriction. If prolonged severe deficiency occurs, complete blindness, dementia, and cardiac arrhythmias may develop (Tanyel and Mancano 1997).

Key Clinical Points

- Many medical conditions can cause chronic encephalopathies.
- It is important to assess medical status when evaluating persons with cognitive impairment.
- A careful history and examination can uncover important clues to the existence of a potentially reversible disorder.
- Patients with cognitive impairment may have more than one contributing factor. Each potential factor suggested by history, examination, or laboratory studies needs to be considered.

References

Ad Hoc Committee on Lupus Response Criteria: Cognition Sub-committee: Proposed response criteria for neurocognitive impairment in systemic lupus erythematosus clinical trials. Lupus 16:418–425, 2007

Aicardi J: The inherited leukodystrophies: a clinical overview. J Inherit Metab Dis 16:733–743, 1993

Amato MP, Portaccio E, Zipoli V: Are there protective treatments for cognitive decline in MS? J Neurol Sci 245:183–186, 2006

American College of Rheumatology: American College of Rheumatology nomenclature for neuropsychiatric lupus syndromes. Arthritis Rheum 42:599–609, 1999a

American College of Rheumatology: Arthritis & Rheumatism: Appendix C: Proposed One-Hour Neuropsychological Battery for SLE. Atlanta, GA, American College of Rheumatology, 1999b. Available at: http://www.rheumatology.org/publications/ar/1999/499apC.asp?aud=mem. Accessed June 8, 2008.

Benedict RH, Fischer JS, Archibald CJ, et al: Minimal neuropsychological assessment of MS: a consensus approach. Clin Neuropsychol 16:381–397, 2002

Benedict RH, Cox D, Thompson LL, et al: Reliable screening for neuropsychological impairment in multiple sclerosis. Mult Scler 10:675–678, 2004

Berek K, Wagner M, Chemelli AP, et al: Hemispheric disconnection in Marchiafava-Bignami disease: clinical, neuropsychological and MRI findings. J Neurol Sci 123:2–5, 1994

Berlit P: Neuropsychiatric disease in collagen vascular diseases and vasculitis. J Neurol 254 (suppl 2):87–89, 2007

Bobholz JA, Rao SM: Cognitive dysfunction in MS: a review of recent developments. Curr Opin Neurol 16:283–288, 2003

Brassington JC, Marsh NV: Neuropsychological aspects of multiple sclerosis. Neuropsychol Rev 8:43–77, 1998

Castillo P, Woodruff B, Caselli R, et al: Steroid-responsive encephalopathy associated with autoimmune thyroiditis. Arch Neurol 63:197–202, 2006

Centers for Disease Control and Prevention: 1993 revised classification system for HIV infection and expanded surveillance case definition for AIDS among adolescents and adults. MMWR Recomm Rep 41 (RR-17):1–19, 1992

Centers for Disease Control and Prevention: West Nile Virus: What You Need to Know. 2006. Available at: http://www.cdc.gov/ncidod/dvbid/westnile/wnv_factsheet.htm. Accessed June 2, 2008.

Chiaravalloti ND, DeLuca J: Cognitive impairment in multiple sclerosis. Lancet Neurol 12:1139–1151, 2008

Damasio AR, Eslinger PI, Damasio H, et al: Multimodal amnestic syndrome following bilateral temporal and basal forebrain damage. Arch Neurol 42:252–259, 1985

Deloire M, Ruet A, Hamel D, et al: Early cognitive impairment in multiple sclerosis predicts disability outcome several years later. Mult Scler 16:581–587, 2010

Duyao M, Ambrose C, Myers R, et al: Trinucleotide repeat length instability and age of onset in Huntington's disease. Nat Genet 4:387–392, 1993

Emori A, Matsushima E, Aihara O, et al: Cognitive dysfunction in systemic lupus erythematosus. Psychiatry Clin Neurosci 59:584–589, 2005

Fallon BA, Nields JA: Lyme disease: a neuropsychiatric illness. Am J Psychiatry 151:1571–1583, 1994

Feinstein A: The Clinical Neuropsychiatry of Multiple Sclerosis. New York, Cambridge University Press, 2007

Filippi M, Rocca MA, Benedict RH, et al: The contribution of MRI in assessing cognitive impairment in multiple sclerosis. Neurology 75:2121–2128, 2010

Glaser CA, Honarmand S, Anderson LJ, et al: Beyond viruses: clinical profiles and etiologies associated with encephalitis. Clin Infect Dis 43:1565–1577, 2006

Hanly JG, Hong C, Smith S, et al: A prospective analysis of cognitive function and anticardiolipin antibodies in systemic lupus erythematosus. Arthritis Rheum 42:728–734, 1999

Harper PS: The epidemiology of Huntington's disease. Hum Genet 89:365–376, 1992

Harrison MJ, Ravdin LD: Cognitive dysfunction in neuropsychiatric systemic lupus erythematosus. Curr Opin Rheumatol 14:510–514, 2002

Hassing L, Wahlin A, Winblad B, et al: Further evidence on the effects of vitamin B12 and folate levels on episodic memory function: a population-based study of healthy very old adults. Biol Psychiatry 45:1472–1480, 1999

Huijbregts SC, Kalkers NF, de Sonneville LM, et al: Differences in cognitive impairment of relapsing remitting, secondary, and primary progressive MS. Neurology 63:335–339, 2004

Huntington's Disease Collaborative Research Group: A novel gene containing a trinucleotide repeat that is expanded and unstable on Huntington's disease chromosomes. Cell 72:971–983, 1993

Ingster-Moati I, Bui Quoc E, Pless M, et al: Ocular motility and Wilson's disease: a study on 34 patients. J Neurol Neurosurg Psychiatry 78:1199–1201, 2007

Ishiko A, Shimizu A, Nagata E, et al: Cerebral autosomal dominant arteriopathy with subcortical infarcts and leukoencephalopathy (CADASIL): a hereditary cerebrovascular disease, which can be diagnosed by skin biopsy electron microscopy. Am J Dermatopathol 27:131–134, 2005

Josephs KA, Silber MH, Fealey RD, et al: Neurophysiologic studies in Morvan syndrome. J Clin Neurophysiol 21:440–445, 2004

Kozora E, Ellison MC, West S: Reliability and validity of the proposed American College of Rheumatology neuropsychological battery for systemic lupus erythematosus. Arthritis Rheum 51:810–818, 2004

Krupp LB, Christodoulou C, Melville P, et al: A multi-center randomized clinical trial of donepezil to treat memory impairment in multiple sclerosis (abstract). Neurology 74 (suppl 2):A294, 2010

Larson EB, Reifler BV, Featherstone HJ, et al: Dementia in elderly outpatients: a prospective study. Ann Intern Med 100:417–423, 1984

Le Ber I, Marié RM, Chabot B, et al: Neuropsychological and 18FDG-PET studies in a family with idiopathic basal ganglia calcifications. J Neurol Sci 258:115–122, 2007

Lovera JF: Memantine for cognitive impairment in multiple sclerosis: a randomized placebo-controlled trial. Mult Scler 16:715–723, 2010

McLaurin EY, Holliday SL, Williams P, et al: Predictors of cognitive dysfunction in patients with systemic lupus erythematosus. Neurology 64:297–303, 2005

Menon S, Jameson-Shortall E, Newman SP, et al: A longitudinal study of anticardiolipin antibody levels and cognitive functioning in systemic lupus erythematosus. Arthritis Rheum 42:735–741, 1999

Meschia JF, Worrall BB: New advances in identifying genetic anomalies in stroke-prone probands. Curr Neurol Neurosci Rep 4:420–426, 2004

Monastero R, Bettini P, Del Zotto E, et al: Prevalence and pattern of cognitive impairment in systemic lupus erythematosus patients with and without overt neuropsychiatric manifestations. J Neurol Sci 184:33–39, 2001

Nance MA, Paulsen JS, Rosenblatt A, et al: A Physician's Guide to the Management of Huntington's Disease, 3rd Edition. New York, Huntington's Disease Society of America, 2011. Available at: http://www.hdsa.org/new-physicians-guide.html. Accessed August 3, 2011.

Perry W, Hilsabeck RC, Hassanein TI: Cognitive dysfunction in chronic hepatitis C: a review. Dig Dis Sci 53:307–321, 2008

Rakheja D, Narayan SB, Bennett MJ: Juvenile neuronal ceroid-lipofuscinosis (Batten disease): a brief review and update. Curr Mol Med 7:603–608, 2007

Relkin N, Marmarou A, Klinge P, et al: Diagnosing idiopathic normal-pressure hydrocephalus. Neurosurgery 57 (suppl 3):S4–S16, 2005

Reynolds N: Revisiting safety of minocycline as neuroprotection in Huntington's disease (letter). Mov Disord 22:292, 2007

Schulz D, Kopp B, Kunkel A, et al: Cognition in the early stages of multiple sclerosis. J Neurol 253:1002–1010, 2006

Selnes OA, Miller EN: Cognitive impairment of HIV infection. AIDS 6:602–604, 1992

Sperling RA, Guttman CRG, Hohol MJ, et al: Regional magnetic resonance imaging lesion burden and cognitive function in multiple sclerosis: a longitudinal study. Arch Neurol 58:115–121, 2001

Sutovsky S, Petrovic R, Chandoga J, et al: Adult onset cerebral form of X-linked adrenoleukodystrophy with dementia of frontal lobe type with new L160P mutation in ABCD1 gene. J Neurol Sci 263:149–153, 2007

Taly AB, Meenakshi-Sundaram S, Sinha S, et al: Wilson disease: description of 282 patients evaluated over 3 decades. Medicine (Baltimore) 86:112–121, 2007

Tanyel MC, Mancano LD: Neurologic findings in vitamin E deficiency. Am Fam Physician 55:197–201, 1997

Tüzün E, Dalmau J: Limbic encephalitis and variants: classification, diagnosis, and treatment. Neurologist 13:261–271, 2007

Ueno S, Maruki Y, Nakamura M, et al: The gene encoding a newly discovered protein, chorein, is mutated in chorea-acanthocytosis. Nat Genet 28:121–122, 2001

UNAIDS: AIDS Epidemic Update. Geneva, Switzerland, Joint United Nations Programme on HIV/AIDS and World Health Organization, 2007. Available at: http://data.unaids.org/pub/epislides/2007/2007_epiupdate_en.pdf. Accessed August 4, 2011.

Vernino SM, Geschwind M, Boeve B, et al: Autoimmune encephalopathies. Neurologist 13:140–147, 2007

Wexler NS, Lorimer J, Porter J, et al: Venezuelan kindreds reveal that genetic and environmental factors modulate Huntington's disease age of onset. Proc Natl Acad Sci USA 101:3498–3503, 2004

Wichowicz HM, Cubala WJ, Saweck J, et al: Wilson's disease associated with delusional disorder. Psychiatry Clin Neurosci 60:758–760, 2006

Zandman-Goddard G, Chapman J, Shoenfeld Y: Autoantibodies involved in neuropsychiatric SLE and antiphospholipid syndrome. Semin Arthritis Rheum 36:297–315, 2007

Zeidler M, Green A: Advances in diagnosing Creutzfeldt-Jakob disease with MRI and CSF 14-3-3 protein analysis. Neurology 63:410–411, 2004

Zhou B, Westaway SK, Levinson B, et al: A novel pantothenate kinase gene (PANK2) is defective in Hallervorden-Spatz syndrome. Nat Genet 28:345–349, 2001

Further Reading

David A, Fleminger S, Kopelman M, et al: Lishman's Organic Psychiatry: A Textbook of Neuropsychiatry. Hoboken, NJ, Wiley-Blackwell, 2009

Lyketsos CG, Lipsey JR, Rabins PV, et al: Psychiatric Aspects of Neurologic Diseases: Practical Approaches to Patient Care. New York, Oxford University Press, 2007

Rosenberg RN, Di Mauro S, Paulson HL, et al: The Molecular and Genetic Basis of Neurologic and Psychiatric Disease. Philadelphia, PA, Lippincott Williams & Wilkins, 2008

PART II

Treatment

12

Treatment of Psychiatric Disorders in People With Dementia

Martin Steinberg, M.D.

Constantine G. Lyketsos, M.D., M.H.S.

In this chapter, we use a case-study approach to discuss five common neuropsychiatric phenomena in persons with dementia: depression, psychosis, apathy, executive dysfunction syndrome, and agitation and aggression. Following each case presentation, we review current understanding of phenomenology and provide guidance regarding clinical assessment and development of a treatment plan.

Supported by the Johns Hopkins Alzheimer's Disease Research Center (NIA P50AG 005146).

Depression

Mrs. Johnson, a 72-year-old woman with moderate Alzheimer disease, is brought by her daughter to Mrs. Johnson's physician because of concerns about behavioral changes. "She seems angry a lot, and is less interested in things. She cries nearly every day," says her daughter. "She used to enjoy helping me with housework, but now she just sits in the living room with the TV on and sulks. She doesn't seem to enjoy anything, even when the grandchildren visit. Twice in the past month, she has said that I'm not her 'real' daughter, that I'm a step-daughter, and that I want to take her money and place her in a nursing home. I'm worried my mother is depressed."

On examination, Mrs. Johnson scores 15 out of 30 on the Mini-Mental State Examination (MMSE; Folstein et al. 1975). She reports that her mood is "fine" and denies all depression symptoms. Her affect is mildly constricted and irritable, but she does occasionally smile and laugh appropriately. "I have no complaints," she says. "I like to take life as it comes." When probed about her concerns regarding her daughter's identity and motives, she smiles tensely and states with a guarded demeanor, "Let's just say she and I have a few disagreements."

Diagnostic Considerations

The diagnosis of depression among patients with dementia is not straightforward. Persons with Alzheimer disease and other dementias may not remember symptoms. Aphasias may also impede the ability of patients to communicate their inner state. For these reasons, obtaining information from a reliable informant is essential. The challenges of diagnosing depression in patients with dementia, however, go beyond patients' difficulties in memory and communication; clinicians and researchers have long realized that depression in patients with dementia differs in some ways from depression in cognitively intact persons. Thus, reliance on DSM-IV-TR criteria (American Psychiatric Association 2000) may result in significant underestimation.

In comparing DSM-III-R (American Psychiatric Association 1987) symptoms in depressed elderly outpatients with and without Alzheimer disease, Zubenko et al. (2003) found differences in the frequency of many symptoms. Patients with Alzheimer disease were less likely to report feelings of worthlessness or guilt, thoughts of death or suicide, and sleep disruption. They were more likely to report diminished concentration, or delusions and hallucinations.

Clinical Assessment

Because dementias cause impairments in memory, expressive skills, and insight, collateral information is crucial in making a diagnosis. Many patients, like Mrs. Johnson, are brought to a clinic by a concerned caregiver; others, especially with milder dementias, may present alone, in which case it is advisable to request permission to speak to a reliable informant. Given the atypical presentation of depression in dementia and the lack of expert consensus diagnostic criteria, use of a rating instrument designed specifically to assess depression in dementia can assist in diagnosis.

The most widely used instrument is the Cornell Scale for Depression in Dementia (Alexopoulos et al. 1988). This 19-item scale was designed to distinguish between symptoms of depression and confounding symptoms that may reflect either the primary dementia process or medical comorbidity. The scale requires that information be obtained from both the patient and a reliable informant. When discrepancy exists, as in Mrs. Johnson's case, the clinician makes a judgment in rating each item after taking all reports into account. A score greater than 7 is commonly accepted as indicating clinically significant depression; a score greater than 11 indicates severe depression.

Although many dementia patients will meet DSM-IV-TR criteria for major depressive disorder (MDD), some will have symptoms warranting intervention without meeting these criteria. Clinicians should also be alert to the potential for other clinical symptoms or syndromes, such as apathy, psychosis, and medical comorbidity, to be confused with depression in dementia.

Apathy is common in Alzheimer disease and other dementias and can co-occur with depression, but it can also be a distinct phenomenon. Apathetic patients lack motivation and initiative but are typically not distressed by their amotivational state. They typically do not display dysphoria, irritability, and delusions. Mrs. Johnson's daughter reported apathy ("she just sits in the living room with the TV on"), but the co-occurrence of tearfulness and irritability suggests more than isolated apathy.

Delusions are common in persons with dementia who are depressed. Compared with psychotic depression in patients without dementia, psychotic symptoms in depression in dementia are typically less severe and more transient. Other mood symptoms, such as tearfulness and irritability, are always present in depression and usually of greater severity than the psychosis. Mrs. Johnson's delusion of her daughter being an imposter is a typical delusion of depression: it is intermittent and occurs in the setting of other depression symptoms. Medical comorbidity can confound a presentation of depression in dementia in two ways: depression can be caused or exacerbated by a variety of medical conditions or medications (e.g., hypothyroidism, use of a β-blocker), and a medical symptom or medication side effect may be misinterpreted as a symptom of depression (e.g., fatigue due to anemia, poor appetite due to gastrointestinal [GI] side effects of a nonsteroidal anti-inflammatory medication). Thus, comprehensive medical evaluation is indicated, including a complete blood count, a comprehensive chemistry profile, and thyroid function tests.

Treatment

Treatment of depression in dementia is individualized and often empirical. In most clinicians' experience, the effectiveness of depression treatments in patients with dementia parallels that in patients without dementia. Both pharmacological and nonpharmacological therapies are available.

Nonpharmacological therapies are of value. For example, Teri et al. (1997, 2003) found that behavioral management and a combination of behavioral management and exercise were useful in alleviating depressive symptoms in persons with Alzheimer disease. Traditional psychotherapies are unlikely to benefit patients with dementia, but these patients do benefit from a supportive relationship with a clinician who can comfort, encourage, and imbue optimism. Caregivers benefit from similar support and from treatment for their own depression, if present. A caregiver's improvement can in turn have positive effects on the patient's own mood. Caregiver education regarding strategies to manage behavioral symptoms (e.g., not arguing or rationalizing) and to encourage stimulation and pleasurable activities can also be of benefit.

For most cases of suspected MDD, an antidepressant should be strongly considered. Data to support efficacy of specific antidepressants or classes of drugs remain limited. In a review of placebo-controlled clinical trials of antidepressants for MDD in dementia patients, Lyketsos and Olin (2002) reported that half of the studies found antidepressants, including selective serotonin reuptake inhibitors (SSRIs), imipramine, and the monoamine oxidase inhibitor moclobemide, to be beneficial. Lyketsos et al. (2003) assigned outpatients with depression in Alzheimer disease to either sertraline or placebo for 12 weeks, and found that sertraline was superior to placebo in treating the depression. Successfully treated patients had less functional decline as well. However, there was no difference between treated and untreated groups at 24 weeks (Weintraub et al. 2010). Published evidence for antidepressants in dementias other than Alzheimer disease is not available.

Because SSRIs are the most widely studied medications in dementia, with several demonstrations of efficacy, they are reasonable first-line antidepressants for most dementia patients (Table 12–1). They are typically begun at at the lowest dosage (e.g., sertraline 25 mg/day), and the dosage is increased as needed. In the Lyketsos et al. (2003) sertraline study, the mean effective dosage was 112 mg/day; thus, it is important to reach a therapeutic dose before concluding that an SSRI is not effective. SSRIs are generally well tolerated; GI side effects are most common. Other side effects include insomnia and increased confusion. The potential for SSRIs to cause the syndrome of inappropriate antidiuretic hormone secretion (SIADH) is a concern in elderly patients, and intermittent monitoring of electrolytes is advisable. Dementia patients are less likely to report or to be distressed by sexual side effects of SSRIs.

Although data are lacking, other antidepressants can be considered as second-line treatments in patients with no response to or poor tolerance of SSRIs. Some antidepressants may even be considered first-line if the clinician believes the side-effect profile is more favorable for a given patient. Such options include venlafaxine, mirtazapine, duloxetine, and bupropion. These antidepressants and their starting doses, maximum dosages, and common side effects are listed in Table 12–1. Two other classes are rarely used as first- or second-line treatments but may be considered in specific cases of poor response or tolerance to other classes. Tricyclic antidepressants such as nortriptyline have the advantage of measurable serum target levels, but their use is limited by the potential for orthostasis, anticholinergic effects, and cardiac effects (e.g., prolonged QT interval). Monoamine oxidase inhibitors have a favorable cardiac profile, but side effects such as hypotension and the low-tyramine diet needed to avoid hypertensive crisis limit their utility.

For severe depression that is resistant to multiple pharmacological trials and that places the patient in physical danger from cachexia due to poor food intake or suicidality, electroconvulsive therapy (ECT) can be considered. Although study of this modality in patients with dementia is very limited, clinical experience suggests that patients with dementia tolerate and respond to ECT similarly to patients without dementia (Steinberg 2008). Particularly close monitoring for treatment-related delirium is indicated; if such delirium is present, treatment frequency can be decreased from three to two times weekly. Despite concern that dementia patients may be at increased risk for permanent cognitive sequelae following ECT, findings from one small study by Rao and Lyketsos (2000) suggest otherwise. In this series of dementia patients (more than half with vascular dementia), half developed delirium during the ECT course, but the mean discharge MMSE score was 1.62 points *higher* than on admission. Like the Lyketsos et al. (2003) sertraline study discussed above, this study suggests that depression treatment in dementia may have favorable cognitive and functional effects beyond treatment of mood symptoms alone.

Update on Mrs. Johnson

After considering the discrepant clinical reports, Mrs. Johnson's clinician concluded that she probably had depression. Her daughter reported multiple symptoms occurring over a several-week period. Although Mrs. Johnson denied most symptoms, she was not deemed a reliable historian due to her dementia. A comment she later made when asked about her memory ("as good as it can be for an old woman") supported the clinician's assessment that she had limited insight. Mrs. Johnson's Cornell Scale score was 10. She began taking sertraline 25 mg/day. The dose was titrated to 75 mg/day with minimal benefit, and the patient reported GI upset and loose stools. She was switched to mirtazapine starting at 7.5 mg at bedtime, but this was stopped after 3 days because of severe sedation. Her clinician then began sustained-release bupropion 100 mg/day, and the patient's symptoms significantly improved at a dosage of 150 mg/day; she did not experience GI or other side effects. Her tearfulness remitted, and she was more active and easier to engage, including cheerfully assisting her daughter with housework. She still occasionally commented that her daughter "is only a stepdaughter," but with less distress, and no longer accused her daughter of stealing.

Psychosis

Mr. Clark's wife calls his physician because she is having difficulty managing his behavior. "He's fine in the morning and early afternoon, but by about 3 P.M., he starts to get moody. He says he needs to 'go home' and see his father, and he

Table 12–1. Antidepressants often used for depression in dementia

Class	Examples	Starting dosage (mg/day)	Maximum dosage (mg/day)	Side-effect concerns
SSRIs	Sertraline	25	150	GI upset, insomnia, confusion, akathisia, SIADH
	Citalopram	10	60	
	Escitalopram	5	20	
	Fluoxetine	10	40	
	Paroxetine	10	40	
SNRIs	Venlafaxine	37.5	300	GI upset, confusion; hypertension with venlafaxine
	Duloxetine	30	60	
		(divided bid)	(divided bid)	
α_1-Adrenergic antagonist	Mirtazapine	7.5	45	Sedation
Dopamine reuptake inhibitor	Bupropion	150 (extended release)	450	GI upset, hypertension, seizure risk

Note.   GI = gastrointestinal; SIADH = syndrome of inappropriate antidiuretic hormone secretion; SNRI = serotonin–norepinephrine reuptake inhibitor; SSRI = selective serotonin reuptake inhibitor.

doesn't believe me when I remind him his father died 30 years ago. By early evening, he asks where the train station is so he can go home. He's even accused me of stealing his ticket. Once, I showed him a picture of his father's headstone to prove he is deceased, and he hit me. I think he needs medicine to calm him down. But I've heard that these medicines can be dangerous and even cause strokes, and you've told me he has a vascular dementia from strokes. Where do I go from here?"

Diagnostic Considerations

In this chapter, the term *psychotic symptoms* refers specifically to delusions and hallucinations. Although they can occur as isolated phenomena, most delusions and hallucinations present along with other neuropsychiatric phenomena, such as depression, agitation and aggression, and irritability (Tractenberg et al. 2003). Delusions and hallucinations can also be caused by delirium due to medical problems and occur frequently in patients with Alzheimer disease.

As with depression, delusions and hallucinations present differently in persons with dementia than in cognitively intact persons. Patients with dementia rarely have thought disorder or loose associations, and they rarely demonstrate the complex, systematized delusions seen in schizophrenia and psychotic depression or mania. Delusions of persons with dementia tend to be simple and nonbizarre. Common delusions include the beliefs that their home is not their home (often expressed as a need to "go home" despite being there), that deceased friends and relatives are still living, and that others (often their spouse or children) are imposters. Patients often believe that items they have misplaced or no longer possess have been stolen, often by their spouse or caregiver.

Whereas auditory hallucinations are more common than visual hallucinations in most psychotic disorders, the reverse is true for dementia. Common visual hallucinations of patients with dementia are of deceased relatives and friends, as well as of young children or other unspecified people. Although people with dementia are frequently distressed by their delusions, they often experience these hallucinations nonchalantly; they may even find these "visits" pleasant. In dementia with Lewy bodies, detailed hallucinations are common and also often cause distress.

Table 12–2 outlines common differences between the delusions and hallucinations of patients with and without dementia. Whereas visual hallucinations often occur as isolated phenomena, delusions are commonly accompanied by

Table 12–2.   Differences between delusions and hallucinations in patients with psychosis with and without dementia

	Patients without dementia	Patients with dementia
Delusions	Systematized	Unsystematized
	Bizarre	Commonplace (children, animals)
Hallucinations	Auditory	Visual

other symptoms, such as depression, irritability, agitation, and occasionally physical aggression.

Clinical Assessment

When evaluating a patient with dementia, the clinician must ascertain whether hallucinations or delusions are present, arrive at a differential diagnosis, and devise a treatment plan based on the probable etiology, taking into account symptom severity and distress caused to the patient and/or caregiver. Patients may not spontaneously report these symptoms, or may not recall them at the time of the interview. Collateral information from a reliable caregiver is crucial, and it is helpful to specifically inquire about the common presentations of psychosis in dementia (e.g., "Does your father ever believe items he cannot locate have been stolen?"). In Mr. Clark's case, his symptoms were of sufficient severity that his wife contacted his physician to discuss them. Typical for dementia patients, his symptoms were limited to delusions, which were of common varieties (e.g., that he needed to "go home" when already at home, that his deceased father was living, and that his train ticket was "stolen").

Once the presence of delusions or hallucinations is ascertained, the clinician must determine whether these reflect an isolated psychosis or whether they are part of another syndrome such as depression or delirium. As discussed in "Depression" above, delusions are commonly observed in dementia patients with depression. Thus, when assessing patients with delusional dementia, clinicians need to consider symptoms related to mood, sleep, appetite, and behavior; if these symptoms are present to a significant degree, the diagnosis of a primary mood syndrome with accompanying delusions should be strongly considered. This distinction may have important implications for pharmacotherapy decisions. If the patient has a primary depressive disorder, the delusions may improve with antidepressant treatment alone, obviating the need for a neuroleptic drug.

Delusions and hallucinations often occur in the context of a delirium. Features suggesting delirium include clouded sensorium, attentional deficits, marked symptom fluctuation, and disruption of the sleep-wake cycle, and these should always be assessed in patients with psychotic dementia.

In Mr. Clark's case, some "moodiness" and irritability are reported, but they appear to be of milder intensity and also to reflect a reaction to his false beliefs (and, as addressed later in this section, to his wife's attempts to correct them). Lack of reported sadness, decreased interest, tearfulness, and sleep or appetite changes argues against a primary depressive disorder. Similarly, lack of sleep disruption or clouded sensorium argues against a delirium. Mr. Clark's delusions fluctuate, with a steady increase in severity from early afternoon until evening. This diurnal symptom pattern occurs with many neuropsychiatric symptoms in dementia and is not pathognomonic of any specific neuropsychiatric syndrome.

Treatment

Once psychotic symptoms have been identified and assessed as unlikely to be part of another neuropsychiatric syndrome, the clinician must decide whether treatment is indicated. Both nonpharmacological and pharmacological options are available. In some cases, no treatment is necessary. For example, the delusions or hallucinations may be mild and intermittent, and may not be distressing to either the patient or caregiver. The clinician may thus need only to educate and reassure the caregiver and/or patient that these symptoms are common in dementia and ensure that the caregiver is responding in an appropriate manner by not arguing or rationalizing with the patient.

More commonly, psychotic symptoms cause some degree of distress for the patient and/or caregiver and intervention is warranted. In such instances, clinicians should attempt nonpharmacological strategies before considering psychotropic intervention, because of the sensitivity that dementia patients may have to neuroleptics, and because of concerns that have arisen about the efficacy and safety of these medications in patients with dementia. Nonpharmacological strategies are typically not aimed at eliminating the delusion and commonly involve brainstorming with the caregiver to implement strategies to lessen the patient's focus on and distress over his or her symptoms.

The first strategy is for caregivers to avoid arguing with or confronting a patient about the delusions. At best, such redirection has only brief benefit (the patient forgets) and can often exacerbate the patient's distress and increase suspiciousness that he or she is being lied to. In the case example, Mrs. Clark's insistence that her husband's father was deceased did not lessen Mr. Clark's delusion; her attempt to use a photo of the father's headstone to "prove" the fact provoked physical aggression. Not rationalizing or correcting is difficult for many caregivers, and they may feel guilty for permitting the patient to believe something false. Education about the goal of responding in ways to lessen distress can be helpful.

Often, caregivers can successfully distract patients distressed by their hallucinations or delusions. Offering a cup of tea together, requesting the patient's assistance with folding laundry or other simple household chores, and changing the topic of conversation are common strategies. A variant of this strategy is to use the content of the patient's delusion to transition onto a less distressing topic. For example, when Mr. Clark expresses concern about not being able to find the train station, his wife may respond by discussing recent construction occurring in town and transition into a conversation about how difficult finding familiar locations has become.

Another technique for caregivers is to discern the emotion underlying the psychotic symptom and respond to that. For example, when a patient such as Mr. Clark insists he needs to see his father, Mrs. Clark, sensing his grief and longing for his father, may respond, "Tell me about your father. What's the favorite thing you did together?" If successful, this strategy can result in redirecting the conversation toward pleasurable reminiscence. When patients are frightened by visual hallucinations, they sometimes respond to reassurance (e.g., "I know these things you see are frightening to you, but I am here and you are safe").

Frequently, these strategies are insufficient and pharmacotherapy is indicated. The mainstays of treatment are neuroleptics. Many clinicians and caregivers understandably worry about instituting neuroleptic treatment. As outlined in Table 12–3, many of the side effects of both typical and atypical neuroleptics are of special concern in fragile elderly patients. Furthermore, a 2003 U.S. Food and Drug Administration (FDA) safety alert warned of increased risk of cerebrovascular events for elderly patients with dementia treated with atypical neuroleptics. In 2005, the FDA issued a public health advisory

Table 12–3.   Neuroleptic side effects

Side effects	More common with atypical than typical neuroleptics	Of special concern in elderly patients with dementia
Sedation	✓	✓
Unsteadiness/falls		✓
Parkinsonism		✓
Anticholinergic side effects		
Dry mouth		
Constipation		✓
Urinary retention		✓
Blurry vision		
Tachycardia		
Akathisia		
Tardive dyskinesia		
Neuroleptic malignant syndrome		
Diabetes risk/exacerbation	✓	✓
Metabolic syndrome	✓	

that elderly patients with dementia treated with atypical neuroleptics are at 1.6–1.7 times increased risk for mortality, most commonly from infectious and cardiovascular causes, and all atypical neuroleptics carry a black box warning to this effect. An independent meta-analysis (Schneider et al. 2005) confirmed this finding and also suggested that typical neuroleptics such as haloperidol are associated with equal or greater mortality risk in this population. Although six double-blind, placebo-controlled clinical trials of risperidone or olanzapine for psychosis found "modest statistical efficacy" (Sink et al. 2005), a recent large, placebo-controlled trial of risperidone, olanzapine, and quetiapine found that although subjects were less likely to stop risperidone or olanzapine due to lack of efficacy, benefit disappeared when subjects who stopped the study medication due to adverse events were taken into account (Schneider et al. 2006).

Nevertheless, neuroleptics have an important role in the treatment of psychosis in dementia, but only in some circumstances. Many patients do not respond adequately to nonpharmacological interventions. Despite concerns about adverse effects, research and clinical experience do indicate that at least a sub-

Table 12–4. Typical initial and maximum doses of neuroleptics for treatment of psychotic symptoms in dementia

Neuroleptic	Typical initial dosage range (mg/day)	Typical maximum dosage range (mg/day)
Haloperidol	0.25–0.5	1–2
Risperidone	0.25–0.5	1–2
Olanzapine	2.5	10–12.5
Quetiapine	12.5–25	150–200

set of dementia patients both benefit from and tolerate neuroleptic treatment. Rabins and Lyketsos (2005) have outlined the three circumstances in which neuroleptic treatment of psychosis in dementia is indicated: 1) when identifiable risk of harm to patient or others is present, 2) when distress caused by symptoms is significant, and 3) when nonpharmacological treatment interventions have been unsuccessful and symptom relief is important.

An open discussion of indications, benefits, risks, and alternatives should occur with the caregiver and/or patient prior to initiating treatment. Starting doses should be low (e.g., haloperidol 0.25 mg/day po; quetiapine 12.5 mg/day po), with slow increases as needed. Table 12–4 indicates common starting and maximum dosages of neuroleptics for which published studies in dementia exist. The need for continued treatment must be reassessed frequently, with regular attempts to taper or stop the medication, or with a clear rationale for continued use.

Update on Mr. Clark

Mr. Clark's physician scheduled an extended appointment with Mrs. Clark to educate her about the nature of delusions in dementia and the importance of not arguing or rationalizing with Mr. Clark when he is delusional. The physician referred her to a geriatric social worker with experience in working with dementia patients to assist in developing strategies to respond to her husband's behavior. During this counseling, Mrs. Clark mentioned that she and her husband used to ballroom dance, and she discovered that putting on music and dancing together in the late afternoon often prevented or minimized the emergence of delusions about needing to "go home" or find the train station. She found reminiscing about his father with a scrapbook a much more effective strategy than trying to convince him that his father was deceased. Sometimes while looking at the scrapbook, he would cry and ask where his father was; she would hold his hand silently until his crying ceased and then announce that it was time for coffee.

Six months later, Mr. Clark's delusions became more severe and were only mildly relieved by the recommended strategies. Several times, he raised his fists at Mrs. Clark in a threatening manner. After a discussion about the risks and benefits of neuroleptic treatment, she and the physician agreed that a trial was warranted. Mr. Clark started taking risperidone 0.25 mg/day po, and at a dosage of 0.75 mg/day po, his symptoms improved and he experienced no side effects. After another 6 months, risperidone was successfully tapered and discontinued, and the previously mentioned nonpharmacological interventions again sufficed.

Apathy

"She just sits in a chair and does nothing all day," says Mr. Benson during a routine follow-up for his wife, who has moderate-stage Alzheimer disease. "I take her out for lunch and shopping, but within a half hour she says she's had enough and is ready to go home. I even tried to enroll her in adult day care, but she refused to get in the van. Her friends say that as long as she seems content, I should respect her decision to just sit around. But my daughter says it hurts to see her mother like this, and that it's as if the joy of life has gone out of her eyes."

Diagnostic Considerations

Apathy is the most common neuropsychiatric symptom of dementia and may be the earliest presenting feature in dementias in the elderly. The apathy syndrome includes a decrease in motivation and initiative, emotional blunting and indifference, and impaired ability to persist in activities (Marin 1991). It can present alone and/or as a symptom of another syndrome (e.g., depression). The lack of interest and motivation from apathy may be interpreted by some as a problem warranting medical assessment; others may see it as a choice to be respected, or as an inevitable and untreatable consequence of the dementia process. It can be challenging for clinicians to decide whether reassurance is more appropriate than pharmacotherapy or behavioral interventions.

Clinical Assessment

Inquiry about depressive symptoms is crucial in the diagnosis of an apathy syndrome. In addition, although depressed patients often appear distressed by their symptoms, apathetic patients often appear content. Mr. Benson's report that his wife appeared content would thus be more supportive of apathy than depression. As commonly occurs with apathy in dementia, he and his children are more distressed by these behaviors than is the patient.

Executive dysfunction syndromes, reviewed in the following section, often include apathy. Many medical conditions cause or contribute to apathy in dementia. Medically frail patients often have low vitality and diminished motivation. The clinician needs to ensure that decreased activity due to pain or discomfort is not mistaken for apathy. The evaluation of a patient with recent onset of apathy should include laboratory studies; anemia, metabolic abnormalities, and hypothyroidism are among the medical conditions that can cause apathy.

Treatment

Often, the most beneficial intervention is education of the caregiver about the nature of apathy as a common feature of dementia. Understanding apathy as a part of the disease process can lessen the caregiver's frustration and bewilderment. In more severe cases, with accompanying risk such as physical deconditioning, treatment trials are warranted. Because of the limited knowledge of effective pharmacotherapies for apathy, nonpharmacological interventions should be attempted first in all but the most severe cases.

Caregivers can benefit from brainstorming with a professional to devise behavioral strategies to encourage increased activity for patients. For example, arguing with or exhorting a dementia patient about the importance of engaging in an activity is rarely helpful and can exacerbate both the patient's and caregiver's distress. Techniques that caregivers may find helpful include offering gentle commands instead of requests (e.g., "You need to come this way. The van (to day care) is waiting," instead of "Won't you please get in the van now?") and offering single instead of multiple options ("I need your help drying the dishes," instead of "Would you prefer to wash or dry the dishes tonight?"). Having an activity set up in advance (e.g., a card table arranged for gin rummy; coat and gloves laid out for the daily walk) can be helpful. Sometimes caregivers will still encounter much resistance. There needs to be a balance between ensuring the patient remains engaged and avoiding persistent, futile prodding. Caregivers are advised to choose their battles wisely (e.g., getting the patient in the day care van, but forgoing help with the dishes), and a nurse or social work counselor with dementia expertise can prove valuable in this regard. Successfully engaging patients in any stimulating activity may in turn have the additional positive effect of decreasing apathy. Politis et al. (2004) found that apathy in dementia patients in long-term care improved with mental stimulation, and the benefit was seen whether patients were assigned to a "mental stimulation kit" intervention or a control "social visit."

Pharmacotherapeutic interventions are difficult to recommend with confidence, but empirical treatment trials may be indicated when behavioral interventions are unsuccessful or the apathy is so severe that the patient refuses to get out of bed.

The most consistent evidence for benefit, and the only evidence based on placebo-controlled studies, is for cholinesterase inhibitors (Mizrahi and Starkstein 2007). Unfortunately, the benefit is typically small, and the positive studies were not designed to measure apathy as a primary outcome. Nevertheless, cholinesterase inhibitors are standard care for many patients with dementia, and some apathetic patients may have the extra benefit of improvement in this behavior. Several other agents have been investigated at the case-study level, although not specifically in patients with dementia. These agents, most of which enhance dopamine transmission (putatively associated with apathy) include amantadine (Marin et al. 1995), bupropion (Corcoran et al. 2004), and methylphenidate (Padala et al. 2007). Potential pharmacological treatments and their dose ranges are displayed in Table 12–5.

Update on Mrs. Benson

Mrs. Benson's physician scheduled a meeting with Mr. Benson and his daughter. At this meeting, it came to light that Mr. Benson himself was not as distressed by his wife's apathy as he initially appeared; rather, he was feeling guilty in the setting of his daughter's frequent implications that he was at fault for "allowing mom to wither away." The neurologist discussed the nature of apathy in dementia and described how apathy is part of the disease course for many patients. Both Mr. Benson and his daughter were receptive to trying suggested behavioral strategies. Mr. Benson discovered that his wife was more amenable to activities when he used gentle commands and avoided giving choices, and

Table 12–5.   Typical starting and maximum doses of putative treatments for apathy in dementia

Agent	Starting dosage (mg/day)	Maximum dosage (mg/day)
Cholinesterase inhibitors		
Donepezil	5	10
Galantamine	8	16–24
Rivastigmine (patch)	4.6	9.5
Amantadine	50	300
Bupropion extended release	150	450
Methylphenidate	2.5–5	20

he was thus able to achieve her going to day care at least three-quarters of the time. A trial of donepezil was begun as part of standard dementia care. Over the next 6 months, Mrs. Benson experienced some slowing of cognitive decline but no improvement in apathy, which remained a persistent but manageable symptom over the next several years.

Executive Dysfunction Syndrome

"He embarrasses me," complains Mrs. Roland to the psychiatrist following her 57-year-old husband with early-stage frontotemporal dementia. "Whenever we go to the store, he makes rude comments to other customers, especially women, about their physical appearance. The night he made a vulgar gesture toward a waitress, I wanted to crawl under the table. The waitress laughed and told me privately that as a 70-year-old woman, she was flattered, but how can I take him anyplace now? At home, he paces a lot, laughs for no reason, and says ridiculous things. Some day, I know he'll need long-term care, but what assisted living facility would even take him like this?"

Overview

Mrs. Roland's description of her husband's sexually inappropriate behavior, disinhibited comments, and frequent pacing suggests an executive dysfunction syndrome. Such syndromes, related to disruption of frontal-subcortical circuits, are less common in dementia than are depression, psychosis, and apathy, although apathy can be a feature of executive dysfunction syndrome. When these syndromes do occur, they distress and embarrass caregivers and can present a safety hazard, and injury from restless pacing or a slap in the face from an offended party may result.

Diagnostic Considerations

Executive dysfunction syndrome can present in a variety of ways and usually involves some combination of disinhibition and stimulus boundedness. Examples of symptoms in this cluster include apathy, sexually inappropriate behavior, pacing, silly comments, ingestion of nonfood objects, and perseverative repetition of phrases. Although executive dysfunction syndrome can occur in all dementias, it is especially common in dementias with prominent frontal-subcortical involvement such as the frontotemporal dementias and Huntington disease. Because these dementias often affect younger persons such as Mr. Roland, the behaviors are sometimes interpreted as volitional and reflecting character traits or moral flaws.

Clinical Assessment

Apathy is the most common symptom, followed by inappropriate, disinhibited behaviors, which frequently co-occur with diminished motivation and initiative. Family members may feel embarrassed and ashamed when discussing patients' disinhibited and inappropriate behavior, particularly when it is sexual in nature. The physician should emphasize that these symptoms are not uncommon in dementia and nearly always relate to the brain disease. The physician should inquire about a wide range of disinhibited and perseverative behaviors, including disinhibited comments and gestures, perseverative behaviors (pacing, repetition of a phrase), physical intrusiveness, stimulus boundedness (reaching for and grabbing at items), and sexually inappropriate behavior. The disinhibited and hypersexual behaviors characteristic of executive dysfunction syndrome can resemble mania or hypomania.

True mania is rare in dementias of the elderly (Lyketsos et al. 2000). Dementias in which mania is more common include Huntington disease and dementia due to HIV. Nevertheless, associated symptoms such as fast or pressured speech, increased vital sense, and grandiosity should raise suspicion for a manic syndrome, particularly in patients with a premorbid history of bipolar affective disorder. Neurosyphilis is another consideration. Hypersexual behavior in the absence of other associated symptoms raises suspicion for a primary disorder of sexual drive instead of a syndrome of executive dyscontrol. Further workup, such as assessing testosterone levels and endocrinological consultation, may be indicated in such circumstances.

Treatment

The approach to treating executive dysfunction is in many ways similar to that for apathy. In both situations, the physician is faced with behaviors that cause significant distress and for which no consistently effective pharmacological or nonpharmacological treatment is available. The physician must assess symptom severity and disruptiveness to determine whether intervention is needed beyond education of the caregiver about the syndrome, including ensuring that the caregiver is aware that these symptoms, while often embarrassing, are not under voluntary control. In Mr. Roland's case, the symptoms are frequent, are disruptive, and cause distress, indicating the appropriateness of further intervention. Given the paucity of evidence for effective pharmacotherapy, nonpharmacological interventions are typically the first approach. For example, if the patient makes inappropriate comments in public, planning a stroll and picnic in a quiet park may be more suitable than dinner in a restaurant followed by a trip to the mall. If the patient touches himself inappropriately, one-piece outfits may decrease this behavior. Patients who pace and wander may benefit from having a secure area where they can pace with minimal risk. Frequent and severe pacing is also an indication to consider a secured living setting, where units are often laid out specifically to address this behavior.

Despite lack of evidence for effective pharmacotherapy, severe symptoms may warrant empirical medication trials. Case reports and some clinic experience suggest benefit in executive dysfunction syndrome from a variety of pharmacological agents (Table 12–6), including SSRIs, mood stabilizers such as valproic acid, stimulants, neuroleptics, and amantadine (Drayton et al. 2004). Antiandrogen therapies (e.g., flutamide) may be helpful in dealing with severe hypersexual behavior.

Update on Mr. Roland

After discussion with the psychiatrist, Mrs. Roland decided to stop taking her husband to public places such as restaurants. She enlisted the help of male friends to watch him so she could continue to socialize on her own. Over the next year, Mr. Roland's behaviors became more severe. His pacing became nearly constant, and the disinhibited sexual comments became coarser and more frequent. Following a counseling session with his tearful wife, the psychiatrist prescribed amantadine, starting at 50 mg/day po. At 100 mg bid, Mr. Roland's pacing and sexual behaviors improved, but the drug was stopped due to severe hallucinations. Mrs. Roland subsequently decided to place her husband in a secured assisted living setting. Over the ensuing months, his sexual behaviors increased further, and he began to inappropriately touch other residents. The evening he was found undressed and aggressively fondling a female resident in her room, he was discharged to an emergency room and from there to an inpatient neuropsychiatry specialty unit. His testosterone level was normal. A trial of flutamide was begun, and Mr. Roland's sexual behaviors abated to the point that he was again manageable in assisted living.

Agitation and Aggression

> Almost immediately after arrival on the nursing home unit, Dr. Smith is approached by a nurse. "A woman named Mrs. Colby was admitted last night. She has dementia and is agitated. She is striking at staff, and last night she punched a resident in the back. She needs something to calm her down."

Diagnostic Considerations

There is no clearly defined "agitation syndrome." These symptoms are typically nonspecific. Potential causes include the primary dementing process, other psychiatric syndromes such as depression and psychosis, a medical problem (e.g., delirium, pain), and provoking factors in the environment or caregiver approach. These causes, with examples and suggested interventions, are listed in Table 12–7.

Clinical Assessment

A systematic process of evaluating agitated dementia patients has been formulated by Rabins et al. (2006) and is referred to as "the 4 Ds": Describe, Decode, Devise, Determine. The physician must first accurately *describe* the behavior. The differential diagnosis and workup for a patient who is tearful, irritable, yelling out, pacing, and suspicious much of the day, for example, will likely be dif-

Table 12–6.   Possibly effective agents for executive dysfunction syndrome

Agent	Starting dosage (mg/day)	Maximum dosage (mg/day)
SSRIs		
Sertraline	25	150
Citalopram	10	60
Escitalopram	5	20
Fluoxetine	10	40
Paroxetine	10	40
Mood stabilizers		
Valproic acid	250 (divided bid)	1,000–1,500
Carbamazepine	50–100	300
Amantadine	50–100	300
Bupropion	150 (extended release)	450
Methylphenidate	2.5–5	20

Note.   SSRI = selective serotonin reuptake inhibitor.

ferent from those of a patient who is usually calm and pleasant but strikes at caregivers when dressed or toileted. Having formulated a precise description of the behavior, the physician attempts to *decode* the cause among the various contributors listed in Table 12–7. Multiple contributing factors are often present. The physician relies on his or her formulation of the likely etiology (or etiologies) to *devise* a treatment plan. Follow-up is crucial to *determine* the effectiveness of the intervention, with adjustments in the patient's care plan as needed.

Treatment

Treatment is guided by the presumed cause(s) of the behavior. If a psychiatric syndrome such as depression or psychosis is suspected, treating these syndromes often results in full remission of the behavior. Similarly, treating the putative medical condition (e.g., using antibiotics for a urinary tract infection or analgesic for pain) can result in similar improvement. When environmental or caregiver approach factors contribute to the behavior, consultation by a clinician with expertise in dementia care can be helpful. Such clinicians can counsel caregivers on ways to modify these provoking factors (see Table 12–7).

If agitation or aggression poses a safety threat to the patient or others, the physician may need to temporarily prescribe a psychotropic medication to manage the behavior while the comprehensive evaluation is under way. Negligible evidence-based guidance exists, but neuroleptics or benzodiazepines at low dosages (e.g., risperidone 0.25 mg/day po or lorazepam 0.25 mg/day) are commonly used. These may be administered as needed or as a standing dose, depending on symptom severity. When no clear etiology is identified or the symptoms persist despite addressing of the presumed cause, empirical trials of pharmacotherapy may be indicated. Neuroleptics are most commonly used, especially for physical aggression. Most of the previously discussed neuroleptic clinical trials included subjects with nonspecific agitation or with psychosis. SSRIs such as citalopram may have benefits similar to neuroleptics in treating these behaviors (Pollock et al. 2007). Anticonvulsants may reduce agitation and aggression in some patients (Porsteinsson et al. 2003), although several clinical trials have not demonstrated this benefit (Tariot et al. 2005). Although cholinesterase inhibitors may decrease agitation (Cummings et al. 2005), this effect is typically mild, and these agents should not be considered first-line treatments for severe agitation or aggression. Benzodiazepines should be avoided because of their association with tolerance and sedation and with increased risk of falls and confusion.

Update on Mrs. Colby

During Dr. Smith's examination, Mrs. Colby was irritable with intermittent tearfulness. She said, "I don't know who you are but get away from me!" Her MMSE score was 13 out of 30. Her physical examination was very limited because she attempted to strike the doctor. Dr. Smith obtained additional history from Mrs. Colby's son, who reported that these behaviors had been increasing over the past week and were similar to those occurring during a bout of pneumonia she had the prior year. Dr. Smith ordered a chemistry panel, complete blood count, chest X ray, and urinalysis and culture. The chest X ray was normal, but her white blood cell count was mildly elevated and the urine culture revealed a urinary tract infection. Dr. Smith began antibiotic treatment and also ordered lorazepam 0.25 mg po or im every 8 hours as needed for severe agitation, with a stop date in 2 weeks for reevaluation. Five days after admis-

Table 12–7. Potential causes of agitation and aggression in dementia

Etiology	Examples	Intervention
Primary disease process	1. Patient swings fists at staff when he cannot express his needs.	1. Provide picture board so patient can point to picture representing his need.
	2. Patient with agnosia is distraught when she sees her reflection in the mirror.	2. Remove or cover mirrors and other reflective surfaces.
Psychiatric syndrome	1. Patient meets criteria for depression of Alzheimer disease.	1. Treat with antidepressant.
	2. Patient is delusional that staff is trying to poison her.	2. Treat with neuroleptic.
Medical problem	1. Patient has urinary tract infection.	1. Treat with antibiotics.
	2. Patient with arthritis of his knees grimaces when walking.	2. Treat with analgesic.
Environmental factors	1. Patient becomes disruptive during shift changes, when there is commotion.	1. Engage her in activity far from nursing station during change of shift.
	2. Patient living at home is restless on days when home health aide is not present.	2. Increase frequency of home health aide visits.
Caregiver approach	1. Patient is physically aggressive with his daughter during morning care. She often rushes him due to time pressure.	1. Provide hands-on caregiver assessment and teaching by expert dementia care nurse.
	2. Caregiver frequently argues with or corrects patient.	2. Provide counseling session with physician to modify caregiver's approach.

sion, Mrs. Colby's son informed staff that he had forgotten to mention that his mother took acetaminophen twice daily for arthritis, and this treatment was reinstituted. When Mrs. Colby was reevaluated by Dr. Smith 2 weeks after admission, her aggression had resolved and she was calm and pleasant. Lorazepam had not been used in the preceding 5 days, and the order was not renewed. Dr. Smith attributed Mrs. Colby's improvement to several factors: treatment of a urinary tract infection that had caused mild delirium, reinstitution of her analgesic, and adjustment to her new living environment.

Key Clinical Points

- Although consistently effective treatments for neuropsychiatric symptoms are currently lacking, clinical experience suggests that most symptoms are treatable.
- Treatment strategies need to be comprehensive, employing nonpharmacological strategies in addition to pharmacotherapy.
- Many neuropsychiatric phenomena, including depression, psychosis, and apathy, may best be classified as syndromes.
- Effective pharmacotherapy for depression and psychosis has been demonstrated in double-blind clinical trials.
- Because of safety concerns, physicians need to carefully weigh risks and benefits of atypical neuroleptics when deciding how to treat patients with dementia.
- Although minimal evidence exists for effective treatments for apathy or executive dysfunction syndrome, a variety of nonpharmacological and pharmacological interventions may be beneficial.
- Agitation and aggression are nonspecific symptoms, and treatment strategies should be guided by the presumed cause of the behavior.

References

Alexopoulos GS, Abrams RC, Young RC, et al: Cornell Scale for Depression in Dementia. Biol Psychiatry 23:271–284, 1988

American Psychiatric Association: Diagnostic and Statistical Manual of Mental Disorders, 3rd Edition, Revised. Washington, DC, American Psychiatric Association, 1987

American Psychiatric Association: Diagnostic and Statistical Manual of Mental Disorders, 4th Edition, Text Revision. Washington, DC, American Psychiatric Association, 2000

Corcoran C, Wong ML, O'Keane V: Bupropion in the management of apathy. J Psychopharmacol 18:133–135, 2004

Cummings JL, Koumaras B, Chen M, et al: Effects of rivastigmine treatment on the neuropsychiatric and behavioral disturbances of nursing home residents with moderate to severe probable Alzheimer's disease: a 26-week, multicenter, open-label study. Am J Geriatr Pharmacother 3:137–148, 2005

Drayton SJ, Davies K, Steinberg M, et al: Amantadine for executive dysfunction syndrome in patients with dementia. Psychosomatics 45:205–209, 2004

Folstein MF, Folstein SE, McHugh PR: "Mini-mental state": a practical method for grading the cognitive state of patients for the clinician. J Psychiatr Res 12:189–198, 1975

Lyketsos CG, Olin J: Depression in Alzheimer's disease: an overview and treatment. Biol Psychiatry 52:243–252, 2002

Lyketsos C, Steinberg M, Tschanz JT, et al: Mental and behavioral disturbances in dementia: findings from the Cache County Study on Memory in Aging. Am J Psychiatry 157:708–714, 2000

Lyketsos CG, DelCampo L, Steinberg M, et al: Treating depression in Alzheimer's disease: efficacy and safety of sertraline therapy, and the benefits of depression reduction: the DIADS. Arch Gen Psychiatry 60:737–746, 2003

Marin RS: Apathy: a neuropsychiatric syndrome. J Neuropsychiatry Clin Neurosci 3:243–254, 1991

Marin RS, Biedrzycki RC, Firinciogullari S: Reliability and validity of the Apathy Evaluation Scale. Psychiatry Res 38:143–162, 1991

Marin RS, Fogel BS, Hawkins J, et al: Apathy: a treatable syndrome. J Neuropsychiatry Clin Neurosci 7:23–30, 1995

Mizrahi R, Starkstein SE: Epidemiology and management of apathy in patients with Alzheimer's disease. Drugs Aging 24:547–554, 2007

Padala PR, Burke WJ, Bhatia SC, et al: Treatment of apathy with methylphenidate. J Neuropsychiatry Clin Neurosci 19:81–83, 2007

Politis AM, Vozella S, Mayer LS, et al: A randomized, controlled clinical trial of activity therapy for apathy in patients with dementia residing in long-term care. Int J Geriatr Psychiatry 19:1087–1094, 2004

Pollock BG, Mulsant BH, Rosen J, et al: A double blind comparison of citalopram and risperidone for the treatment of behavioral and psychotic symptoms of dementia. Am J Geriatr Psychiatry 15:942–952, 2007

Porsteinsson AP, Tariot PN, Jakmiovich LJ, et al: Valproate therapy for agitation in dementia: open-label extension of a double-blind trial. Am J Geriatr Psychiatry 11:434–440, 2003

Rabins PV, Lyketsos CG: Antipsychotic drugs in dementia: what should be made of the risks? JAMA 294:1963–1965, 2005

Rabins PV, Lyketsos CG, Steele CD: Practical Dementia Care, 2nd Edition. New York, Oxford University Press, 2006

Rao V, Lyketsos CG: The benefits and risks of ECT for patients with primary dementia who also suffer from depression. Int J Geriatr Psychiatry 15:729–735, 2000

Schneider LS, Dagerman KS, Insel P: Risk of death with atypical antipsychotic drug treatment for dementia: meta-analysis of randomized placebo-controlled trials. JAMA 294:1934–1943, 2005

Schneider LS, Tariot PN, Dagerman KS, et al: Effectiveness of atypical antipsychotic drugs in patients with Alzheimer's disease. N Engl J Med 355:1525–1538, 2006

Sink KM, Holden KF, Yaffe K: Pharmacological treatment of neuropsychiatric symptoms of dementia: a review of the evidence. JAMA 293:596–608, 2005

Steinberg M: Alzheimer's disease, in Psychiatric Aspects of Neurological Diseases: Practical Approaches to Patient Care. Edited by Lyketsos CG, Rabins PV, Lipsey J, et al. New York, Oxford University Press, 2008, pp 217–233

Tariot PN, Raman R, Jakimovich L, et al: Divalproex sodium in nursing home residents with possible or probable Alzheimer disease complicated by agitation: a randomized clinical trial. Am J Geriatr Psychiatry 13:942–949, 2005

Teri L, Logsdon RG, Uomoto J, et al: Behavioral treatment of depression in dementia patients: a controlled clinical trial. J Gerontol B Psychol Sci Soc Sci 52:P159–P166, 1997

Teri L, Gibbons LE, McCurry SM, et al: Exercise plus behavioral management in patients with Alzheimer's disease. JAMA 290:2015–2022, 2003

Tractenberg RE, Weiner MF, Patterson MB, et al: Comorbidity of psychopathological domains in community-dwelling persons with Alzheimer's disease. J Geriatr Psychiatry Neurol 16:94–99, 2003

U.S. Food and Drug Administration: Risperdal (risperidone). Dear Healthcare Professional Letter, April 16, 2003. Available at: http://www.fda.gov/Safety/MedWatch/SafetyInformation/SafetyAlertsforHumanMedicalProducts/ucm168933.htm. Accessed November 4, 2011.

U.S. Food and Drug Administration: Public Health Advisory: Deaths with antipsychotics in elderly patients with behavioral disturbances. April 11, 2005. Available at: http://www.fda.gov/Drugs/DrugSafety/PostmarketDrugSafetyInformationforPatientsandProviders/DrugSafetyInformationforHeathcareProfessionals/PublicHealthAdvisories/ucm053171.htmAccessed November 4, 2011.

Weintraub D, Rosenberg PB, Drye LT, et al: Sertraline for the treatment of depression in Alzheimer disease: week-24 outcomes. Am J Geriatr Psychiatry 18:332–340, 2010

Zubenko GS, Zubenko WN, Mcpherson S, et al: A collaborative study of the emergence and clinical features of major depressive syndrome of Alzheimer disease. Am J Psychiatry 160:857–866, 2003

Further Reading

McCurry SM: When a Family Member Has Dementia: Steps to Becoming a Resilient Caregiver. Westport, CT, Greenwood Publishing Group, 2006

Rabins PV, Lyketsos CG, Steele CD: Practical Dementia Care, 2nd Edition. New York, Oxford University Press, 2006

13

Pharmacological Treatment of Neuropsychiatric Symptoms

Roy Yaari, M.D., M.A.S.

Pierre N. Tariot, M.D.

Danielle F. Richards

Up to 90% of patients with dementia will develop significant behavioral problems in the course of their illness (Tariot et al. 1993). These behavioral changes are major features of dementia and require a thoughtful appreciation of their phenomenology, assessment, and management. Examples of the behavioral manifestations of dementia are features suggestive of depression, mania, anxiety, psychosis, apathy, and agitation. There have been efforts to propose syndromal criteria for "psychosis" (Jeste and Finkel 2000) and "depression" of Alzheimer disease, but these proposed criteria have not been validated. Cohen-Mansfield and Billig (1986) defined agitation as "inappropriate verbal, vocal, or motor activity unexplained by apparent needs or confusion" (p. 712). This pragmatic definition emphasizes the clinician's responsibility to presume that the behaviors have some meaning. Shouting or striking out during care should not be dismissed as "agitation" that mandates psychotropic therapy when a specific behavioral intervention might be identified. The behavioral changes seen in dementia tend to occur in clusters that may vary among patients and within patients over time, presumably reflecting the complex interaction between cognitive deficits and environmental variables. These clusters can be used as guides in the selection of appropriate therapy. No pharmacological therapy, however, has been approved by the U.S. Food and Drug Administration (FDA) for treatment of psychopathology associated with dementia; clinicians must approach these symptoms on a case-by-case basis.

A Rational Approach to Evaluation

Articulating a logical approach to the evaluation and management of psychopathology in dementia is by itself therapeutic, because it offers reassurance to families and caregivers that a confusing situation can be clarified, understood, and helped. The approach proposed here is summarized in Figure 13–1 (Tariot 1999).

Nonpharmacological Interventions

Nonpharmacological interventions can include making efforts to cue or reorient the person in a manner that is not frustrating; ensuring that the environment is comfortable and permits safe physical activity while providing visual cues; avoiding excessive stress or demands; maintaining a regular schedule of pleasant events; and optimizing interpersonal variables (e.g., by simplifying language, avoiding negative statements, and avoiding confrontation). Cohen-Mansfield (2001) offered an overview of approaches, such as including music, pet therapy, massage, recordings of familiar persons' voices, and walking programs. Most physicians are not accustomed to implementing these approaches, which do require a degree of familiarity and need to be tailored to each situation. It is therefore helpful to partner with others to assist in formulating a care plan and to learn how to formulate the plan more independently over time. The collaborating health professionals may vary depending on the community and the specific need and can include nurses, social workers, psychologists or neuropsychologists, occupational therapists, speech therapists, or physical therapists. Psychiatrists have historically functioned well as members of interdisciplinary teams; dementia care affords an ideal opportunity for this type of collaborative care.

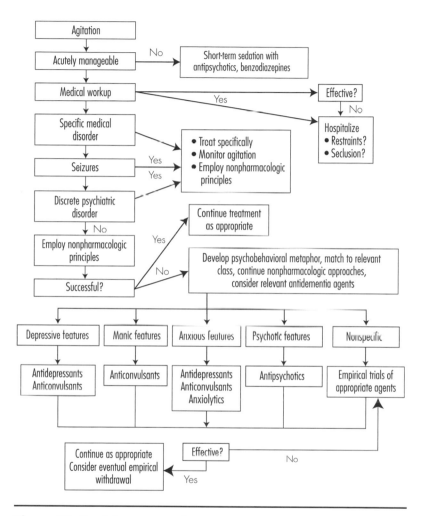

Figure 13–1. Management of agitation in dementia.

Source. Reprinted from Tariot PN: "Treatment of Agitation in Dementia." *Journal of Clinical Psychiatry* 60 (suppl 8):11–20, 1999. Copyright 2009, Physicians Postgraduate Press, Inc. Used with permission.

Pharmacological Interventions

General Precepts

When working with patients who have nonemergent problems for which non-pharmacological interventions have been exhausted, we begin with a definition of a target symptom pattern analogous to a drug-responsive syndrome. We then match the dominant target symptoms to the most relevant drug class. This approach reflects consensus guidelines (Alexopoulos et al. 2004) but has not been established empirically.

We select a medication with at least some empirical evidence of efficacy and with the highest likelihood of tolerability and safety. We employ low dosages and escalate slowly, assessing target symptoms as well as toxicity. If a psychotropic is helpful, an empirical trial is often performed in reverse at an appropriate time and the patient is monitored for recurrence of the problem, an approach mandated in the nursing home setting in the United States by federal regulations created in 1987 (Health Care Financing Administration 1992). Sometimes several medications need to be tried in series before a successful one is identified, sometimes combinations are warranted, and sometimes no medication is helpful.

Antipsychotic Medications

Within the context of the symptomatic approach, antipsychotics would be used first for treatment of agitation with psychotic features. There are two main classes of antipsychotics: so-called conventional antipsychotics and the newer atypical agents.

Conventional Antipsychotics

Schneider et al. (1990) published a meta-analysis of clinical trials of conventional antipsychotics in patients with dementia, finding that, on average, 59% of patients treated with active medication showed behavioral improvement versus 41% of those receiving placebo, only an 18% drug-placebo difference. Lanctôt et al. (1998) performed a more recent meta-analysis of studies of conventional agents and reported an average therapeutic effect (antipsychotic vs. placebo) of 26% above placebo response rates, ranging from 19% to 50%. Side effects, which were reported to occur more often with drug than placebo (mean difference=25%), included akathisia, parkinsonism, tardive dyskinesia, sedation, peripheral and central anticholinergic effects, postural hypotension, cardiac conduction defects, and falls.

Lonergan et al. (2002), in a pooled analysis of five randomized trials of haloperidol versus placebo, found decreased aggression but not significant improvement in agitated symptoms overall among the haloperidol group. This group also had a significant increase in adverse side effects such as rigidity and bradykinesia compared to the placebo group.

FDA warning about cerebrovascular adverse events and increased mortality with conventional antipsychotics. In view of the considerable toxicity of conventional agents, there was great hope that atypical antipsychotics would have special utility in patients with dementia. However, in April 2005, the FDA issued warnings regarding side effects of and mortality risk from atypical antipsychotics in patients with dementia, as discussed in the following section. Since that time, two studies have reported similar risks for dementia patients with conventional antipsychotic drugs, leading the FDA (U.S. Food and Drug Administration 2008) to issue a warning for these compounds. Gill et al. (2007) performed a retrospective cohort study of 27,259 persons with dementia age 66 years and older. The authors reported that atypical antipsychotics were associated with increased mortality as compared with no antipsychotic use as early as 30 days and persisting until study end at 180 days. The investigators found that conventional antipsychotic use showed a marginally higher risk of death compared with atypical antipsychotic use. Schneeweiss et al. (2007) performed a retrospective analysis of 37,241 persons, age 65 and older, who were prescribed conventional (12,882) or atypical (24,359) antipsychotic medications for any reason. The investigators compared the 180-day all-cause mortality rate with use of a conventional antipsychotic versus an atypical antipsychotic. They found that the risk of death in the group of patients who had been treated with conventional antipsychotic medications was comparable to, or possibly greater than, the risk of death in the group of patients treated with atypical antipsychotic medications.

Atypical Antipsychotics

Clozapine. Clozapine is the prototype atypical drug for treatment of schizophrenia, with arguably the lowest rate of motor toxicity and with established efficacy in patients who are refractory to other therapies. However, only case series have been reported for patients with dementia (Rosenquist et al. 2000; Tariot 1999). These studies suggest a starting dosage of about 12.5 mg/day, with maintenance dosages of 12.5–50 mg/day. The limited literature emphasizes potential side effects such as sedation, ataxia, falls, and delirium. Clozapine has a significant risk of agranulocytosis (about 1%), which is more common in elderly than in younger patients, and regular monitoring of blood counts is required at least weekly for the first 6 months of continuous treatment, every other week for the following 6 months, and every 4 weeks thereafter if blood counts remain acceptable. Clozapine has also been associated with an increased risk of diabetes and worsening lipid profiles in younger people, but data are not available for elderly adults (American Diabetes Association et al. 2004). The risk of toxicity, the need for monitoring white blood cell counts, and the lack of efficacy data limit the utility of this agent in patients with dementia, although it does have a role in patients with movement disorders who have not had any response to other agents (Parkinson Study Group 1999).

Risperidone. Risperidone has been studied more extensively than other psychotropics in patients with dementia. Preliminary studies of dosages from 0.5 to 5 mg/day suggested that dosages of 0.5–2 mg/day might be tolerated best. Three placebo-controlled trials have been conducted in nursing home patients. The first two trials were 3 months in duration and included patients with Alzheimer disease and/or vascular dementia who experienced agitation, psychotic features, or both.

The first compared risperidone at dosages of 0.5, 1, and 2 mg/day with placebo (Katz et. al. 1999). Extrapyramidal features emerged in approximately 22% of subjects at the dosage of 2 mg/day, with a trend toward peripheral edema and dose-related sedation, and apparently good tolerability and safety. Using an a priori definition of clinical response as a 50% reduction in the total score on a behavioral rating scale, Katz and colleagues (1999) found that 33% of patients in the placebo group improved, as did a similar percentage of patients receiving 0.5 mg/day, 45% of those receiving 1 mg/day, and 50% of those receiving 2 mg/day. The treatment effects were statistically significant for the 1- and 2-mg/day dosages. Subscale scores indicated beneficial effects on both measures of psychosis and measures of verbal and physical aggression.

The second trial compared placebo with risperidone or haloperidol given in flexible doses (0.5–4 mg/day) in nursing home residents with dementia accompanied by agitation and/or psychosis (De Deyn et al. 1999). The mean total daily doses used were 1.1 mg of risperidone and 1.2 mg of haloperidol. No significant difference was found between the treatments on a global measure of psychopathology. Secondary analyses showed no effect for either of the active treatments relative to placebo on measures of psychosis, although a positive effect was found for both active treatments on measures of aggression. Incidence of extrapyramidal adverse events was 11% for patients receiving placebo, 15% for those taking risperidone, and 22% for those taking haloperidol. Sedation occurred more frequently for patients taking haloperidol (18.3%) and risperidone (12.2%) than for those given placebo (4.4%).

Brodaty et al. (2003) conducted a randomized, double-blind, placebo-controlled trial in nursing home patients with Alzheimer disease, vascular dementia, or mixed dementia with significant aggressive behaviors. Patients were randomly assigned to receive placebo or flexible dosing of risperidone solution up to a maximum of 2 mg/day for 12 weeks. The mean total daily dose was 1 mg. Significant improvement in the risperidone group was seen in scores on the Cohen-Mansfield Agitation Inventory (Cohen-Mansfield 1986) and on secondary measures, including the Clinical Global Impression—Severity (CGI-S) and Clinical Global Impression—Change (CGI-C) scales (Guy 1976). Common adverse events were somnolence and urinary tract infection in risperidone-treated patients and agitation in placebo-treated patients.

Subsequent reviews yielded similar results. An 18-week randomized, double-blind, crossover comparison of risperidone and haloperidol in Korean patients with dementia and behavioral disturbances showed that risperidone had a favorable efficacy and tolerability profile (Suh et al. 2004). A post hoc analysis of this study found that risperidone was more effective than haloperidol in treating aggression. Researchers also found that risperidone was significantly more effective in treating physical sexual advances, pacing, wandering, intentional falling, hoarding, verbal and physical repetition, and general negativism (Suh et al. 2006). Overall, the efficacy of risperidone appears to be equivalent to that of haloperidol.

Olanzapine.   Street et al. (2000) reported a 6-week, randomized, parallel-group, multicenter study in nursing home residents who had dementia complicated by agitation, psychosis, or both, and who were treated with olanzapine 5, 10, or 15 mg/day versus placebo for 6 weeks. In patients receiving 5 or 10 mg/ day, significant improvement compared with placebo was seen, as defined by >50% reduction from the baseline sum of the Agitation/Aggression, Hallucinations, and Delusions items of the Neuropsychiatric Inventory—Nursing Home version. Sedation and postural instability were observed at all dosages in at least 25% of subjects.

Meehan et al. (2002) studied acute treatment of agitation with intramuscular olanzapine in inpatients or nursing home residents with Alzheimer disease and/or vascular dementia. Patients were given up to three injections of olanzapine 2.5 mg or 5.0 mg, lorazepam 1.0 mg or 0.5 mg, or placebo and assessed within a 24-hour period. Olanzapine was superior to placebo in treating agitation at 2 hours and 24 hours. Lorazepam was superior to placebo at 2 hours but not at 24 hours. Adverse events were not significantly different between groups.

De Deyn et al. (2004) randomly assigned Alzheimer patients with delusions or hallucinations to receive placebo or fixed-dose olanzapine (1.0, 2.5, 5.0, or 7.5 mg/day) in a 10-week double-blind study. Significant improvement in psychotic symptoms was seen in the 7.5-mg olanzapine group compared with the placebo group. On the CGI-C, the greatest improvement was seen in the 2.5-mg olanzapine group. The olanzapine groups had significant differences in increased weight, anorexia, and urinary incontinence, but no significant difference in extrapyramidal symptoms compared with placebo.

Quetiapine.   Quetiapine is widely used in patients with dementia because of its relative lack of extrapyramidal effects. A 10-week multicenter placebo-controlled trial of quetiapine versus haloperidol was conducted in elderly nursing home patients with psychosis (Tariot et al. 2006). Most subjects had dementia. Flexible doses of the medication were permitted; the mean total daily dose of haloperidol was 2 mg at endpoint, whereas that of quetiapine was about 120 mg. None of the treatment groups differed with respect to reduction in measures of psychosis, which was the primary outcome of the trial. One of the secondary measures of agitation showed improvement with both the haloperidol and the quetiapine treatments. Rates of somnolence were 25.3% for quetiapine, 36.2% for haloperidol, and 4.1% for placebo. Serious adverse events occurred in approximately 15% of participants in the quetiapine, haloperidol, and placebo groups. Parkinsonian features were most prevalent in the haloperidol group; other safety and tolerability measures differed little among groups.

This study led to a second placebo-controlled trial of quetiapine in agitated nursing home residents with dementia (Zhong et al. 2007). In this 10-week double-blind study, patients were randomly assigned to a fixed-dose trial of quetiapine 100 or 200 mg/day. Titration was relatively rapid, with 100 mg/day achieved by day 4 and 200 mg/day by day 8. Quetiapine at 200 mg/day was associated with significant improvement on the Excitement Component subscale of the Positive and Negative Syndrome Scale (Kay et al. 1987), the primary outcome, as well as on several secondary outcomes; at the 100-mg/day dosage, no significant improvement was seen on the primary outcome. Incidents of cerebrovascular adverse events, postural hypotension, and falls were similar among groups.

Ballard et al. (2005) performed a 26-week randomized, double-blind, placebo-controlled trial assessing quetiapine and rivastigmine in institutionalized patients with dementia and severe agitation. Neither quetiapine nor rivastigmine was effective. In another randomized, double-blind, placebo-controlled clinical trial involving patients with dementia, agitation, and parkinsonism, Kurlan et al. (2007) found that quetiapine (mean total daily dose = 120 mg) was well tolerated and did not worsen parkinsonism but did not show significant benefits for treating agitation or psychosis.

Ziprasidone.   Rocha et al. (2006) conducted a 7-week open-label trial testing the effects of low-dose ziprasidone on agitation and other behavioral symptoms of dementia in 25 patients. By the end of the trial, only 15 patients remained; the main reasons for discontinuation were numerous adverse events, including somnolence, gastrointestinal symptoms, and parkinsonism. The mean total Neuropsychiatric Inventory (NPI; Cummings et al. 1994) score fell significantly, and the NPI score for caregiver burden showed significant improvement in distress. These limited data are insufficient to inform practice.

Aripiprazole.   In a 10-week placebo-controlled trial of aripiprazole for outpatients meeting clinical criteria for psychosis of Alzheimer disease (Jeste and Finkel 2000), dosages ranged from 2 to 15 mg/day; the mean total daily dose at endpoint was about 10 mg (De Deyn 2005). Titration occurred slowly over a period of weeks. The primary outcome, the NPI Psychosis subscale rating, did not show a difference between drug and placebo, although there was a suggestion of behavioral benefit on some secondary measures. The medication was generally well tolerated, with numerically more frequent sedation in the active treatment group.

Two placebo-controlled studies of aripiprazole have been published. The first was a placebo-controlled study of fixed-dose aripiprazole conducted in nursing home residents with dementia and psychotic features (Mintzer et al. 2007). The only significant effect on measures of psychosis was found at the 10-mg/day dosage. The second placebo-controlled flexible-dose study, by Streim et al. (2008), involved nursing home residents with dementia. This study found no difference between aripiprazole at a mean total daily dose of 8.6 mg and placebo. Details are lacking from these studies regarding safety and secondary measures.

Meta-analysis of atypical antipsychotics.   The meta-analysis of Schneider et al. (2006b) included results from both published and publicly presented unpublished placebo-controlled studies. These 15 trials were generally 6–12 weeks long and included participants with dementia of varying types complicated by agitation and/or aggression and/or psychosis. The overall response rates for patients undergoing active treatment were 48%–65%, versus 30%–48% for those given placebo. On average, there was an incremental treatment benefit of about 18% for active drug over placebo; about 1 in 5 patients experienced significant improvement. Atypical antipsychotics were about three times as likely as placebo to cause adverse events, the most common being somnolence, falls with or without injury, syncope, parkinsonism, bruising, peripheral edema, and infections. The weight gain and metabolic concerns with use of atypical agents in younger populations have not been seen in the relatively brief studies conducted thus far in the elderly.

In a separate meta-analysis analyzing adverse events of atypical antipsychotics in patients with dementia, Schneider et al. (2006a) found that 1.9% of those who received the atypical drug reported cerebrovascular adverse events, versus 0.9% of those given placebo. In a meta-analysis of nine placebo-controlled trials of atypical antipsychotic agents, Ballard et al. (2006) found improved aggressive behavior with olanzapine versus placebo, but patients given olanzapine also had a significantly higher rate of cerebrovascular events and extrapyramidal effects.

In a pooled analysis of five double-blind randomized trials, Lee et al. (2004) compared two atypical antipsychotics (risperidone and olanzapine) with haloperidol and placebo in a total of 1,570 institutionalized patients, mostly with Alzheimer disease. Three trials found a statistically superior efficacy for drug to placebo. Two trials comparing risperidone with haloperidol found no statistically significant difference in efficacy. Substantial adverse events were also reported, including extrapyramidal symptoms and somnolence.

FDA warning about cerebrovascular adverse events and increased mortality with atypical antipsychotics. In October 2002, Health Canada issued a letter, based on four placebo-controlled trials of risperidone, stating that risperidone use may be associated with cerebrovascular adverse events in elderly patients with dementia (Wooltorton 2002). The data revealed that 4% (29 of 764) of risperidone-treated patients versus 2% (7 of 466) of patients receiving placebo had a cerebrovascular adverse event, defined as either a transient ischemic attack or stroke, including four deaths among risperidone-treated patients and one among placebo-treated patients. The effect was seen in only two of the four studies.

The FDA (U.S. Food and Drug Administration 2003) later issued a similar warning for risperidone use in patients with dementia. Studies also have shown an increase of cerebrovascular events from use of aripiprazole, olanzapine, and risperidone. In 2004, Eli Lilly released a warning of increased risk of cerebrovascular events in dementia patients treated with olanzapine. They found the incidence with olanzapine (1.3%) to be triple that with placebo (0.4%), with a concomitant increase in mortality (3.5% vs. 1.5%) (U.S. Food and Drug Administration 2004).

In placebo-controlled trials of aripiprazole in psychosis of Alzheimer disease (two flexible-dose trials and one fixed-dose study), an increased incidence of stroke and transient ischemic attack, including fatalities, was seen in patients whose mean age was 84 years ("Abilify Prescribing Information" 2011). Although not directly reported in the prescribing information, data from a "Dear Doctor" letter from Bristol-Myers Squibb (2005) indicated that cerebrovascular events had occurred in 1.3% of aripiprazole-treated patients versus in 0.6% of placebo-treated patients. In the fixed-dose study, there was a statistically significant dose-response relationship for cerebrovascular events.

Data on quetiapine use for patients with dementia are limited compared with those on use of risperidone, olanzapine, or aripiprazole. No specific warning has been released for quetiapine.

Later, the FDA reviewed 17 placebo-controlled trials performed with olanzapine, aripiprazole, risperidone, and quetiapine in elderly patients with dementia and behavioral disorders. A 1.6- to 1.7-fold increase in all-cause mortality rate was found. In 2005, the FDA required that the producers of olanzapine, aripiprazole, risperidone, quetiapine, clozapine, and ziprasidone provide black box warnings on packaging (U.S. Food and Drug Administration 2005). These results are consistent with the meta-analysis by Schneider et al. (2005) of randomized placebo-controlled trials of aripiprazole, olanzapine, quetiapine, and risperidone. The overall death rate was 3.5% for atypical antipsychotics versus 2.3% for placebo.

Other studies have shed further light on the possible link between atypical antipsychotics and increased mortality and cerebrovascular events, and have also addressed the question of conventional agents. In a population-based retrospective cohort study, Herrmann et al. (2004) failed to show a significant increase in the risk of stroke among patients receiving olanzapine or risperidone when compared with those initiating therapy with typical antipsychotics. Herrmann and Lanctôt (2005) conducted post hoc analyses of pooled data from 11 randomized controlled trials of risperidone and olanzapine in patients with dementia. The authors reported an increased risk of cerebrovascular adverse events in those taking atypical antipsychotics compared with placebo, but they added that some of the risk could be attributed to nonspecific events unrelated to strokes. Johnson & Johnson Pharmaceutical Research and Development collected data from six Phase II and III double-blind trials in elderly patients to analyze the mortality rate among the participants taking risperidone versus placebo. The mortality was 4.0% with risperidone versus 3.1% with placebo from trial initiation to within 30 days after discontinuation. No significant relationship was found between risperidone dose and mortality. In each trial, common adverse events associated with mortality were pneumonia, cardiac failure, and cerebrovascular disorder. Overall, a nonsignificant increase in mortality occurred during treatment with risperidone. Such inconclusive data have been echoed in numerous other studies (Haupt et al. 2006).

In a population-based retrospective cohort study, participants receiving atypical antipsychotics showed no increased risk of ischemic stroke compared with those receiving conventional antipsychotics (Gill et al. 2007).

Raivio et al. (2007) assessed the impact of atypical and conventional antipsychotics on mortality. The use of atypical antipsychotics (risperidone, olanzapine) showed a lower risk of mortality (32.1%) compared with conventional antipsychotics (45.3%) and no neuroleptic (49.6%). Therefore, neither the use of conventional antipsychotics nor the use of atypical antipsychotics increased mortality.

These warnings should be interpreted cautiously. The fact that deaths seem to occur for many different reasons suggests that any type of medication-induced impairment in elderly patients with dementia could tip the scales from vulnerability to death.

Clinical Antipsychotic Trials of Intervention Effectiveness—Alzheimer's Disease. In the Clinical Antipsychotic Trials of Intervention Effectiveness—Alzheimer's Disease (CATIE-AD) study, outpatients with Alzheimer disease and symptoms of psychosis and/or aggression were randomly assigned to treatment with olanzapine, risperidone, quetiapine, or placebo (Schneider et al. 2006b). The primary measure of effectiveness, time to discontinuation, did not differ significantly across the treatment conditions (approximately 5–8 weeks). The median time to discontinuation due to lack of efficacy was significantly longer with olanzapine and risperidone (22.1 and 26.7 weeks, respectively) than with quetiapine and placebo (9.1 and 9.0 weeks, respectively). Compared with placebo, the atypical antipsychotics were associated with a shorter time to discontinuation due to adverse events or intolerability. Intolerability accounted for discontinuations in 24% of patients receiving olanzapine, 18% receiving risperidone, 16% receiving quetiapine, and 5% receiving placebo.

Antidepressants

Trazodone

Case series and open trials suggest the benefit of trazodone, at dosages ranging from 50 to 400 mg/day, in treating behavioral and psychological symptoms in patients with dementia (Rosenquist et al. 2000). Symptoms of irritability, anxiety, restlessness, sleeplessness, and depressed affect have been reported to improve, although trazodone has side effects, including sedation, orthostatic hypotension, and occasional delirium. In a 9-week crossover study, Sultzer et al. (1997) compared trazodone at a mean total daily dose of 220 mg with haloperidol at a mean total daily dose of 2.5 mg in 28 patients. Agitation improved equally in both groups, with better tolerability in the trazodone group. A prior expert consensus guideline (Alexopoulos et al. 2004) had favored use of trazodone primarily to treat sleep disturbance, relegating it to second- or third-line use for "mild" agitation. A typical starting dosage would be 25 mg/day, with maximum dosages usually of 100–250 mg/day.

Selective Serotonin Reuptake Inhibitors

Trials of selective serotonin reuptake inhibitors for agitation in patients with dementia have had mixed results. Nyth and Gottfries (1990) reviewed controlled studies of citalopram in patients with various dementia diagnoses and found some beneficial behavioral effects. A double-blind, placebo-controlled study compared citalopram and perphenazine with placebo in patients with various dementia diagnoses and at least one symptom of psychosis or behavioral disturbance (Pollock et al. 2002). After 3 days of dose escalation, hospitalized patients were treated with citalopram 20 mg/day or perphenazine 0.1 mg/kg per day for up to 14 days. In both the citalopram and perphenazine groups, there was significant improvement in Neurobehavioral Rating Scale (Levin et al. 1987) scores for agitation, lability, and psychosis compared with placebo. Side effects were similar in the three treatment groups.

Pollock et al. (2007) tested citalopram versus risperidone in the treatment of psychosis and agitation in patients with dementia. Dementia patients who had been hospitalized for behavioral symptoms were randomly assigned in this 12-week study. There was no difference between citalopram and risperidone on the primary behavioral outcome measure, the NPI; agitation and psychotic symptoms decreased in both treatment groups. Significantly greater side effects, especially sedation, occurred with risperidone than with citalopram. Comparable increases in extrapyramidal symptoms were seen in the two groups.

In a review of 29 double-blind, randomized, placebo-controlled trials or meta-analyses, Sink et al. (2005) found that among five trials of antidepressants, only one study of citalopram in dementia patients showed improvement in neuropsychiatric symptoms other than depression.

No benefit has been reported for fluoxetine or fluvoxamine. Only anecdotal findings are available regarding other serotonergic agents. Despite the lack of clinical trial data regarding their effectiveness, serotonergic agents are used widely. Their use may be due in part to familiarity with this class of agents for depression, as well as basic, preclinical, and clinical evidence linking impulsivity to disordered serotonergic function (Coccaro 1996). The side-effect profile of this class includes gastrointestinal symptoms, sedation or insomnia, sexual dysfunction, hyponatremia, and occasional neuromuscular signs, with rare anecdotes of paradoxical agitation.

Benzodiazepines

Most studies of benzodiazepine use for treatment of patients with dementia, which are older and were conducted in ill-defined populations and usually not placebo controlled, tended to demonstrate an average reduction in agitation with short-term therapy. A study by Coccaro et al. (1990) was the most methodologically rigorous. Oxazepam 10–60 mg/day was compared with low-dose haloperidol in patients with mixed dementia diagnoses. Five percent of patients in the benzodiazepine group improved, versus 24% of those in the haloperidol group. A double-blind randomized controlled trial comparing intramuscular lorazepam with intramuscular olanzapine showed that lorazepam was equal to olanzapine in efficacy at 2 hours but inferior at 24 hours (Meehan et al. 2002). However, at this time, no studies have compared benzodiazepines to one another, and no data are available concerning their efficacy after 8 weeks.

Compared with antipsychotics, benzodiazepines may have more side effects and a lower likelihood of benefit (Coccaro et al. 1990; Meehan et al. 2002). Benzodiazepine side effects include ataxia, falls, confusion, anterograde amnesia, and sedation. Benzodiazepines are not recommended beyond a brief period of use because of risks of dependence, tolerance, sedation, insomnia, cognition deterioration, disinhibition, and delirium. These agents have also been associated with respiratory suppression during sleep.

For these reasons, use of benzodiazepines is typically limited to agitation associated with procedures or time-limited acute or as needed use, with chronic use only in those patients for whom other agents have proven ineffective. Benzodiazepines are recommended for use with only minimum effective doses, given that side effects are dose related. Also, because of withdrawal risks, agents that are prescribed for an extended period should not be stopped abruptly. Drugs with simpler metabolism and relatively short half-lives, such as lorazepam 0.5 mg 1–4 times daily, are selected most often; long-acting agents such as diazepam, clonazepam, flurazepam, and nitrazepam are generally avoided. In elderly patients, agents such as clonazepam, with long half-lives and long-lived metabolites, may take up to several weeks to reach steady levels, and therefore are not generally recommended.

Buspirone

Buspirone treatment for patients with dementia has been reported only in case series and small clinical trials (Cooper 2003; Herrmann and Eryavec 1993). The medication requires twice-daily dosing, is generally well tolerated, and can require several weeks to achieve maximal clinical benefit. The level of evidence supporting use of this agent is very weak. Consensus statements (e.g., Alexopoulos et al. 2004) suggest a possible role for buspirone for patients with mild agitation associated with anxiety or irritability, with the dosage starting at 5 mg bid and increasing to a potential maximum of 40–60 mg/day.

Anticonvulsants

Carbamazepine

Carbamazepine is not recommended for use with dementia patients because of side effects, such as rashes, sedation, hematological abnormalities, hepatic dysfunction, and altered electrolytes. Also, it has considerable potential for significant drug-drug interactions.

Valproic Acid

Valproic acid, also known generically as valproate and available as the enteric-coated derivative divalproex sodium, has been approved by the FDA for acute mania associated with bipolar disorder. The first placebo-controlled study of this agent for agitation in dementia was 6 weeks in duration (Porsteinsson et al. 2001). Divalproex sodium at a mean dosage of 826 mg/day (mean level = 46 µg/dL) was assessed in agitated nursing home residents with dementia. The primary measure of agitation did not show benefit, although the trend was sufficient to warrant proceeding to a larger trial. Serious adverse events occurred at a rate of 10% in both the drug and placebo groups; milder side effects, consisting chiefly of sedation, gastrointestinal distress, and ataxia, occurred more frequently in the drug group, and the expected decrease in average platelet count was about 20,000/mm^3.

A multicenter, 6-week, randomized placebo-controlled study of divalproex sodium in agitated nursing home residents with dementia (who also met criteria for secondary mania) incorporated a rapid dosing and titration protocol with a target dosage of 20 mg/kg per day at 10 days (Tariot et al. 2001). This titration rate and dose resulted in sedation in about 20% of the drug-treated group and a high dropout rate, leading to premature discontinuation of the study. No significant drug-placebo differences in manic features were found, but the drug had a significant effect on agitation. Sedation occurred in 36% of the drug group versus 20% of the placebo group, and mild thrombocytopenia occurred in 7% of the patients in the drug group and none of the placebo-treated patients.

A 6-week placebo-controlled trial of divalproex, using an average total daily dose of about 750 mg, in agitated nursing home residents with dementia showed no drug-placebo difference in any behavioral measures (Tariot et al. 2005). Side effects were as described in the preceding paragraphs.

Finally, a randomized, double-blind, placebo-controlled, crossover study of valproate 480 mg/day for 3 weeks was conducted in patients with dementia and aggressive behavior (Sival et al. 2002). No significant impact on aggressive behavior was seen according to the primary outcome measure, although trends toward improvement were found on measures of aggression and of dependent and suspicious behaviors. No drug-placebo differences were found in rate or type of adverse events.

If valproate is used, the available evidence suggests a starting dosage of about 125 mg po bid, increasing in 125- to 250-mg increments every 5–7 days, with a maximal dose determined by clinical response or, when there is uncertainty, a serum level of about 60–90 μg/mL. We typically aim for a target dosage of about 10–12 mg/kg per day. The utility of the new once-daily extended-release formulation has not been established in the elderly population.

We know of no controlled studies of the newer anticonvulsants, including lamotrigine, gabapentin, and topiramate, in older patients with dementia. In the meantime, consensus statements suggest a limited role for anticonvulsants in view of the limited and mixed evidence regarding efficacy and safety (Alexopoulos et al. 2004).

Antidementia Therapies

Antidementia agents, addressed in Chapter 14, "Pharmacological Treatment of Alzheimer Disease and Mild Cognitive Impairment," can play an important role in the medical treatment of psychopathology associated with dementia. Few trials have prospectively assessed the behavioral efficacy of these agents; therefore, the evidence from clinical trials addressing their efficacy comes primarily from secondary analyses of behavioral outcomes. Because it is clinically appropriate to consider a treatment trial of a cholinesterase inhibitor and/or memantine at some point in treating most patients with Alzheimer disease, we routinely use these medications to try to mitigate such psychopathology.

Conclusion

Clinical trials show that the overall treatment effect for drugs used to reduce the behavioral manifestations of dementia is about 20%, which is nearly the same rate as the likelihood of significant side effects. Some patients can be helped without being harmed, some gain no benefit, and some are only harmed. Clinicians should be familiar with evidence addressing efficacy and toxicity of available treatments; determine whether a particular treatment is justified, including explicitly assessing the degree of subjective distress, functional impairment, dangerous resistance to personal care, and risk of harm to self or others; and evaluate the patient's risk profile in view of the treatment being considered. Whether the risks and benefits warrant use of a particular treatment is a judgment that needs to be made on a case-by-case basis. This justification should be explained to the relevant stakeholders and documented accordingly. Patients should be monitored adequately, and treatment that is ineffective or harmful should be stopped. Given the relatively low likelihood of achieving benefit without harm in using medication, nonpharmacological interventions should be used when possible.

Key Clinical Points

- Behavioral and psychological disturbances require thoughtful appreciation of their phenomenology, assessment, and management.
- Best practice precepts emphasize careful clinical evaluation and dementia diagnosis, assessing for pain and delirium, and employing nonpharmacological approaches first.
- Pharmacological therapy is guided by the "psychobehavioral metaphor": define a target symptom pattern analogous to a drug-responsive syndrome, and then match the dominant target symptoms to the most relevant drug class.
- Clinicians should employ low medication dosages, escalate slowly, assess target symptoms and toxicity, and discontinue medication if harmful or ineffective.
- Atypical antipsychotics have a benefit of about 18% over placebo (about 1 in 5 patients experience significant improvement).

- Use of atypical antipsychotics is associated with slightly increased risk for cerebrovascular adverse events and all-cause mortality.
- In considering whether to use an antipsychotic, the clinician should weigh the risk of not treating a morbid complication of the illness against the risks of active treatment.
- Evidence for efficacy and lack of toxicity is largely lacking or inconclusive for nonantipsychotic psychotropic medications.
- Antidementia therapies, which are clinically appropriate in the treatment of Alzheimer disease, may benefit behavioral features.

References

Abilify (aripiprazole) prescribing information. 2011. Available at: http://www.abilify.com/pdf/pi.aspx. Accessed August 4, 2011.

Alexopoulos GS, Streim J, Carpenter D, et al; Expert Consensus Panel for Using Antipsychotic Drugs in Older Patients: Using antipsychotic agents in older patients. J Clin Psychiatry 65 (suppl 2):5–99, 2004

American Diabetes Association, American Psychiatric Association, American Association of Clinical Endocrinologists, et al: Consensus Development Conference on Antipsychotic Drugs and Obesity and Diabetes. Diabetes Care 27:596–601, 2004

Ballard C, Margallo-Lana M, Juszczak E, et al: Quetiapine and rivastigmine and cognitive decline in Alzheimer's disease: randomised double blind placebo controlled trial. BMJ 330:874, 2005

Ballard C, Waite J, Birks J: Atypical antipsychotics for aggression and psychosis in Alzheimer's disease. Cochrane Database of Systematic Reviews 2006, Issue 1. Art. No.: CD003476. DOI: 10.1002/14651858.CD003476.pub2.

Bristol-Myers Squibb: Labeling change for Abilify on risk of CVA in elderly. Bristol-Myers Squibb Medical Letter, February 10, 2005

Brodaty H, Ames D, Snowdon J, et al: A randomized placebo-controlled trial of risperidone for the treatment of aggression, agitation, and psychosis of dementia. J Clin Psychiatry 64:134–143, 2003

Coccaro EF: Neurotransmitter correlates of impulsive aggression in humans. Ann NY Acad Sci 794:82–89, 1996

Coccaro EF, Kramer E, Zemishlany Z, et al: Pharmacologic treatment of noncognitive behavioral disturbances in elderly demented patients. Am J Psychiatry 147:1640–1645, 1990

Cohen-Mansfield J: Agitated behaviors in the elderly, II: preliminary results in the cognitively deteriorated. J Am Geriatr Soc 34:722–727, 1986

Cohen-Mansfield J: Nonpharmacologic interventions for inappropriate behaviors in dementia: a review, summary, and critique. Am J Geriatr Psychiatry 9:361–381, 2001

Cohen-Mansfield J, Billig N: Agitated behaviors in the elderly, I: a conceptual review. J Am Geriatr Soc 34:711–721, 1986

Cooper JP: Buspirone for anxiety and agitation in dementia (letter). J Psychiatry Neurosci 28:469, 2003

Cummings JL, Mega M, Gray K, et al: The Neuropsychiatric Inventory: comprehensive assessment of psychopathology in dementia. Neurology 44:2308–2314, 1994

De Deyn PP, Rabheru K, Rasmussen A, et al: A randomized trial of risperidone, placebo, and haloperidol for behavioral symptoms of dementia. Neurology 53:946–955, 1999

De Deyn PP, Carrasco MM, Deberdt W, et al: Olanzapine versus placebo in the treatment of psychosis with or without associated behavioral disturbances in patients with Alzheimer's disease. Int J Geriatr Psychiatry 19:115–126, 2004

De Deyn PP, Jeste DV, Swanink R, et al: Aripiprazole for the treatment of psychosis in patients with Alzheimer's disease: a randomized, placebo-controlled study. J Clin Psychopharmacol 25:463–467, 2005. Erratum in: J Clin Psychopharmacol 25:560, 2005

Gill SS, Bronskill SE, Normand SL, et al: Antipsychotic drug use and mortality in older adults with dementia. Ann Intern Med 146:775–786, 2007

Guy W: ECDEU Assessment Manual for Psychopharmacology—Revised (DHHS Publ No ADM 91-338). Rockville, MD, U.S. Department of Health and Human Services, 1976

Haupt M, Cruz-Jentoft A, Jeste D: Mortality in elderly dementia patients treated with risperidone. J Clin Psychopharmacol 26:566–570, 2006

Health Care Financing Administration: State Operations Manual. Baltimore, MD, U.S. Department of Health and Human Services, 1992

Herrmann N, Eryavec G: Buspirone in the management of agitation and aggression associated with dementia. Am J Geriatr Psychiatry 1:249–253, 1993

Herrmann N, Lanctôt KL: Do atypical antipsychotics cause stroke? CNS Drugs 19(2):91–103, 2005

Herrmann N, Mandami M, Lanctôt KL: Atypical antipsychotics and risk of cerebrovascular accidents. Am J Psychiatry 161:1113–1115, 2004

Jeste DV, Finkel SI: Psychosis of Alzheimer's disease and related dementias: diagnostic criteria for a distinct syndrome. Am J Geriatr Psychiatry 8:29–34, 2000

Katz IR, Jeste DV, Mintzer JE, et al: Comparison of risperidone and placebo for psychosis and behavioral disturbances associated with dementia: a randomized, double-blind trial. J Clin Psychiatry 60:107–115, 1999

Kay SR, Fiszbein A, Opler LA: The Positive and Negative Syndrome Scale (PANSS) for schizophrenia. Schizophr Bull 13:261–276, 1987

Kurlan R, Cummings J, Raman R, et al: Quetiapine for agitation or psychosis in patients with dementia and parkinsonism. Neurology 68:1356–1363, 2007

Lanctôt KL, Best TS, Mittmann N, et al: Efficacy and safety of neuroleptics in behavioral disorders associated with dementia. J Clin Psychiatry 59:560–561, 1998

Lee PE, Gill SS, Freedman M, et al: Atypical antipsychotic drugs in the treatment of behavioural and psychological symptoms of dementia: systematic review. BMJ 329:75, 2004

Levin HS, High WM, Goethe KE, et al: The Neurobehavioral Rating Scale: assessment of the behavioural sequelae of head injury by the clinician. J Neurol Neurosurg Psychiatry 50:183–193, 1987

Lonergan E, Luxenberg J, Colford J, et al: Haloperidol for agitation in dementia. Cochrane Database of Systematic Reviews 2002, Issue 2. Art. No.: CD002852. DOI: 10.1002/14651858.CD002852.

Meehan KM, Wang H, David SR, et al: Comparison of rapidly acting intramuscular olanzapine, lorazepam, and placebo: a double-blind, randomized study in acutely agitated patients with dementia. Neuropsychopharmacology 26:494–504, 2002

Mintzer JE, Tune LE, Breder CD, et al: Aripiprazole for the treatment of psychoses in institutionalized patients with Alzheimer dementia: a multicenter, randomized, double-blind, placebo-controlled assessment of three fixed doses. Am J Geriatr Psychiatry 15:918–931, 2007

Nyth AL, Gottfries CG: The clinical efficacy of citalopram in treatment of emotional disturbances in dementia disorders: a Nordic multicentre study. Br J Psychiatry 157:894–901, 1990

Parkinson Study Group: Low-dose clozapine for the treatment of drug-induced psychosis in Parkinson's disease. N Engl J Med 340:757–763, 1999

Pollock BG, Mulsant BH, Rosen J, et al: Comparison of citalopram, perphenazine, and placebo for the acute treatment of psychosis and behavioral disturbances in hospitalized, demented patients. Am J Psychiatry 159:460–465, 2002

Pollock, BG, Mulsant BH, Rosen J, et al: A double-blind comparison of citalopram and risperidone for the treatment of behavioral and psychotic symptoms associated with dementia. Am J Geriatr Psychiatry 15:942–952, 2007

Porsteinsson AP, Tariot PN, Erb R, et al: Placebo-controlled study of divalproex sodium for agitation in dementia. Am J Geriatr Psychiatry 9:58–66, 2001

Raivio MM, Laurila JV, Strandberg TE, et al: Neither atypical nor conventional antipsychotics increase mortality or hospital admissions among elderly patients with dementia: a two-year prospective study. Am J Geriatr Psychiatry 15:416–424, 2007

Rocha FL, Hara C, Ramos MG, et al: An exploratory open-label trial of ziprasidone for the treatment of behavioral and psychological symptoms of dementia. Dement Geriatr Cogn Disord 22:445–448, 2006

Rosenquist K, Tariot PN, Loy R: Treatments for behavioral and psychological symptoms in Alzheimer's disease and other dementias, in Dementia. Edited by Ames D, Burns A, O'Brien J. London, Chapman and Hall, 2000, pp 571–601

Schneeweiss S, Setoguchi S, Brookhart A, et al: Risk of death associated with the use of conventional versus atypical antipsychotic drugs among elderly patients. CMAJ 176:627–632, 2007

Schneider LS, Pollock VE, Lyness SA: A metaanalysis of controlled trials of neuroleptic treatment in dementia. J Am Geriatr Soc 38:553–563, 1990

Schneider LS, Dagerman KS, Insel P: Risk of death with atypical antipsychotic drug treatment for dementia: meta-analysis of randomized placebo-controlled trials. JAMA 294:1934–1943, 2005

Schneider LS, Dagerman K, Insel PS: Efficacy and adverse effects of atypical antipsychotics for dementia: meta-analysis of randomized, placebo-controlled trials. Am J Geriatr Psychiatry 14:191–210, 2006a

Schneider LS, Tariot PN, Dagerman KS, et al: Effectiveness of atypical antipsychotic drugs in patients with Alzheimer's disease. N Engl J Med 355:1525–1538, 2006b

Sink KM, Holden KF, Yaffe K: Pharmacological treatment of neuropsychiatric symptoms of dementia: a review of the evidence. JAMA 293:596–608, 2005

Sival RC, Haffmans PM, Jansen PA, et al: Sodium valproate in the treatment of aggressive behavior in patients with dementia: a randomized placebo controlled clinical trial. Int J Geriatr Psychiatry 17:579–585, 2002

Street JS, Clark WS, Gannon KS, et al: Olanzapine treatment of psychotic and behavioral symptoms in patients with Alzheimer disease in nursing care facilities: a double-blind, randomized, placebo-controlled trial. Arch Gen Psychiatry 57:968–976, 2000

Streim JE, Porsteinsson AP, Breder CD, et al: A randomized, double-blind, placebo-controlled study of aripiprazole for the treatment of psychosis in nursing home patients with Alzheimer disease. Am J Geriatr Psychiatry 16:537–550, 2008

Suh GH, Son HG, Ju YS, et al: A randomized, double-blind, crossover comparison of risperidone and haloperidol in Korean dementia patients with behavioral disturbances. Am J Geriatr Psychiatry 12:509–516, 2004

Suh GH, Son HG, Ju YS, et al: Comparative efficacy of risperidone versus haloperidol on behavioural and psychological symptoms of dementia. Int J Geriatr Psychiatry 21:654–660, 2006

Sultzer DL, Gray KF, Gunay I, et al: A double-blind comparison of trazodone and haloperidol for treatment of agitation in patients with dementia. Am J Geriatr Psychiatry 5:60–69, 1997

Tariot PN: Treatment of agitation in dementia. J Clin Psychiatry 60 (suppl 8):11–20, 1999

Tariot PN, Podgorski CA, Blazina L, et al: Mental disorders in the nursing home: another perspective. Am J Psychiatry 150:1063–1069, 1993

Tariot PN, Schneider L, Mintzer J, et al: Safety and tolerability of divalproex sodium in the treatment of signs and symptoms of mania in elderly patients with dementia: results of a double-blind, placebo-controlled trial. Curr Ther Res 62:51–67, 2001

Tariot PN, Raman R, Jakimovich L, et al: Divalproex sodium in nursing home residents with possible or probable Alzheimer disease complicated by agitation: a randomized, controlled trial. Am J Geriatr Psychiatry 13:942–949, 2005

Tariot PN, Schneider L, Katz IR, et al: Quetiapine treatment of psychosis associated with dementia: a double-blind, randomized, placebo-controlled clinical trial. Am J Geriatr Psychiatry 14:767–776, 2006

U.S. Food and Drug Administration: Risperdal (risperidone). April 2003. Available at: http://www.fda.gov/Safety/MedWatch/SafetyInformation/SafetyAlertsforHumanMedicalProducts/ucm153478.htm. Accessed August 4, 2011.

U.S. Food and Drug Administration: Safety Alert: Zyprexa (olanzapine). March 2004. Available at: http://www.fda.gov/Safety/MedWatch/SafetyInformation/SafetyAlertsforHumanMedicalProducts/default.htm. Accessed August 4, 2011.

U.S. Food and Drug Administration: Atypical antipsychotic drugs. April 11, 2005. Available at: http://www.fda.gov/Safety/MedWatch/SafetyInformation/SafetyAlertsforHumanMedicalProducts/ucm150688.htm. Accessed August 4, 2011.

U.S. Food and Drug Administration: Information for healthcare professionals: conventional antipsychotics. June 16, 2008. Available at: http://www.fda.gov/Drugs/DrugSafety/PostmarketDrugSafetyInformationforPatientsandProviders/ucm124830.htm. Accessed August 4, 2011.

Wooltorton E: Risperidone (Risperdal): increased rate of cerebrovascular events in dementia trials (letter). CMAJ 167:1269–1270, 2002

Zhong KX, Tariot PN, Mintzer J, et al: Quetiapine to treat agitation in dementia: a randomized, double-blind, placebo-controlled study. Curr Alzheimer Res 4:81–93, 2007

Further Reading

Agronin ME, Maletta GJ: Geriatric Psychiatry. Baltimore, MD, Lippincott Williams & Wilkins, 2011

Jacobson SA, Pies RW, Katz IR: Clinical Manual of Geriatric Psychopharmacology. Washington, DC, American Psychiatric Publishing, 2007

14

Pharmacological Treatment of Alzheimer Disease and Mild Cognitive Impairment

Martin R. Farlow, M.D.

Malaz Boustani, M.D., M.P.H.

In this chapter, we review the drugs currently approved in the United States for treatment of cognitive symptoms of dementing disorders. None of the drugs have yet been approved for mild cognitive impairment (MCI), but many physicians treat individuals with MCI using the medications that are available for Alzheimer disease (AD). We focus primarily on drugs for which there are double-blind, placebo-controlled studies, but we consider a few widely used drugs for which less rigorous evidence for efficacy is available. Drugs aimed primarily at improving cognitive deficits may also have an impact on behavioral and psychiatric symptoms (Cummings 2000). In this chapter, we also present the cognitive and behavioral effects of the drugs used to treat cognitive symptoms in AD.

These effects are also discussed in Chapter 12, "Treatment of Psychiatric Disorders in People With Dementia," and Chapter 13, "Pharmacological Treatment of Neuropsychiatric Symptoms."

General Principles

The rational use of drugs for treating cognitive deficits is aided by an accurate diagnosis; by knowledge of patients' past medical history, including prescription and nonprescription drug use; and by a complete physical and neurological examination to detect potentially reversible causes of cognitive impairment. Other comorbid illnesses must also be considered for their potential to be negatively affected by the medications commonly prescribed for dementia (e.g., peptic ulcer disease, obstructive pulmonary disease, arrhythmias). Medical, social, and psychological histories are also important because they may indicate one or more factors precipitating the presenting symptoms, such as a change of environment, as indicated in the following case example.

> The daughter-in-law of Mrs. Alden, an elderly woman with AD enrolled in a cognitive-enhancer study, called and expressed alarm that Mrs. Alden initially had had a good response to the drug but had suddenly worsened. When asked to describe what had happened, she told the physician that Mrs. Alden had been living with her and her husband for about 1 month. They had gone to the apartment where Mrs. Alden had formerly resided to pack up more of her possessions. While there, Mrs. Alden suddenly became very confused and no longer recognized her son. They took her back to their home, where she sat on her bed crying out for her own mother. The physician reassured the daughter-in-law that Mrs. Alden had experienced a catastrophic response to the emotional stimulus of giving up her apartment and her former lifestyle, and that with a day or two to adjust, her symptoms would probably improve. The daughter-in-law called the next morning to say that indeed all was well again.

Many medical conditions have the potential to worsen cognition in dementing illnesses. This is especially important in late-stage dementia patients who are unable to report their physical symptoms.

Having ruled out or treated medical conditions that may precipitate or worsen cognitive symptoms, the physician should also review a patient's medications for drugs that may produce confusion or alter mood. In some cases, eliminating a medication or reducing the dosage of a drug may be more effective than adding a cognitive enhancer. Certain classes of drugs should be avoided or used at the minimum dosage needed. For example, the cholinergic deficit of AD makes individuals highly susceptible to further impairment from taking anticholinergic drugs or drugs with anticholinergic side effects. Thus, the use of antihistamines, such as diphenhydramine (Benadryl), or strongly anticholinergic antidepressant medications, such as amitriptyline (Elavil), is relatively contraindicated. Although the bladder relaxants oxybutynin (Ditropan) and tolterodine (Detrol) primarily have peripheral cholinergic effects, they also can act centrally and worsen cognition; therefore, they also should be used with caution (Katz et al. 1998). Physicians caring for patients with late-stage dementia must weigh these medications' potential deleterious effects versus their beneficial effects in treating urinary incontinence. Arginine vasopressin can sometimes be substituted for the anticholinergic drugs for nighttime urinary incontinence.

Cholinergic Augmentation

Acetylcholine precursors, cholinomimetics, and anticholinesterases have been used to treat AD based on the observations that cholinergic neurons are selectively reduced in AD (Davies and Maloney 1976) and that anticholinergic drugs have deleterious effects on memory (Drachman and Leavitt 1974). Also, physostigmine is used because it has been found to have direct memory-enhancing effects in humans (Davis et al. 1987). On the basis of these findings, three main approaches have been investigated to increase cholinergic transmission: increasing substrate available for the biosynthesis of acetylcholine, using cholinomimetics to augment acetylcholine activity, and blocking the degradation of acetylcholine to prolong its activity at receptor sites.

Acetylcholine Precursors

Acetylcholine is produced in the brain by the acetylation of choline through the action of the enzyme choline acetyltransferase and the cofactor coenzyme A. Lecithin (whose primary constituent is phosphatidylcholine) is ineffective, makes patients malodorous, and does not improve the cognitive deficits in AD. Acetyl-L-carnitine, marketed in Italy as Nicetile for treatment of cognitive impairment, is also available in the United States as a food supplement. It is a naturally occurring substance that may help in the formation of acetyl coenzyme A, acetylcholine, or both. It has been used in AD and vascular dementia, but there is no evidence of its effectiveness (Thal et al. 1996).

Cholinomimetics

The cholinomimetic approach to AD, including the use of drugs such as carbachol, milameline, and xanomeline, has been largely abandoned because of drug toxicity, including induction of depression by the cholinergic agonist oxotremorine (Davis et al. 1987).

Anticholinesterases

The anticholinesterases (Table 14–1) have been the most successful cognitive enhancers for AD. Tacrine (Cognex) was introduced in 1993, donepezil (Aricept) in 1997, rivastigmine (Exelon) in 2000, and galantamine (Reminyl, now called Razadyne) in 2001. All four drugs are reversible inhibitors of acetylcholinesterase; rivastigmine also reversibly inhibits butyrylcholinesterase. Galantamine has additional effects in modulating nicotinic receptors. The therapeutic and side effects of all these drugs are very similar except that tacrine causes hepatotoxicity. Although the cholinergic system appears to be integrally involved in the encoding of memory, the effects of anticholinesterases in AD appear to be more general, augmenting executive functioning as well as memory, and are likely to alter positively the complex interactions between cholinergic, noradrenergic, and dopaminergic systems (Robbins and Roberts 2007).

Tacrine

Tacrine, an aminoacridine derivative, was the first U.S. Food and Drug Administration (FDA)–approved treatment for AD in the United States and is now mostly of historical interest. Because of its tolerability issues, frequency of dosing, and the need for close monitoring of liver functions, use of tacrine has largely been abandoned.

Donepezil

Donepezil, a piperidine-based reversible acetylcholinesterase inhibitor, reaches peak plasma concentrations 2–4 hours after an oral dose. It is 100% bioavailable, and food has no effect on its absorption. The drug is more than 90% protein bound. Plasma concentrations increase linearly with dosage increase.

Table 14–1. Dosages of cholinesterase inhibitors

Generic name	Trade name	Initial dosage (mg/day)	Optimal dosage (mg/day)	Dose frequency
Tacrine	Cognex	40	40	Four times daily
Donepezil	Aricept	5	10	Every morning
Rivastigmine	Exelon	3	6	Twice daily with food
	Exelon patch	4.6	9.5	Every morning
Galantamine	Razadyne	8	8–12	Twice daily
	Razadyne ER	8	24	Every morning with food

Note. Dosages should be increased no sooner than 4 weeks. ER=extended release.

The half-life of the drug is approximately 70 hours. At 5 mg/day, donepezil produces 64% red blood cell cholinesterase inhibition (Crismon 1998). A relationship has been shown between the cognitive effect of donepezil and the degree of plasma acetylcholinesterase inhibition, but a plateau of acetylcholinesterase inhibition was reached at plasma concentrations greater than 50 ng/mL (Rogers and Friedhoff 1996). Levels of cholinesterase inhibition in brain may lag, however, and be considerably less than in red blood cells or plasma. In the initial pivotal 24-week, double blind, placebo-controlled study, roughly 80% of patients receiving donepezil 5 or 10 mg showed no cognitive worsening in evaluation at at least one follow-up time point, compared with 42% of the placebo group (Rogers et al. 1998). On a measure of global function, approximately 25% of the donepezil-treated group (5 or 10 mg) improved, compared with 11% of the placebo group. Thus, the overall effect of the drug was to maintain patients at their baseline level of symptomatic functioning for approximately 24 weeks, whereas those receiving placebo declined below baseline.

A large 48-week, double-blind, placebo-controlled, randomized donepezil study withdrew patients from the blinded portion of the study if they deteriorated in their activities of daily living (ADL). By study end, 51% of patients with AD taking donepezil had not deteriorated in terms of ADL, versus 36% in the placebo group (Mohs et al. 2001). In another randomized, double-blind trial, patients with mild to moderate AD were treated with donepezil 5–10 mg/day versus placebo for 1 year (Winblad et al. 2006). In this study, the patients who were taking donepezil maintained cognitive scores near baseline, whereas the placebo group deteriorated significantly. In the longest (3-year) placebo-controlled study (Courtney et al. 2004), cognitive scores were slightly better at the end in the donepezil group than in the placebo group, but there was no difference in scores on disability scales or rates of institutionalization.

Several reports have indicated that donepezil is of value in late-stage AD (Feldman et al. 2005). A 24-week study of subjects in assisted living or nursing homes compared donepezil 10 mg/day with placebo (Winblad et al. 2006). The subjects' Mini-Mental State Examination (MMSE; Folstein et al. 1975) scores ranged from 1 to 10. At 24 weeks, patients taking active drug showed greater improvement on a test of cognitive function and less decline on a measure of ADL than did those given placebo. The differences were small but significant. A second 24-week placebo-controlled study included subjects with MMSE scores ranging from 1 to 12 (Black et al. 2007). Although the donepezil and placebo groups had essentially no improvement in performance of ADL, small but significant differences on cognitive and global measures favored donepezil.

Common side effects of donepezil are nausea, vomiting, diarrhea, muscle cramps (due to nicotinic effects), mild stimulation, and vivid dreams at night that are sometimes frightening. Other, less common side effects include muscarinic cholinomimetic effects, such as urinary urgency or incontinence, sweating, rhinorrhea, and syncope. The more common gastrointestinal adverse effects are usually transient and respond to a short-term holiday from the drug or lowering of the dose. Although slightly greater efficacy occurs at 10 mg/day than at 5 mg/day, significantly greater side effects also occur at that dosage. Titration from 5 to 10 mg is recommended after 4–6 weeks; earlier increases in dosage are associated with more frequent side effects. Drug-drug interactions are unlikely. Although the manufacturer recommends dosing the medication at bedtime to minimize gastrointestinal effects, the stimulating effects of the drug (including vivid dreams) may be better tolerated with morning administration.

Recently, a higher (23-mg) dose of donepezil was tested in moderate- to severe-stage patients with AD who had previously been taking a stable 10-mg dose of the drug for at least 3 months. In this double-blind, 24-week study, the comparison group included patients continuing to take the 10-mg dose of donepezil (Farlow et al. 2010). The 23-mg group had significantly improved cognitive but not global functioning compared with the 10-mg group. Nausea, vomiting, and anorexia side-effect rates were increased in the 23-mg group versus the 10-mg group, usually in the first month after up-titration. The 23-mg dose is now available as another treatment option as the illness progresses.

Rivastigmine

Rivastigmine, a carbamate, reversibly inhibits both acetylcholinesterase and butyrylcholinesterase. It is rapidly absorbed when taken orally and has a bioavailability of 36%, but it is only 40% protein bound. Elimination half-life is approximately 2 hours. The drug covalently binds to cholinesterases, and breaking of these bonds converts rivastigmine to an inactive metabolite. The parent compound is not metabolized by the liver (Jann 2000). Rivastigmine's effects are dose dependent. In a double-blind, placebo-controlled study in patients with AD, rivastigmine at two dosage ranges (1–4 and 6–12 mg/day) was compared with placebo over 26 weeks (Corey-Bloom et al. 1998). Dose was titrated upward weekly until the maximum tolerable total daily dose was reached. Only 55% of the persons in the high-dose group achieved the maximum rivastigmine dosage of 12 mg/day. At 26 weeks, the high-dose rivastigmine group remained cognitively above baseline, whereas the placebo group had worsened. On an ADL scale, 25% of high-dosage rivastigmine-treated patients had clinically meaningful improvement, compared with 15% of persons in the placebo group. There was no difference in outcome between the low-dose rivastigmine and placebo groups. Rösler et al. (1999) described similar difficulty in achieving the highest dosage of rivastigmine. In both studies, the incidence of treatment-related side effects increased with rivastigmine dosage increases and decreased with dosage reduction.

Rivastigmine was originally available in capsules of 1.5, 3, 4.5, and 6 mg to be administered twice daily with food. Fewer side effects are encountered with dose titration at 4-week intervals, and the current recommendation is that the medication be taken after a full meal. Even with these modifications, dosing is limited by nausea, vomiting, and diarrhea. For this reason, a transdermal patch has been developed that has much lower cholinergic gastrointestinal side effects than the capsules. A 24-hour transdermal patch is now available in doses of 4.6 and 9.5 mg/24 hours. This preparation has few gastrointestinal side effects, and skin irritation is relatively uncommon. No delay between doses is required when transitioning from an oral dose of 1.5–3 mg bid to the 4.6-mg patch. Patients receiving an oral dose of 4.5–6 mg bid can readily be switched to the 9.5-mg patch. The patch has largely replaced the use of rivastigmine capsules in clinical practice.

Galantamine

Galantamine, an alkaloid derived from the bulbs of the snowdrop variety of daffodil, reversibly and competitively inhibits acetylcholinesterase (Bores et al. 1996). It is well absorbed and has absolute bioavailability of about 90%. It has a terminal elimination half-life of 7 hours and has linear pharmacokinetics at dosages from 8 to 32 mg/day. It is 18% protein bound. The drug is metabolized by the hepatic cytochrome P450 (CYP) isoenzymes and by glucuronidation, and it is also excreted unchanged in the urine.

A 6-month, randomized, placebo-controlled trial was undertaken in subjects with mild to moderate AD (Raskind et al. 2000). Patients were randomly assigned to receive either placebo or escalating doses of galantamine up to a dosage of 24 or 32 mg/day. Compared with patients receiving placebo, patients receiving galantamine at either dosage had significantly improved cognitive scores, and both drug groups had significantly better scores than the placebo group on the Clinician's Interview-Based Impression of Change plus Caregiver Input (CIBIC-Plus; Schneider et al. 1997). After patients had been taking galantamine 24 mg/day for 12 months, their cognitive scores and daily function showed no deterioration from baseline. Wilcock et al. (2001) reported on a double-blind, placebo-controlled study of galantamine for persons with mild to moderate AD. The dosage of galantamine was escalated weekly over 3–4 weeks to 24 or 32 mg/day. At 6 months, cognitive scores were significantly improved for the drug groups compared with the placebo group. Apolipoprotein E genotype had no effect on outcome. Titration was at monthly intervals in a study by Tariot et al. (2000); there were significant differences favoring galantamine in scores on the CIBIC-Plus, on ADL, and on behavioral symptoms. Adverse events in all studies were primarily gastrointestinal symptoms. On the basis of these studies, the manufacturer recommends titrating galantamine to 16 or 24 mg/day (8- or 12-mg capsules twice daily) at 1-month intervals.

Galantamine has been available in 4-, 8-, and 12-mg capsules that are administered twice daily. In a study investigating use of 8-mg, 16-mg, and 24-mg extended-release capsules dosed once per day, the effective area under the curve was similar to that of twice-daily dosing, with half-life extended to 4.4 hours (Zhao et al. 2005). The adverse effects and efficacy of galantamine in this study were comparable to those of the immediate-release form of the medication. An extended-release form is now available that allows once-daily dosing of 8, 12, or 24 mg, usually in the morning. The manufacturer suggests that the extended-release capsules be taken with food. The extended-release once-daily form of galantamine has largely replaced the immediate-release form in clinical practice.

Head-to-Head Comparisons

A number of head-to-head comparisons have been made between cholinesterase inhibitors and have shown essentially no difference in efficacy. For example, in a 52-week parallel-group study, galantamine was compared with donepezil. Galantamine was started at 4 mg bid, and the dosage was titrated up to 12 mg bid if tolerated. The dosage of donepezil was titrated to 10 mg/day if tolerated. At study end, there were no differences between study groups on an ADL scale (Wilcock et al. 2003).

Switching Anticholinesterases

Patients who do not tolerate or who appear to be losing ground taking one cholinesterase inhibitor may benefit from change to another drug of the same class. For example, a 6-month open-label study evaluated the safety and efficacy of rivastigmine in patients with AD who had failed to benefit from donepezil (80% due to lack of efficacy, 11% due to tolerability problems, and 9% due to both) (Auriacombe et al. 2002). At the end of the study, 56% of patients had responded to rivastigmine on both global and cognitive measures. Contrary to the clinical experience of others, these investigators found that having had side effects from donepezil did not predict similar problems with rivastigmine. In general, trying a second cholinesterase inhibitor is reasonable if the family, patient, or clinician believes the first drug is ineffective; if the benefits from the medication are failing; or if the patient is having significant adverse effects. Results with the second drug may be better, the same, or worse than with the first. When progressive disease with worsening symptoms obscures any beneficial effects, a consensus decision among the patient, family or caregiver, and physician should be made regarding the cost and benefits of therapy and whether to continue it.

Anticholinesterases for Behavioral and Psychological Symptoms

Cummings (2000) suggested that acetylcholinesterase inhibitors should be used as psychotropic drugs because loss of input from cholinergic neurons in the basal forebrain to the limbic and paralimbic regions and to the cerebral cortex might be the underlying mechanism connecting behavioral and psychiatric symptoms to the cholinergic system.

Mega et al. (1999) studied community-dwelling patients with AD who were treated with donepezil 5 mg/day for 4 weeks, followed by treatment with 10 mg/day for 4 weeks. Based on global scores on the Neuropsychiatric Inventory (NPI; Cummings et al. 1994), behavioral improvement was seen in 41% and behavioral worsening in 28% of patients. Patients who showed behavioral responses had worse initial scores on the following NPI subscales: Delusions, Agitation, Depression, Anxiety, Apathy, Disinhibition, and Irritability. Cummings (2000) contrasted a group of patients with AD who were treated with donepezil for 6 months with a group of patients who were not taking the drug. Patients taking donepezil were significantly less likely to be threatening, destroy property, or talk loudly, and fewer were receiving sedatives. Weiner et al. (2000) performed a prospective 12-month study of donepezil in patients with AD compared with a reference group of community-dwelling patients with AD who were not receiving anticholinesterase treatment. Using the Consortium to Establish a Registry for Alzheimer's Disease (CERAD) Behavior Rating Scale for Dementia (CBRSD; Tariot et al. 1995), the authors found that the donepezil-treated group showed improvement in CBRSD total scores at 3 months and in depression and behavioral dysregulation scores at 4 months. The donepezil group's CBRSD total, depression, and behavioral dysregulation scores returned to baseline at 12 months, whereas the reference group's CBRSD scores worsened minimally over the 12 months.

In an open-label study of rivastigmine in persons diagnosed clinically with dementia with Lewy bodies, NPI item scores fell after 12 weeks of treatment by 73% for delusions, 63% for apathy, 45% for agitation, and 27% for hallucinations. Of the 11 persons treated, 5 had not responded to prior treatment, including treatment with low-dose neuroleptics. Furthermore, parkinsonian symptoms tended to be improved. The mean dose of rivastigmine was 9.6 mg/day (range=3–12 mg/day) (McKeith et al. 2000a). Another double-blind, placebo-controlled study was conducted over 20 weeks in 120 patients with dementia with Lewy bodies. The mean total daily dose of rivastigmine was 9.4 mg at the end of the 8-week titration period. The maximum total daily dose of 12 mg was achieved by 56% of the 48 completers; most (92%) were able to tolerate at least 6 mg/day. Patients taking rivastigmine had no change in extrapyramidal symptoms. At 20 weeks, patients receiving rivastigmine were significantly less anxious and apathetic and had fewer delusions and hallucinations than control subjects (McKeith et al. 2000b). Ringman and Simmons (2000) reported successful treatment of three cases of rapid eye movement sleep behavior disorder with donepezil.

Although there have been reports of salutary behavior effects from cholinesterase inhibitors, these are generally from uncontrolled case series or retrospective subanalyses. These patients often had little behavioral disturbance at baseline, and the clinical significance of any apparent improvements is not clear. The responsiveness of the persons with greater symptoms may be a function of having scores high enough on behavioral instruments to be detected, and their improvement as regression to their mean level of disturbance (Cummings et al. 2004).

Real-World Therapy Using Anticholinesterases

Cholinesterase inhibitors should be used with caution in persons with complete heart block or sinus bradycardia and in the presence of active peptic ulcer disease, asthma, or chronic obstructive pulmonary disease. However, drug-drug interactions are uncommon. Patients and their families do need to be counseled about the concomitant use of highly anticholinergic drugs such as diphenhydramine, oxybutynin, and dicyclomine.

We offer cholinesterase inhibitors to patients whom we believe to be in the prodromal stage of AD and to patients with mild, moderate, or severe AD. We also offer these drugs to patients who appear to have a vascular component to their symptoms in addition to AD. Both vascular dementia and mixed vascular dementia and AD groups treated with galantamine showed beneficial treatment responses (Erkinjuntti et al. 2002). In our experience, vascular or mixed dementia subjects invariably have at least moderate Alzheimer pathology at autopsy. We generally attempt to reach the maximum dosage suggested by the manufacturer in all dementia subjects, regardless of the specific diagnosis, because the beneficial effects of these drugs are dose related. Our hope is to maintain each patient's level of function in ADL as long as possible. In dealing with families, we emphasize that mild improvement, stabilization, and slowing of progression are all good outcomes.

How long treatment should be continued is difficult to know, because it is difficult to distinguish loss of drug effect from progression of the disease, and symptoms may worsen with discontinuance of therapy. When the decision is made to discontinue a cholinesterase inhibitor, downward dose titration seems appropriate; our experience is that rapid withdrawal is often followed by an exacerbation of cognitive and behavioral symptoms. If symptoms worsen with withdrawal, we restart or continue the cholinesterase inhibitor. In the later stages of dementia, when patients no longer know or interact in a meaningful way with family or caregivers, we believe the medication no longer has any meaningful benefits to the patient or the family, and with the family's consent, we discontinue therapy.

NMDA Receptor Antagonists

Memantine

Memantine, an N-methyl-D-aspartate (NMDA) receptor antagonist marketed as Namenda, blocks the actions of glutamate at the NMDA receptor, thereby improving synaptic transmission and/or preventing calcium release, which may provide neuroprotection. Memantine is well absorbed and has a 70-hour or greater half-life, but is still given twice per day because that was the dosage scheme used prior to and during studies establishing efficacy.

In a 12-week multicenter European study, nursing home patients with moderate- to severe-stage Alzheimer dementia or vascular dementia were treated with placebo or memantine 10 mg/day. The memantine-treated patients demonstrated delay in symptomatic cognitive and functional deterioration and were significantly less dependent on nursing staff (Winblad and Poritis 1999). In a large 28-week, double-blind, placebo-controlled U.S. study of memantine 20 mg/day in patients with moderate- to severe-stage AD, similar benefits of memantine were seen in delaying cognitive loss and deterioration in functioning in ADL (Reisberg et al. 2003). Memantine-treated patients also required significantly less caregiver time. In clinical practice, memantine is helpful in patients with moderate- and severe-stage AD, with the dosage started at 5 mg/day and titrated up by 5 mg/day each week to a final dosage of 10 mg bid. There may be transient confusion or sedation during the titration phase, but memantine generally has had fewer adverse effects than the cholinesterase inhibitors (Table

14–2). Two large double-blind, placebo-controlled studies of memantine in patients with mild-stage AD have shown minimal or borderline results in efficacy assessments (Bakchine and Loft 2008; Peskind et al. 2006). Nonetheless, memantine is frequently used in these patients, with variable efficacy. A major issue is often the cost of this off-label use of the drug.

Combination Therapy With Cholinesterase Inhibitors and Memantine

Because cholinesterase inhibitors and memantine have different mechanisms of action, the rationale is strong that combination therapy may provide additional benefits. Tariot et al. (2004) conducted a large double-blind, placebo-controlled trial of memantine in subjects who had been taking established stable dosages of donepezil for an average of 24 months. Compared to subjects given stable dosages of donepezil plus placebo, patients taking donepezil plus memantine were more likely to complete the trial, had fewer gastrointestinal adverse effects, and had improved global functioning, cognition, function in ADL, and behavior. Open-label studies of galantamine or rivastigmine plus memantine have had similar outcomes. Combination of a cholinesterase inhibitor with memantine has become the preferred treatment in clinical practice for patients with moderate to severe AD, except as limited by adverse effects or financial burden.

Serotonin Augmentation

Cell loss in AD often occurs in the dorsal raphe nucleus of the brain stem, the site of serotonergic innervation of the forebrain. As a result, brain serotonin metabolites are reduced by 30%–40% (Gottfries et al. 1983). The relationship between the serotonergic system and cognition in AD is unclear, but clinical experience suggests that serotonergic augmentation may modestly increase functional performance, as well as reduce symptoms of depression and anxiety.

The most successful serotonergic strategy has been the use of selective serotonin reuptake inhibitors (SSRIs). This class of drugs includes fluoxetine (Prozac), sertraline (Zoloft), citalopram (Celexa), and escitalopram (Lexapro). Paroxetine (Paxil), another member of this class, should be avoided due to anticholinergic side effects. SSRIs are the most commonly prescribed class of an-

Table 14–2. Percentage of adverse events (5% or over) associated with the use of cholinesterase inhibitors and memantine in patients with Alzheimer disease

Adverse event[a]	Donepezil oral (n=747)	Rivastigmine oral (n=1,189)	Rivastigmine transdermal (n=291)	Galantamine oral (n=1,040)	Memantine oral (n=940)
Abdominal pain		13		5	
Accident	7	10			
Anorexia		17		9	
Anxiety		5			
Asthenia		6			
Confusion		8			6
Constipation		5			5
Depression		6		7	
Diarrhea	10	19	6	9	
Dizziness	8	21		9	7
Dyspepsia		9		5	
Fatigue	5	9		5	
Headache	10	17		8	6
Insomnia	9	9		5	
Malaise		5			
Muscle cramps	6				

Table 14–2.   Percentage of adverse events (5% or over) associated with the use of cholinesterase inhibitors and memantine in patients with Alzheimer disease (continued)

Adverse event[a]	Donepezil oral (n=747)	Rivastigmine oral (n=1,189)	Rivastigmine transdermal (n=291)	Galantamine oral (n=1,040)	Memantine oral (n=940)
Nausea	11	47	7	24	
Pain	9				
Somnolence		5			
Urinary tract infection		7		8	
Vomiting	5	31	6	13	
Weight decrease				7	

Note.   Information from manufacturers' package inserts.
[a]The numbers represent adverse events reported in at least 5% of the patients receiving drug and at a higher frequency than placebo-treated patients. (The 10 most frequently occurring adverse events for each drug are indicated in bold.) Because of differences in trial design, the percentages of adverse events for each drug should not be directly compared to each other but provide a perspective on which adverse events are more likely with each drug.

tidepressants in elderly subjects because of their relative lack of life-threatening or other unpleasant side effects and once-daily dosing. These drugs are administered in the morning because of their mild stimulating effects. Transient side effects that may occur with all drugs of this class include increased anxiety, sleeplessness, loss of appetite, diarrhea, and sexual dysfunction (inhibited orgasm or ejaculation, loss of libido).

Fluoxetine is virtually devoid of anticholinergic, antihistaminic, and antiadrenergic side effects. It does occasionally have antidopaminergic actions that can be associated with extrapyramidal adverse effects in some patients. It has been widely used in elderly patients, but has been associated with weight loss in nursing home patients (Brymer and Winograd 1992) and with the syndrome of inappropriate antidiuretic hormone secretion (SIADH) (Druckenbrod and Mulsant 1994). Sleep disturbance and increased agitation have also been reported. Its long half-life (1–3 days), the presence of an active metabolite, and its potent inhibition of CYP 2D6 and intermediate inhibition of CYP 3A4 can result in drug accumulation. Therefore, low doses or less than daily dosing should be considered in treating very frail elderly patients with dementia. Fluoxetine is typically administered at a dosage of 5–20 mg/day, but if the drug is overly stimulating, the patient can take one capsule every other day or fluoxetine concentrated solution.

Sertraline has a 24-hour half-life. It is a weak inhibitor of CYP 3A4 and CYP 2D6. Transient nausea may occur with its use. The drug appears to be well tolerated by elderly patients (Cohn et al. 1990). Dosing in older outpatients is either 50 or 100 mg/day, starting at 50 mg/day; in frail elders, dosing begins at 25 mg/day. Little evidence indicates that dosages greater than 100 mg/day are more effective. Dose escalation often is desirable over time to avoid adverse effects.

Citalopram and its S-isomer escitalopram are the most serotonin-selective of the SSRIs (Owens and Rosenbaum 1997). These drugs are well tolerated in elderly subjects with AD. Citalopram is initiated at 20 mg/day, and escitalopram at 10 mg/day.

Serotonin Syndrome

Serotonin syndrome may be seen occasionally with any of the SSRIs (Isbister et al. 2007). It is rare but occurs more commonly when combinations of drugs are employed. Combinations of monoamine oxidase inhibitors (MAOIs) and tricyclic antidepressants, MAOIs and SSRIs, and MAOIs and venlafaxine (Effexor) are the most commonly reported causes. The full-blown serotonin syndrome includes mental status changes, agitation or restlessness, myoclonus, hyperreflexia, diaphoresis, tremor, shivering, incoordination, autonomic dysfunction, hyperthermia, and muscular rigidity. Myoglobinuria and renal failure may result, as may seizures or disseminated intravascular coagulation. Treatment of serotonin syndrome entails withdrawal of the precipitating drug.

SSRI Withdrawal

Withdrawal symptoms are common when SSRIs are discontinued, even when they are tapered slowly. Such symptoms tend to be more common with short-acting SSRIs, such as paroxetine, than with sertraline or fluoxetine. The symptoms persist up to 21 days and most commonly include dizziness, lethargy, paresthesia, nausea, vivid dreams, irritability, and depressed mood. Symptoms are relieved, usually within 24 hours, by restarting the medication (Lader 2007) and are not relieved by benzodiazepines.

Antioxidants

Evidence of possible central nervous system damage due to lipid peroxidation and oxidative injury led to a trial of vitamin E (α-tocopherol) and the MAOI selegiline in a double-blind, placebo-controlled trial in persons with moderate to severe AD (Sano et al. 1997). The trial, conducted over 2 years, compared α-tocopherol (2,000 IU/day), selegiline (10 mg/day), α-tocopherol plus selegiline, and placebo. The primary outcome measure (endpoint) was time to death, institutionalization, loss of ability to perform basic ADL, or severe dementia. After adjustment for severity of illness at the beginning of the study, selegiline was associated with time to endpoint of 655 days; α-tocopherol, 670 days; and selegiline and α-tocopherol combined, 585 days. No difference was found between groups in cognitive measures or in overall side effects. The most important contraindication to high-dose vitamin E is the use of warfarin (Coumadin) as an anticoagulant. For many years, 2,000 IU of vitamin E was widely prescribed in patients with MCI and AD. However, recent studies have suggested an increase in potential for abnormal blood clotting in patients taking >1,000 IU of vitamin E (Petersen et al. 2005). For this reason, use of vitamin E as a neuroprotective agent in treating MCI and AD has declined. Similarly, a 1-year double-blind, placebo-controlled transdermal patch study of high-dose selegiline failed to show any benefit over placebo in patients with AD (Farlow et al. 1999).

Ginkgo Biloba

Flavonoid extracts of the leaves of the *Ginkgo biloba* (maidenhair) tree are available on a nonprescription basis throughout the world for a variety of nonspecific indications, including an implicit claim of improving memory in healthy persons as well as people with disorders affecting memory. The substance may have antioxidant and anti-inflammatory properties. Double-blind, placebo-controlled studies have been performed for up to 1 year using dosages up to 240 mg/day (Solomon et al. 2002). In the largest study, Schneider et al. (2005) performed a double-blind, placebo-controlled trial in 600 patients with mild-to moderate-stage AD. No benefits were seen over the 6-month course of the study in cognition, ADL, or behavior.

Although *Ginkgo biloba* is still widely used by elderly patients with and without memory problems, as well as by patients with AD, the evidence suggests modest to no effects on cognitive function. On the positive side, this herbal substance appears to cause very few side effects.

Treatment of Mild Cognitive Impairment

A recent review found three published and five unpublished randomized, double-blind, placebo-controlled trials of acetylcholinesterase inhibitors in MCI patients; three studies were with donepezil, two with rivastigmine, and three with galantamine (Raschetti et al. 2007). The trials ranged from 24 weeks to 3 years. Over these periods of time, no significant difference occurred in the probability of conversion from MCI to dementia between the active treatment groups and placebo groups. MCI has not been accepted by the FDA as a treatment indication, primarily because of ambiguity regarding the specificity of the diagnosis. In practice, many physicians treat MCI as the mildest stage of AD and offer cholinesterase inhibitor therapy as a possible choice for their patients.

Conclusion

The cholinesterase inhibitors mildly improve cognition and functioning in ADL across mild to severe stages of AD. They tend to be most effective at their maximum tolerated dosages, which are typically limited by adverse gastrointestinal effects. Their actions are symptomatic. Benefits may not be seen in many patients. Memantine, a partial antagonist at the NMDA receptor, has been demonstrated to mildly improve cognition and ADL in subjects with AD and moderate- to severe-stage dementia, and these benefits may be additive to the effects of cholinesterase inhibitors. Other commonly used drugs, such as antidepressants and *Ginkgo biloba*, have much less secure evidence supporting their use. Other therapeutic approaches, such as exercise, reducing body weight, or aggressively treating the metabolic syndrome, are increasingly being recommended by physicians to reduce vascular disease and AD, although objective evidence that these efforts will be effective is years away. For now, treatment with a cholinesterase inhibitor and/or memantine and with psychotropic drugs added as needed to treat behavioral symptoms remains the approach most likely to achieve best clinical outcome in patients with AD or related dementias.

Key Clinical Points

- The two classes of U.S. Food and Drug Administration (FDA)–approved cognitive enhancers for Alzheimer disease (AD) are acetylcholinesterase inhibitors and N-methyl-D-aspartate (NMDA) antagonists.
- The various cholinesterase inhibitors in the current dosage forms are comparable in efficacy and adverse effect rates.
- Acetylcholinesterase inhibitors and NMDA antagonists have modest efficacy and have not been shown to delay progression of the illness.
- Careful attention must be paid to comorbid conditions and titration when initiating therapy with acetylcholinesterase inhibitors and NMDA antagonists.

References

Auriacombe S, Pere JJ, Loria-Kanza Y, et al: Efficacy and safety of rivastigmine in patients with Alzheimer's disease who failed to benefit from treatment with donepezil. Curr Med Res Opin 18:129–138, 2002

Bakchine S, Loft H: Memantine treatment in patients with mild to moderate Alzheimer's disease: results of a randomized, double-blind, placebo-controlled 6-month study. J Alzheimers Dis 13:97–107, 2008

Black SE, Doody RS, Li H: Donepezil preserves function and global function in patients with severe Alzheimer disease. Neurology 69:459–469, 2007

Bores GM, Huger FP, Petko W, et al: Pharmacological evaluation of novel Alzheimer's disease therapeutics: acetylcholinesterase inhibitors related to galantamine. J Pharmacol Exp Ther 277:728–738, 1996

Brymer C, Winograd CH: Fluoxetine in elderly patients: is there cause for concern? J Am Geriatr Soc 40:902–905, 1992

Cohn CK, Shrivastava R, Mendels J, et al: Double-blind, multicenter comparison of sertraline and amitriptyline in elderly depressed patients. J Clin Psychiatry 51:28–33, 1990

Corey-Bloom J, Anand R, Veach J: A randomized trial evaluating the efficacy and safety of ENA 713 (rivastigmine tartrate), a new acetylcholinesterase inhibitor, in patients with mild to moderately severe Alzheimer's disease. International Journal of Geriatric Psychopharmacology 1:55–65, 1998

Courtney C, Farrell D, Gray R, et al; AD2000 Collaborative Group: Long-term donepezil treatment in 565 patients with Alzheimer's disease (AD2000): randomised double-blind trial. Lancet 363:2105–2115, 2004

Crismon ML: Pharmacokinetics and drug interactions of cholinesterase inhibitors administered in Alzheimer's disease. Pharmacotherapy 18(2):47–54, 1998

Cummings JL: Cholinesterase inhibitors: a new class of psychotropic compounds. Am J Psychiatry 157:4–15, 2000

Cummings JL, Mega M, Gray K, et al: The Neuropsychiatric Inventory: comprehensive assessment of psychopathology in dementia. Neurology 44:2308–2314, 1994

Cummings JL, Tractenberg RE, Gamst A, et al: Regression to the mean: implications for clinical trials of psychotropic agents in dementia. Curr Alzheimer Res 1:323–328, 2004

Davies P, Maloney AJF: Selective loss of central cholinergic neurons in Alzheimer's disease (letter). Lancet 2:1403, 1976

Davis KL, Hollander E, Davidson M, et al: Introduction of depression with oxotremorine in patients with Alzheimer's disease. Am J Psychiatry 1445:468–471, 1987

Drachman DA, Leavitt J: Human memory and the cholinergic system. Arch Neurol 30:113–121, 1974

Druckenbrod R, Mulsant BH: Fluoxetine-induced syndrome of inappropriate antidiuretic hormone secretion: a geriatric case report and a review of the literature. J Geriatr Psychiatry Neurol 7:254–256, 1994

Erkinjuntti T, Kurz A, Gauthier S, et al: Efficacy of galantamine in probable vascular dementia and Alzheimer's disease combined with cerebrovascular disease: a randomized trial. Lancet 359:1283–1290, 2002

Farlow MR, Tariot P, Hochadel T, et al: Disease stage severity at baseline influenced progression rate in a 48-week selegiline Alzheimer's disease treatment trial. Neurology 52 (suppl 2):S172–S173, 1999

Farlow MR, Salloway S, Tariot PN, et al: Effectiveness and tolerability of high-dose (23 mg/d) versus standard-dose (10 mg/d) donepezil in moderate to severe Alzheimer's disease: a 24-week, randomized, double-blind study. Clin Ther 32:1234–1251, 2010

Feldman H, Gauthier S, Hecker J, et al: Efficacy and safety of donepezil in patients with more severe Alzheimer's disease: a subgroup analysis from a randomized, placebo-controlled trial. Int J Geriatr Psychiatry 20:559–569, 2005

Folstein MF, Folstein SE, McHugh PR: "Mini-mental state": a practical method for grading the cognitive state of patients for the clinician. J Psychiatr Res 12:189–198, 1975

Gottfries CG, Adolfsson R, Aquilonius SM, et al: Biochemical changes in dementia disorders of the Alzheimer type (AD/SDAT). Neurobiol Aging 4:261–271, 1983

Isbister GK, Buckley NA, Whyte IM: Serotonin toxicity: a practical approach to diagnosis and treatment. Med J Aust 187:361–365, 2007

Jann MW: Rivastigmine: a new-generation cholinesterase inhibitor for the treatment of Alzheimer's disease. Pharmacotherapy 20:1–12, 2000

Katz IR, Sands LP, Bilker W, et al: Identification of medications that cause cognitive impairment in older people: the case of oxybutynin chloride. J Am Geriatr Soc 46:8–13, 1998

Lader M: Pharmacotherapy of mood disorders and treatment discontinuation. Drugs 67:1657–1663, 2007

McKeith I, Del Ser T, Spano P, et al: Efficacy of rivastigmine in dementia with Lewy bodies: a randomised, double-blind, placebo-controlled international study. Lancet 356:2031–2036, 2000a

McKeith IG, Grace JB, Walker Z, et al: Rivastigmine in the treatment of dementia with Lewy bodies: preliminary findings from an open trial. Int J Geriatr Psychiatry 15:387–392, 2000b

Mega MS, Masterman DM, O'Connor SM, et al: The spectrum of responses of cholinesterase inhibitor therapy in Alzheimer's disease. Arch Neurol 56:1388–1393,
1999

Mohs RC, Doody RS, Morris JC, et al: A 1-year, placebo-controlled preservation of
function survival study of donepezil in AD patients. Neurology 57:481–488, 2001

Owens MJ, Rosenbaum JF: Escitalopram: a second generation SSRI. CNS Spectr 7:34–
39, 1997

Peskind ER, Potkin SG, Pomara N, et al: Memantine treatment in mild to moderate
Alzheimer disease: a 24-week randomized, controlled trial. Am J Geriatr Psychiatry
14:704–715, 2006

Petersen RC, Thomas RG, Grundman M, et al: Vitamin E and donepezil for the
treatment of mild cognitive impairment. N Engl J Med 352:2379–2388, 2005

Raschetti R, Albanese E, Vanacore N, et al: Cholinesterase inhibitors in mild cognitive
impairment: a systematic view of randomized trials. PLoS Med 4:818–826, 2007

Raskind MA, Peskind ER, Wessel T, et al: Galantamine in AD: a 6-month randomized,
placebo-controlled trial with a 6-month extension. Neurology 54:2261–2268, 2000

Reisberg B, Doody R, Stoffler A, et al: Memantine in moderate-to-severe Alzheimer's
disease. N Engl J Med 348:1333–1341, 2003

Ringman JM, Simmons JH: Treatment of REM sleep behavior disorder with donepezil:
a report of three cases. Neurology 55:870–871, 2000

Robbins TW, Roberts AC: Differential regulation of fronto-executive function by the
monoamines and acetylcholine. Cereb Cortex 17 (suppl 1):151–160, 2007

Rogers SL, Friedhoff LT: The efficacy and safety of donepezil in patients with Alzheimer's disease: results of a U.S. multicentre, randomized, double-blind, placebo-
controlled trial. Dementia 7:293–303, 1996

Rogers SL, Farlow MR, Doody RS, et al: A 24-week, double-blind, placebo-controlled
trial of donepezil in patients with Alzheimer's disease. Neurology 50:136–145, 1998

Rösler M, Anand R, Cicin-Sain A, et al: Efficacy and safety of rivastigmine in patients
with Alzheimer's disease: international randomised controlled trial. BMJ
318:633–638, 1999

Sano M, Ernesto C, Thomas RG, et al: A controlled trial of selegiline, alpha-tocopherol,
or both as treatment for Alzheimer's disease. The Alzheimer's Disease Cooperative
Study. N Engl J Med 336:1216–1222, 1997

Schneider LS, Olin JT, Doody RS, et al: Validity and reliability of the Alzheimer's
Disease Cooperative Study–Clinical Global Impression of Change. Alzheimer Dis
Assoc Disord 11 (suppl 2):S22–S32, 1997

Schneider LS, DeKosky ST, Farlow MR, et al: A randomized, double-blind, placebo-
controlled trial of two doses of Ginkgo biloba extract in dementia of the Alzheimer's type. Curr Alzheimer Res 2:541–551, 2005

Solomon PR, Adams F, Silver A, et al: Ginkgo for memory enhancement: a randomized controlled trial. JAMA 288:835–840, 2002

Tariot PN, Mack JL, Patterson MB, et al: The Behavior Rating Scale for Dementia of the Consortium to Establish a Registry for Alzheimer's Disease. The Behavioral Pathology Committee of the Consortium to Establish a Registry for Alzheimer's Disease. Am J Psychiatry 152:1349–1357, 1995

Tariot PN, Solomon PR, Morris JC, et al: A 5-month randomized, placebo-controlled trial of galantamine in AD. The Galantamine USA-10 Study Group. Neurology 54:2269–2276, 2000

Tariot PN, Farlow MR, Grossberg GT, et al: Memantine treatment in patients with moderate to severe Alzheimer's disease already receiving donepezil: a randomized controlled trial. JAMA 291:317–324, 2004

Thal LJ, Carta A, Clarke WR, et al: A 1-year multicenter placebo-controlled study of acetyl-L-carnitine in patients with Alzheimer's disease. Neurology 47:705–711, 1996

Weiner MF, Martin-Cook K, Foster BM, et al: Effects of donepezil on emotional/behavioral symptoms in Alzheimer's disease patients. J Clin Psychiatry 61:487–492, 2000

Wilcock GK, Lilienfeld S, Gaens E: Efficacy and safety of galantamine in patients with mild to moderate Alzheimer's disease: multicentre randomised controlled trial. BMJ 321:1445–1449, 2001

Wilcock GK, Howe I, Coles H, et al: A long-term comparison of galantamine and donepezil in the treatment of Alzheimer's disease. Drugs Aging 20:777–789, 2003

Winblad B, Poritis N: Memantine in severe dementia: results of the 9M-Best study (benefit and efficacy in severely demented patients during treatment with memantine). Int J Geriatr Psychiatry 14:135–146, 1999

Winblad B, Kilander L, Eriksson S, et al: Donepezil in patients with severe Alzheimer's disease: double-blind, parallel-group, placebo-controlled study. Lancet 367:1057–1065, 2006

Zhao Q, Janssens L, Verhaeghe T, et al: Pharmacokinetics of extended-release and immediate-release formulations of galantamine at steady state in healthy volunteers. Curr Med Res Opin 21:1547–1554, 2005

Further Reading

Fillit HM, Smith-Doody R, Binaso K, et al: Recommendations for best practices in the treatment of Alzheimer's disease in managed care. Am J Geriatr Psychiatry 15:953–960, 2007

Hake AM, Farlow MR: Dementia, in Practical Neurology, 3rd Edition. Edited by Biller J. Philadelphia, PA, Lippincott-Raven, 2008

Katona C, Livingston G, Cooper C, et al: International Psychogeriatric Association consensus statement on defining and measuring treatment benefits in dementia. Int Psychogeriatr 19:345–354, 2007

Matthews FE, McKeith I, Bond J, et al: Reaching the population with dementia drugs: what are the challenges? Int J Geriatr Psychiatry 22:627–631, 2007

Tinklenberg JR, Kraemer HC, Yaffe K, et al: Donepezil treatment and Alzheimer disease: can the results of randomized clinical trials be applied to Alzheimer disease patients in clinical practice? Am J Geriatr Psychiatry 15:953–960, 2007

15

Supporting Family Caregivers

Kristin Martin-Cook, M.S., C.C.R.C.

Myron F. Weiner, M.D.

In the long-term management of patients with dementia, the clinician's primary relationship is with the patient's family, especially when patients lack self-awareness, as in many cases of Alzheimer disease and almost all cases of Pick disease, or when patients are cognitively compromised to the point that they can no longer make reasonable decisions. In these situations, family members must learn to substitute their judgment for that of the patient. They must assume the responsibility for managing a patient's person and property in accordance with his or her previously expressed wishes, if possible. And they must do so in a way that does not demean or demoralize. Therefore, after the clinician makes a diagnosis and institutes appropriate medical treatment, the most important issues to address are the education and emotional and physical support of family caregivers.

Education About the Illness

Caregivers need to and usually want to learn about the cognitive and behavioral effects of dementing illness, its anticipated course, available treatments, and the social and financial consequences of the illness. Different caregivers require different information and differing styles of presenting the information. Some caregivers cope best by being fully informed; others are overwhelmed by the changes in their relationship to their loved ones and can deal only with small amounts of information that have immediate relevance. We generally do not push family members to read caregiver- or dementia-oriented books that describe the full course of illnesses such as Alzheimer disease. We encourage them instead to live day by day, and to deal with issues such as incontinence and wandering when they arise, if they arise. We offer participation in our monthly support group to reduce the family's sense of isolation and provide practical advice and management strategies. We also offer brief, relevant handouts, mostly from the Alzheimer's Association, that focus on specific behavioral and legal issues. We explain that more information can be obtained as issues arise or whenever the caregiver feels it is needed. For those who are information seekers, many lay-directed guides are available for families of dementia patients, especially those with Alzheimer disease. The best resource is the fourth edition of *The 36-Hour Day* (Mace and Rabins 2006). The appendix of this book lists additional sources of information.

Family members need to understand that their loved one has a reduced capacity to encode, process, integrate, communicate, act on information, and in some cases, regulate his or her behavior. These changes in turn impair the individual's ability to act appropriately in response to certain situations or information.

Medical jargon should be avoided if possible, and when it is used, the clinician needs to explain it. For example, we explain the term *dementia* as shorthand for describing a decrement in level of function sufficient to interfere with daily activities, and comment that having a dementing illness does not necessarily mean that a person is already demented.

Day-to-day fluctuations in self-awareness, cognitive functioning, and behavior often leave family members puzzled about the patient's abilities and inabilities and, very often, about the diagnosis. As one wife said,

> My husband could remember what I was telling him yesterday but today seems utterly confused. Is he deliberately not paying attention? Sometimes it

seems he is deliberately ignoring me or seeking attention by asking the same questions over and over.

Cognitive or behavioral fluctuations are hard for families to understand. We explain to families that just as normal persons have changes in their ability to understand and to cope, persons with brain compromise experience the same fluctuations but with greater intensity because of their brain damage or disease.

If there are positive findings, it is sometimes useful to show brain images to families (e.g., magnetic resonance images), because it helps caregivers view cognitive loss in the context of a brain disease. Also, concrete examples of how cognitive symptoms may affect daily functioning are important.

Your husband becomes lost when trying to find his way to the bathroom at night. This is frequent in dementing illness. Because his memory is impaired, he has to rely on his eyesight to help him make up for that loss. When he can't see well, his memory is no longer good enough to guide him.

Your mother probably burns food on the stove because she is having difficulty with her concentration and her memory. Her attention wanders easily, and she forgets what she is doing. She gives the appearance of carelessness when she is actually performing as well as she can.

Sometimes the cognitive impairment is best conveyed by analogizing the patient's inability to reason or understand to that of a small child—including a child's need for simple directions and for direction by example.

You tell me that you deal with your young children by showing them how to do something instead of telling them what to do. Instead of telling your mother to stir the soup so that it won't burn, show her how you want the soup stirred, help her to do it for a few moments, and then let her do it on her own. When she gets confused on the way to the bathroom, guide her to it. If you tell her where the bathroom is, she won't remember. She'll be less irritable if she's helped to do what you want her to do or what she wants to do instead of being told what not to do or that what she's doing is wrong.

Because disturbing behaviors, even more than cognitive dysfunction, lead families to seek diagnosis and treatment, the clinician needs to address these symptoms and to explain the link between these symptoms and the dementing illness. Irritability, for example, requires an explanation similar to that for disorientation.

You find that your father is more irritable. Irritability often goes along with his illness. His irritability is partly from his inability to suppress minor irritation as you and I do when we get upset over something that we know is trivial. It is also partly from his anger with himself because he is unable to concentrate and remember.

Disinhibition also needs to be explained, so that a cognitively impaired person who accidentally exposes his genitals in a long-term-care facility is not believed to be a sexual predator, making it possible for staff to deal with such acts through simple redirection into other activities.

Depression, too, is often a concern of families. The apathy inherent in most dementing illnesses is frequently misinterpreted as depression. In fact, many families and primary care physicians postpone treatment for dementing illness in the hope or belief that the patient is "just depressed." Clinicians need to help families understand that withdrawal often represents an adaptive disengagement from activities that are too challenging.

The clinician can bring each patient's specific cognitive problems to light by including caregivers in the patient's mental status examination and by reviewing the examination with them afterward. The digit span test can be used to show caregivers that the patient's defects in concentration make it difficult to remember and that information must be presented in small increments. Testing of remote memory and immediate recall can demonstrate that recall is the type of memory that is most seriously affected and that what was encoded long ago may be partially intact. Understanding that there are different types of memory helps caregivers to deal with the logical inconsistency that the patient can easily remember something from long ago and not something that happened only a few minutes ago. The clinician can demonstrate a patient's impairment of judgment by asking simple questions involving social judgment. Caregivers' observations of the clinician's management of the patient's irritability or inappropriate social behavior can be translated into useful management strategies.

Families often want to know what element of cognitive functioning or behavior will be affected next and whether there is a predictable pattern of loss. In the case of progressive dementing illnesses, families can be told that there will be progressive impairment of the ability to learn new skills and ideas, so that patients will have to rely increasingly on what they already know how to do. Families can also be told to expect impairment of reasoning ability.

Your wife's impaired judgment is likely to show up in the car. She will probably continue to stop at red traffic lights and go when they turn green, but she may not take into account that somebody may still be crossing the street or that a car is entering the intersection from another direction.

Families of patients with Alzheimer disease in particular are becoming more sophisticated and educated, thanks largely to the Alzheimer's Association and the ready access to information provided by the Internet. Many families want to discuss the pathophysiology of the illness and to find out what areas of the brain and what neurotransmitters are involved. We use a brain model for this purpose. Families learn that anticholinergic drugs are prone to cause delirium in patients with Alzheimer disease, and learn to guard these patients from antihistamines and other medications with significant anticholinergic properties. Educating families about the potentially toxic side effects of medications is also helpful. They need not be given a list of delirium-producing medications. Instead, they can be asked to always consider the possibility that a new medication or a dosage increase of a long-standing medication may be responsible for a change in mental status. Families also need to be cautioned about the potential paradoxical excitatory effects of minor tranquilizers in patients with all forms of dementing illness.

Families can be taught that patients' difficulty with new learning makes it unwise to introduce their loved ones into new situations and that the wiser action is to involve them in familiar activities in familiar places. Caregivers can be taught not to remind patients of their deficits, and to serve as memory and a social buffer.

Prognosis

Prognosis is a very important issue for families, from both practical and emotional points of view. Families want to know the anticipated course of the illness. Most families can tolerate being told that a disease is expected to progress but that the exact course cannot be predicted. They can be told that there may be long periods of no apparent decline. They generally appreciate being told both the worst and the best possible outcomes. Generally speaking, it seems unwise to suggest that the course of the illness may at any time involve agitation or violence. Such a suggestion can make a family wary of the loved one and may cause them to overreact to trivial events. In cases of patients with vascular dementia, the family may be offered the hope that progression may be slowed by the use of aspirin or antiplatelet drugs, but they should also be told that a good likelihood remains that the dementia will progress and that plans should be made accordingly. In cases of Alzheimer disease, families can be told that the disease will progress, that its rate of progression is uncertain, and that medications are available to slow progression. When families ask about the ultimate outcome of Alzheimer disease, they can be told that if the patient lives long enough, this disease may result in complete inability to communicate or perform self-care. However, they should also be told that few people live out the entire course of illness.

Our general policy is to suggest to families that they live one day at a time rather than live in anticipation of symptoms or behaviors that may never arise. When patients ask us when nursing home care will be needed, we indicate that need for such care depends on several factors, but that the ability of families to deal with and to tolerate behaviors such as wandering and incontinence is often the impetus, and families generally know when their tolerance has been exceeded.

Family Risk

Some dementing illnesses involve risk to family members. In the case of Huntington disease and Alzheimer disease, the risks are genetic. Because the former expresses in midlife, the pattern of dominant inheritance poses a serious threat to siblings and offspring; great sensitivity is needed in dealing with the issue of heritability. The situation in Alzheimer disease is similar for dominantly inherited early-onset Alzheimer disease but not for late-onset disease. We respond to concern about the heritability of Alzheimer disease by stating that not enough is currently known to enable sound counseling but that the risk increases for siblings and children of affected persons, although we are unable to predict the exact risk for individuals. In the instances of familial Alzheimer disease with onset as early as the fifth decade, families can be reasonably counseled that the risk approaches 50% for offspring of an afflicted person should they live to the age of usual disease onset in the family. When presenting data concerning the heritability of illness, clinicians need to be alert to the impact of this information on family members. An open-ended discussion following the communication of this information usually brings to light fears, misgivings, and potential negative effects.

When counseling about infectious disorders such as Creutzfeldt-Jakob disease or AIDS, the clinician indicates that these diseases can be communicated only from body fluid to body fluid and that, therefore, appropriate precautions are necessary. In the case of Creutzfeldt-Jakob disease, blood-to-blood transmission would be likely only in the event that a caregiver punctured himself or herself with a needle contaminated with the patient's blood. With AIDS, contact with blood and seminal fluid is to be avoided.

Other Major Issues

The family of a patient with dementia has many questions and issues to consider. Who will be the primary caregiver and conduit of information to and from the patient and family? The designated primary caregiver, in consultation with the clinician, the patient, and the rest of the family, needs to consider what supervision is necessary and how supervision is to be arranged. If the person is living independently, is that living situation feasible or desirable? If it is, how independent is the person? Can the patient be allowed to continue driving? Buy groceries? Cook? Must eating and personal hygiene be supervised? In many instances, persons with cognitive impairment can continue to live in their own accustomed residence, with once- or twice-daily supervision by friends, relatives, and neighbors. If independent living is not feasible from the standpoint of safety or convenience, where can the person best be served and accommodated? Could the person live with a friend or relative? Would a day care program ease the burden? Would assisted living be appropriate? Is a special care facility needed?

Families attempt to balance these quality-of-life issues with safety issues. Because many patients have impaired awareness and insight, their families are often left to make decisions regarding the level of independence the patient will maintain—a situation that many patients resent and resist.

For patients with more advanced disease, the issue of nursing home care arises. For near-terminal patients in nursing homes, one issue is whether to institute tube feeding. Financial and legal issues must be raised. Has a will been made? If not, is the patient able to indicate his or her true wishes? Is the patient able to transact business or enter contracts, such as for the sale of property? Does another family member have the type of power of attorney that can be used when the patient is no longer able to direct his or her own affairs? Is guardianship necessary to ensure impartial supervision of the patient's assets? If guardianship is needed, should it be full or partial?

In anticipation of the need for Medicaid coverage of possible prolonged nursing home placement, is it best that the patient's property be transferred to other family members? Although for specific questions we typically refer families to financial consultants specializing in issues related to the elderly population, clinicians can provide some general information regarding financial issues. Many people believe that Medicare will provide for the health care needs of patients. The clinician should explain that custodial care of persons with dementing illnesses is not covered by Medicare, so families need to make plans accordingly.

Imparting a Psychological Point of View

Clinicians should make an effort to impart a psychological point of view to caregivers. Family members are often confused by daily fluctuations in cognitive ability and behavior and tend to see cognitively impaired persons as arbitrarily deciding to forget and consciously manipulating others. Typically, however, what appear to be willful, negatively perceived behaviors are actually attempts to avoid becoming overwhelmed, based on each person's own style of coping with or adapting to stress.

Caregivers often see persons with cognitive impairment as unreasonably irritable and fail to recognize how frustrating it is to be unable to reason, to remember, and to perform simple activities of daily living. When caregivers' attempts at orienting a patient are met with apparent indifference, the caregivers must be reminded that this appearance of indifference is both a product of the disease and a psychological protection against overwhelming anxiety, rather than indifference to the caring of others.

Family members, out of their own needs and their inability to conceive of the impact of the brain changes that are taking place, often prefer to see loved ones with cognitive impairment as intact persons who are concealed behind a confused exterior. Caregivers can be told that although fragments of their loved one may exist intact, changes in cognition necessitate adjusting and readjusting to a new person with different needs, interests, perceptions, and abilities throughout the course of the dementing illness. Nevertheless, persons with cognitive impairment should be shown the same respect as human beings as cognitively intact persons are shown. Attention must also be given to certain prominent mechanisms of defense in dementia.

Dealing With Denial and Projection

Two of the most important psychological mechanisms of defense in dementing illness are denial and projection. Clinicians need to explain these mechanisms to caregivers as normal means of dealing with the emotionally overwhelming situation of literally losing one's mind and control over one's behavior. Clinicians need to tell caregivers how frightening it is for people to be unable to maintain a sense of self, how all persons use denial to avoid dealing with their own mortality, and how blaming others helps each person avoid full awareness of his or her deficits or limitations.

Caregivers often need to respect a patient's need for denial while addressing his or her realistic inability to cope with certain aspects of the environment. For example, it may be better for a caregiver to say that the car is being repaired or has been borrowed by another family member than to tell a person with cognitive impairment that he or she may no longer drive. One woman dealt with her concern about her husband's driving by telling him that she wanted him to supervise her driving.

Projection is more difficult for caregivers to tolerate than denial because they are usually the object of the projection. When a wallet or purse, house keys, or items of clothing cannot be found, caregivers are usually the ones blamed. We tell caregivers that rather than arguing that they have not borrowed or stolen a particular object, they should institute a search for what is missing, accompanied by the patient if he or she is willing. Another useful tactic is to note where commonly used objects or possessions are kept and to see that they are kept in those places if at all possible.

Delusional projection is even more difficult for caregivers because it frequently ties in with their own wishes and concerns. A cognitively impaired person may express concern that caregivers are trying to steal his or her money. Perhaps the family is attempting to control spending so that the person will not lose all of his or her financial resources, or maybe the beneficiaries are trying to protect their inheritance. Their own emotional entanglement may lead caregivers into vigorous denials that further heighten mutual suspicion.

Caregivers typically cope more easily when instead of being blamed themselves, they are told that strange-looking little people are entering the house and stealing money. When something specific is missing, caregivers need only institute a matter-of-fact search and produce what is missing, if they can. Many times, missing items have been concealed by the patient, who can no longer remember where they are. For that reason, it may be useful to periodically search the environment to find such hiding places. When accusations are made by the patient that cannot be controverted, such as "I know you are stealing my money," it is best to give a brief assurance to the contrary and then to engage the patient in a distracting activity. A reasonable reply to the foregoing accusation would be, "No, I'm not stealing your money. Breakfast is ready. Let's eat." If the delusional projection does not abate and results in great perturbation for the patient or family, the use of antipsychotic medication may be temporarily indicated.

At times, clinicians may suspect that the patient's suspicions of family members or other caregivers are well founded. If the family is suspected of financial or other abuse, Adult Protective Services can be contacted to investigate the situation. The family or proper agencies can be notified if abuse by professional caregivers is suspected.

Maintaining Self-Esteem

Individuals in the early stages of a dementing illness have difficulty maintaining their self-esteem because they can no longer live up to their own notion of who they ought to be and at what level they ought to function. They also recognize that they cannot do for themselves what they have been able to do since childhood: perform simple calculations, follow directions, maintain orientation in time and space, button garments, tie shoelaces, and so on. As cognitive impairment progresses, the capacity for self-awareness and communication diminishes, and maintenance of self-esteem becomes less of a problem, both in terms of patients' self-assurance and their ability to communicate concern about themselves.

Many persons define who they are by what they do. Loss of capacity to work or to carry out one's usual activities leads to a sense of uselessness. It is therefore useful for families to help persons with milder cognitive impairment to find activities at which they can feel competent. These may include activities as simple as dusting the furniture or helping to fold the laundry. Persons who enjoy and are kept occupied by housekeeping chores can be encouraged to do those chores daily—it makes little difference whether the house needs cleaning again or whether the laundry really needs to be folded again. Playing simple games such as bingo can be pleasurable. Each person is unique in the activities that are meaningful to him or her. Helping to discover those activities can be a positive experience for both caregiver and patient.

Caregivers often need to redefine their notion of an activity and to reevaluate their view of the loved one's abilities. Caregivers frequently come to the clinic saying that their care recipient "can't do anything anymore" simply because he or she can no longer engage in his or her previous activities. The clinician should suggest examples of everyday activities that may be enjoyable and esteem-maintaining, and propose ways to initiate these activities. For example, less impaired persons might organize a drawer in the kitchen, whereas more impaired persons can sort items in a drawer, sharpen pencils, test pens, or sort coins. Whatever the activity, it is important to help caregivers view an activity as a series of smaller, more manageable tasks, and to focus on the process of doing the activity rather than on the end product. The Pleasant Events Schedule (Teri and Logsdon 1991) is useful for discovering more activities.

Impact of Dementia on the Family

Dementing illness affects various families and family members in many different ways. It affects spouses, companions, children, grandchildren, and sometimes parents. Family members experience denial, bargaining, anger, depression, and acceptance—the stages of adjustment to disability and grief—many times throughout the course of the illness. These emotional reactions are especially prominent at diagnosis, placement in long-term care, and death, but also when patients have major declines in functioning or changes in personality. This process of adjustment and readjustment is complicated by the progression of the disease, and practical lifestyle changes and medical management are needed. Generally, a theme or focus seems to exist for caregiving in different stages of dementing illness, and a task must be negotiated for each stage. Like the staging of dementing illness, however, the staging of caregiving is imprecise, and the challenges that are prominent at one stage also may continue to exist in another stage.

During the stage at which patients are experiencing mild cognitive impairment, the challenge for caregivers is to become aware that something is happening. Once caregivers become aware of cognitive issues, their task is to obtain a diagnosis. This is often not an easy task. Caregivers may have to deal with conflicting views of the individual's functioning from the patient himself or herself, from other family members, and sometimes from the patient's primary care physician. Caregivers often are ambivalent about receiving a diagnosis. They are validated by the acknowledgment that something is wrong, yet are terrified to face the implications of a diagnosis. Mild declines are frequently unnoticed or glossed over by spouses of elderly persons. In many well-functioning couples, one person automatically compensates for the other's deficits. A husband will begin cooking as the wife becomes less competent in the kitchen, or the wife will take over household repairs from the husband. In our experience, it is not unusual for one member of a couple to be physically handicapped but cognitively intact, whereas the other spouse is cognitively impaired and physically intact. In this situation, the physically disabled member guides the cognitively disabled person in doing the daily chores. Often, the first person to comment on the cognitive deficit of an elderly person with dementia is a son or daughter who lives at a distance and visits infrequently. Many times, it is difficult for the adult children to convince the intact parent that the cognitively impaired parent needs medical evaluation.

The challenge or focus of caregivers of patients with early dementing illness is acceptance, which is necessary for planning to begin. Acceptance involves grieving for the loss of the person, the relationship with that person, life as it was (normalcy), and dreams of the future. When the cognitive impairment of one spouse begins to markedly reduce a couple's quality of life, the unaffected spouse or partner feels frustration, anger, sadness, and sometimes frank depression. A common reaction in elders is a sense of having been robbed of one's golden years. Many elders have postponed pleasures earlier in life for the sake of their careers or their children, in the expectation that retirement would bring comfortable leisure. They become frustrated at their inability to enjoy a time when they are no longer burdened by work or family responsibilities, angry at having lost the opportunity, and sad for their spouse's loss of quality of life. They become depressed as they look forward to their situation deteriorating further and eventually losing their spouse as a person.

As the patient's cognitive function continues to deteriorate, the caregiver's challenge or focus is to adjust his or her own role to fit the caregiving task at hand (financial manager, social coordinator, housekeeper). The personal challenge during the late stages of dementing illnesses is disengagement from the role of spouse or adult child and assumption of the role of physical caregiver. The work involved in this stage is feeding, maintaining hygiene, and helping the patient to find his or her way and to ambulate. Caregivers at this stage often make comments such as "This person is not my wife" or "My mom is already gone."

Spousal caregivers experience difficulties in many areas. Although many persons with a dementing illness are indifferent to their loss of cognitive function, others strive to maintain their premorbid level of functioning and autonomy. A key area of conflict for many couples is driving. For example, a wife might note that her husband's judgment is becoming impaired. He not only becomes lost while driving but also changes lanes without looking or makes left turns from the right lane. Although she does not want her husband to feel less of a person, she fears for his and others' safety. Furthermore, she does not wish to engage in the endless arguments that arise from intensely emotional issues such as relinquishing driving. In situations in which one spouse has difficulty preventing the other from driving, we often suggest that the blame be assigned to the physician (e.g., by saying, "The doctor doesn't want you to drive right now"). Our female patients frequently insist that they can still cook, despite their forgetting how to follow simple recipes and ignoring food burning on a stovetop. Strategies employed in such cases might include turning off the gas supply or electricity to the stove unless there is someone who can directly supervise the cooking process.

Another key area of difficulty for spouses is coping with suspiciousness or outright delusional blaming. Being constantly accused of stealing and lying is demoralizing at best. Although spouses can be educated not to challenge suspicions and delusions, it is difficult for them not to feel unappreciated.

In our experience, two situations most often precipitate nursing home admission. They are the advent of total incontinence and the caregiver's inability to get adequate sleep. Spouses seem able to tolerate occasional urinary incontinence. They are often able to manage toileting their spouse frequently, restricting fluid intake after supper to prevent "accidents," or using incontinence pads. Prolonged fecal incontinence is not well tolerated. The emotional transition from spouse to nurse often cannot be accomplished. When persistent incontinence appears to be a result of the dementing illness and not a result of factors such as urinary tract infection, bladder prolapse, fecal impaction, or improper diet, we begin raising the question of institutionalization with the now-exhausted spouse. The same is true when the dementia patient's nighttime agitation or wandering makes it impossible for the caregiver to sleep.

Dementing illness affects both adult children and grandchildren. The adult children who are particularly compromised are those still raising their own children. They are sandwiched between caring for the generations ahead of and behind them. Our experience suggests that daughters and daughters-in-law are frequently affected more than sons or sons-in-law. Brody (1989) suggests that this is because women have more nurturing expectations of themselves than men do, but also men are more often employed full time outside the home.

Adult children often have problems adjusting when their parents become less competent. For many adult children, having an active, decisive parent is so important that they want to continue following that parent's judgment and have difficulty substituting their own judgment for that of their parent. A surprisingly large number of adults continue to be emotionally and financially dependent on their parents and experience the onset of a dementing illness in a parent as a threat to their own integrity. Some children who want to protect parents from the consequences of dementia have parents whose suspiciousness or need for autonomy is so great that they reject help with nutrition or proper clothing. Many of our patients are widows who have lived and managed on their own for many years and are fiercely independent. In this situation, we try to help the children achieve a reasonable balance between safeguarding their parents and interfering with their parents' much-needed sense of autonomy. Adult children are understandably upset that meals delivered to a parent's home are uneaten, that ice cream and cookies are preferred to a balanced diet, that clothing goes unwashed, or that the house is not kept clean. Our general stance is that persons who strongly value their independence and can maintain their nutrition and personal hygiene fairly well will have a better quality of life living on their own than in an institution, and it may be worth risking their safety in exchange for maintaining their quality of life.

Tensions also develop between the adult children of parents with cognitive impairment. Ordinarily, one adult child assumes the majority of the burden of care. This primary nonspousal caregiver is usually self-selected and is most often the child who has maintained the strongest attachment to the parents over the years. At times, the role of primary caregiver falls to the child who is geographically closest or who is not employed outside the home. The primary caregiver's closeness to the parent is often envied by other siblings, who may deal with their envy by criticizing the primary caregiver's quality of care. He or she is seen as too domineering, too harsh, or too easy on the affected parent. Despite their willingness to criticize, envious siblings who act out their rivalry by criticism are often difficult to engage as helpers.

Grandchildren are generally not strongly affected unless the grandmother or grandfather comes to live with them. At times, there is a comfortable relationship, with the grandparent enjoying the interaction with grandchildren and the grandchildren tolerating a grandparent's deficits well. Often, however, grandparents with dementia regress and feel competitive with grandchildren for their parents' attention. Children, in turn, may have difficulty with their grandparents' incapacity and may claim that the elders are faking. Children who feel deprived of nurturing by the presence of a grandparent in the house may also act against the older person and attempt to discredit him or her or drive him or her out of the house.

Dementing illness in an adult child also poses problems for parents. Many parents appreciate the opportunity to do what they can for a child of any age. Others feel that their freedom from child rearing has been hard won and resent intrusion on their middle-age or late-life style of living. They feel a wish to care for their children, as well as guilt because they would now like to conserve some of their energy for themselves. Having reached adulthood, many children are resentful of parents reentering their lives in a decision-making capacity. This is especially true for immature adults or adults for whom autonomy from parents has been a significant and poorly resolved struggle.

Caregiver Stress

Living with or coping with cognitively impaired persons can be extremely stressful. In fact, a large body of literature exists on caregiver stress in Alzheimer disease (Light and Lebowitz 1989). Many supportive community resources exist, including support groups, respite care, elder companions, and adult day care. Interestingly, institutionalization of patients does not totally relieve caregiver strain (George 1984). Families maintain their supportive activities even when loved ones are institutionalized (Martin-Cook et al. 2001). They visit nursing homes frequently, interact with nursing personnel, help with feeding, feel sad about their loved one's condition, and feel guilty because of their inability to maintain their loved one at home. They often feel helpless to complain about suboptimal care for fear that staff will retaliate against their loved one.

As cognitive impairment progresses in Alzheimer disease, most persons appear to lose awareness of their deficits and experience less concern. To the family, the deficits become increasingly apparent as they result in a heavier work and emotional load. Despite the heavy emotional burden and frequent signs of emotional and physical overload, several questionnaire studies show no strong relationship between duration or severity of illness and indexes of caregiver burden (George and Gwyther 1986). Patient and caregiver factors such as health status and problem solving seem to have greater impact on burden (Zarit and Teri 1992). Dysphoria is extremely common. In a survey of primary caregivers, Rabins et al. (1982) found that 87% reported chronic depression, fatigue, and/or anger.

Time with the family is needed to identify their particular stressors before means can be recommended to partially relieve caregivers' physical and emotional distress. In the setting of our dementia clinic, this process begins during the initial interview with the physician, in which the family is seen apart from the patient by both the physician and the clinic nurse. Caregiver stress is also assessed at the reporting interview, to which all concerned family members are invited. In addition to diagnosing the patient and providing direct treatment recommendations, our clinic team tries to help family members arrive at a management plan that is optimal for them and the patient. We state that our aim is to maintain the highest quality of life for all members of the family and that planning for a person's care involves balancing that person's needs against the needs of the rest of the family. On occasions, we recommend supportive counseling or active psychiatric treatment for a family member. We also support professional caregivers doing home care, usually by telephone. They are vulnerable to intense buffering between family members with divergent points of view and often stand between an irritable, nonunderstanding spouse and the patient. Frequently, elderly spouses are only slightly less cognitively impaired than the primary patient and therefore cannot fathom why the husband or wife cannot understand. We offer continued advice and support by telephone and through regular revisits, and we suggest active involvement with the educational programs and support groups of the local Alzheimer's Association and other sources of community support (see appendix at end of book).

Driving

Some cognitively impaired persons who are aware of their deficits will spontaneously curtail or relinquish driving, even when they still have the capacity to drive. Those with little or no insight often put up a fierce battle to stay behind the wheel, citing the many years they have driven and their clean driving record, despite forgotten or ignored accidents and misjudgments. There are many potential strategies for dealing with the latter situation. The easiest method for physicians is to ask patients to stop driving until they have adapted to their new medications, hoping that within several months the patients will become reconciled to having someone else take the wheel. With persons who still maintain the ability to reason, family and physician can state that given a diagnosis such as Alzheimer disease, they would not be covered by their insurance if in an accidental collision and could lose their home and savings if sued. Persons with minimal to moderate insight can be asked to take a driving test at the state Department of Motor Vehicles or be graded on a driving simulator, frequently available in hospital departments of occupational therapy. We have at times notified the Department of Public Safety and requested that a person's license not be renewed. Unfortunately, persons with little insight are often not deterred by having no license. When patients do not respond to threats or to reasoning, further steps may be taken, including removing the person's vehicle from his or her home, often with the excuse that the car is in the shop or has been loaned to one of the grandchildren. In the worst-case scenario, removing the car keys or disabling the car's ignition may be necessary. As always, there are exceptions. In dealing with elderly widows who live alone in the country, we tend to be lenient because they need their own transportation if they are to maintain independent living, their driving is limited to the grocery and beauty shop, and the local law enforcement officers are aware of the situation. As expected, family caregivers are more lenient with their own family members than they would be with others in the same situation because of the physical inconvenience they would experience and their loved ones' anger (Hebert et al. 2002).

Sexuality

The need for affection and intimacy persists in persons with dementing illness (Davies et al. 1992). In some instances, especially with frontotemporal dementing illnesses (Joseph 1999), individuals become hypersexual. Although losing sexual intimacy compounds the sense of loss (Svetlik et al. 2005), sexual involvement with a partner who no longer provides an intimate relationship becomes uncomfortable or aversive. In most couples for whom dementia onset is after age 70, sexual involvement has already diminished and does not present a major problem; however, for younger couples with active sex lives, problems do occur. Spouses report that as they assume a caregiver role in relation to their spouse and become more of a parent than a partner in the relationship, their sexual desire decreases. Some even report feelings of revulsion because it feels as though they are committing incest with their "child." These feelings can cause great conflict, guilt, and frustration for spouses, who are often not comfortable bringing up these issues with professionals. Therefore, the responsibility lies with the professional to address this aspect of the disease and its impact on the relationship.

Volicer et al. (1988) suggest that caregivers be taught how to distract or gently dissuade sexually persistent spouses. In our experience, some spouses cannot be dissuaded behaviorally, and their sexual drive cannot be reduced through use of tranquilizers or antipsychotics. Medroxyprogesterone has been found to be useful in reducing inappropriate sexual aggression in men with cognitive impairment (Weiner et al. 1991), but no effective treatment has been found for female patients. Although anecdotal reports suggest that selective serotonin reuptake inhibitors (SSRIs) have been effective in reducing sexual disinhibition, it is too early to conclude that SSRIs should be considered the treatment of choice in elderly patients (Hashmi et al. 2000).

Long-Term-Care Placement

Decisions regarding placement in long-term-care facilities are usually made by the family and are implemented when the primary caregiver becomes physically and emotionally overwhelmed (Chenoweth and Spencer 1986). In our experience, long-term-care placement is the result of a process in which the needs of both the caregiver and the care recipient are considered. It con-

cludes with the decision that placement is best for each. The process can require caregivers to deal with their guilt over "abandoning" their loved one
(usually a spouse whom they have promised never to institutionalize) and to
accept their own physical, emotional, and financial limitations. An important
obstacle to nursing home placement of persons with frontotemporal dementias is their unawareness of their impaired judgment and behavioral dyscontrol. Families are usually counseled to follow the path that offers the greatest
quality of life to those able to appreciate that quality. Here again, an analogy
to early childhood may be useful: a patient with severe dementia can be lik-
ened to an infant in that both are unable to recognize the source of caregiving
but are in need of being cared for. The source of the caregiving is far less important than that caregiving is provided.

Family scapegoating may become a difficulty in deciding about long-
term-care placement. Family members living at a distance often tell the family
member managing the patient how unfair it is to institutionalize the patient.
The physician can help to undercut this process by adding the weight of medical opinion to the decision.

Families also need to be counseled that once a nursing home placement is
made, the length and frequency of visits should be such that the patient comes
to accept the long-term-care facility as a permanent place of residence. Thus,
families are urged not to visit daily or to visit for hours at a time. Instead, they
are encouraged to visit a few times a week and for brief periods. Once the patient accepts transition to the facility, brief outings can be arranged. In our experience, the transition to full-time long-term-care placement is facilitated by
enrolling patients in day care at the facility, later using the facility for respite
care, and finally using it for full-time care.

Ethical Issues for Caregivers

The primary ethical issues that arise in dealing with persons who have cognitive impairment are related to following their wishes with regard to independence and maintenance of life. Many persons who eventually develop
dementing illnesses express the desire to be cared for at home in the event of a
debilitating illness. Their loved ones agree. However, the time comes when the
patient becomes an impossible burden for the primary caregiver, often because
the caregiver has become physically incapacitated. At that point, the family

weighs practical necessity against the earlier expressed wishes of the patient and decides whether that person's experienced quality of life is more important than state of health or length of life or whether the needs of other family members take precedence. The family may decide that the patient's quality of life would not be measurably diminished by nursing home placement, whereas the quality of life of the now-disabled caregiver might be immeasurably improved. Many persons with cognitive impairment who live alone do not want to leave their homes despite their inability to adequately maintain themselves. In some cases, these individuals are a danger to themselves. In other cases, they are a danger to both themselves and others. If failure to institutionalize would lead to the person's near-term death by starvation, it is unlikely that society at large would condone such inaction. In the eventuality that a severely impaired person living alone refuses needed institutionalization, Adult Protective Services can assist in arranging involuntary long-term-care placement. If a person living alone in an apartment has inadvertently started several fires and has flooded the building on several occasions by stuffing inappropriate objects in the toilet, long-term care may be required based on danger to self and others if adequate supervision cannot be provided.

The conflict between length of life and quality of life also arises when dementia progresses to the point that the person is no longer capable of self-feeding and does not swallow spoon-fed food. Some individuals will have previously expressed a preference concerning sustenance by artificial means. If they have expressed a preference not to be so sustained, and the family agrees, it is permissible to offer food and water at appropriate intervals and let nature take its course. The court in *In re Conroy* (1985) determined that every person has a right to make a decision regarding what medical interventions can be performed on him or her that continues after the person is no longer competent, as long as the person's previous competently expressed wishes can be ascertained. In the same case, the court held that when a patient with dementia has expressed no preference, the family and physician have the right to decide, based on their knowledge of that individual's interests and preferences, what he or she would have wanted. A decision to discontinue life-extending treatment was based, by another court, on the spouse's testimony concerning his wife's independent nature and dislike of physicians (*In re Colyer* 1983). When there has been no clear statement of the patient's wishes concerning maintenance of life support and when that person's probable wishes cannot be clearly inferred, decisions can be made based on what appears to be in the best interest of the patient. To continue life support using the best interests of the patient as a guide, the generally accepted formula is that the benefits the patient derives from life should outweigh the burden of the treatment (Cantor 1987). The actual weighing of these factors is highly subjective and should involve discussion between physician and family, in consultation with a legal advisor familiar with the law in that particular jurisdiction. The U.S. Supreme Court has ruled that individuals have the right to terminate life-sustaining treatment or may designate a person to represent their wishes (*Cruzan v. Director, Missouri Department of Health et al.* 1990).

Conclusion

Because no cures are currently available for most dementing illnesses, an important role for health care professionals is family support. Educating families about the disease process helps reduce stress and anxiety, as does introducing families to a dynamic view of a loved one's behavior. Referrals to other agencies encourage interaction of the families with others and help to reduce feelings of isolation. Providing concrete management suggestions for specific behaviors and help with decisions about placement is also necessary as part of family support. Addressing family issues can also be important. Being available to listen to complaints and validate emotions when there is no specific intervention or solution to a problem is also important for caregivers. Through discussion and addressing specific questions, the physician and co-workers can assess, enhance, and support family members' knowledge, emotional comfort, and decisions.

Key Clinical Points

- The process of caregiving is one of continual change and adaptation by caregivers.
- Caregivers need education about their loved one's illness.
- Caregivers require emotional support and support in decision making, including the timing of long-term care and hospice care.
- Many community resources are available for both education and support.

References

Brody B: The family at risk, in Alzheimer's Disease Treatment and Family Stress: Directions for Research. Edited by Light E, Lebowitz B. Rockville, MD, U.S. Department of Health and Human Services, 1989, pp 2–49

Cantor NL: Legal Frontiers of Death and Dying. Bloomington, Indiana University Press, 1987

Chenoweth B, Spencer B: Dementia: the experience of family caregivers. Gerontologist 26:267–272, 1986

Cruzan v Director, Missouri Department of Health et al, 110 S. Ct. 2841 (1990)

Davies HD, Zeiss A, Tinklenberg JR: 'Til death do us part: intimacy and sexuality in the marriages of Alzheimer's patients. J Psychosoc Nurs Ment Health Serv 30:5–10, 1992

George LK: Dynamics of Caregiver Burden. Durham, NC, Center for the Study of Aging and Human Development, 1984

George LK, Gwyther LP: Caregiver well-being: a multidimensional examination of family caregivers of demented adults. Gerontologist 26:253–259, 1986

Hashmi FH, Krady AI, Qayum F, et al: Sexually disinhibited behavior in the cognitively impaired elderly. Clin Geriatr 8:61–68, 2000

Hebert K, Martin-Cook K, Svetlik DA, et al: Caregiver decision making and driving: what we say versus what we do. Clin Gerontol 26:17–30, 2002

In re Colyer, 660 P2d 738, 748 (1983)

In re Conroy, 486 A2d 1209 (NJ 1985)

Joseph R: Frontal lobe psychopathology: mania, depression, confabulation, catatonia, perseveration, obsessive compulsions, and schizophrenia. Psychiatry 62:138–172, 1999

Light E, Lebowitz B: Alzheimer's Disease Treatment and Family Stress: Directions for Research. Washington, DC, Department of Health and Human Services, 1989

Mace NL, Rabins PV: The 36-Hour Day: A Family Guide to Caring for People With Alzheimer Disease, Other Dementias, and Memory Loss in Later Life, 4th Edition. Baltimore, MD, Johns Hopkins University Press, 2006

Martin-Cook K, Hynan L, Chaftez P, et al: Impact of family visits on agitation in residents with dementia. Am J Alzheimers Dis Other Demen 16:1–4, 2001

Rabins PV, Mace NL, Lucas MJ: The impact of dementia on the family. JAMA 248:333–335, 1982

Svetlik DS, Dooley WK, Weiner MF, et al: Declines in satisfaction with physical intimacy predict caregiver perceptions of overall relationship loss: a study of elderly caregiving dyads. Sex Disabil 23:65–79, 2005

Teri L, Logsdon R: Identifying pleasant activities for individuals with Alzheimer's disease: the Pleasant Events Schedule–AD. Gerontologist 31:124–127, 1991

Volicer L, Fabiszewski K, Rheaume Y, et al: Clinical Management of Alzheimer's Disease. Rockville, MD, Aspen, 1988

Weiner MF, Denke M, Williams K, et al: Intramuscular medroxyprogesterone acetate for sexual aggression in elderly men (letter). Lancet 339:1121–1122, 1991

Zarit SH, Teri L: Interventions and services for family caregivers, in Annual Review of Gerontology and Geriatrics, Vol 11. Edited by Schaie K, Lawton MP. New York, Springer, 1992, pp 287–310

Further Reading

Coon DW, Gallagher-Thompson D, Thompson LW (eds): Innovative Interventions to Reduce Dementia Caregiver Distress: A Clinical Guide. New York, Springer, 2003

Schulz RC (ed): Handbook on Dementia Caregiving: Evidence-Based Interventions for Caregivers. New York, Springer, 2000

Resources

National Agencies

Administration on Aging (AOA),
U.S. Department of Health and Human Services
One Massachusetts Avenue NW
Washington, DC 20001
Mailing address: Administration on Aging, Washington, DC 20201
1-800-677-1116
www.aoa.gov
E-mail: aoainfo@aoa.hhs.gov

The AOA supports a nationwide network providing services to the elderly, especially to enable them to remain independent. AOA supports some 240 million meals for the elderly each year, including home-delivered "meals on wheels"; helps provide transportation and at-home services; supports ombudsman services for the elderly; and provides policy leadership on aging issues.

Alzheimer's Association (National Office)
225 N. Michigan Avenue, Floor 17
Chicago, IL 60601-7633
1-800-272-3900 or 1-312-335-8700; fax: 1-866-699-1246
www.alz.org
E-mail: info@alz.org

The Alzheimer's Association is a privately funded national voluntary organization with chapters nationwide. The national office can be contacted for information on many issues regarding Alzheimer disease, as well as referral to the nearest local chapter.

Alzheimer's Disease Education and Referral (ADEAR) Center
P.O. Box 8250
Silver Spring, MD 20907-8250
1-800-438-4380
www.nia.nih.gov/Alzheimers
E-mail: adear@nia.nih.gov

This agency is contracted through the National Institute on Aging. ADEAR maintains an online database and functions as a clearinghouse for publications and information on Alzheimer disease. Publications from the federally funded Alzheimer's Disease Centers and other sources can be ordered through the ADEAR Web site.

American Association of Retired Persons (AARP)
601 E Street, NW
Washington, DC 20049
1-888-687-2277
www.aarp.org
E-mail: member@aarp.org

AARP distributes resource kits consisting of several publications about aging and caregiving.

American Parkinson Disease Association (APDA)
135 Parkinson Avenue
Staten Island, NY 10305
1-800-223-2732 or 1-718-981-8001; fax: 1-718-981-4399
www.apdaparkinson.org
E-mail: apda@parkinson.org

APDA supports research and produces educational materials, including a newsletter and various pamphlets covering issues such as nutrition in Parkinson disease and mobility aids.

Association for Frontotemporal Degeneration (AFTD)
Radnor Station Building 2, Suite 320
290 King of Prussia Road
Radnor, PA 19087

1-866-507-7222 or 1-267-514-7221

www.theaftd.org

AFTD is a national voluntary organization providing support and services to patients and families regarding frontotemporal dementia, Pick disease, primary progressive aphasia, and others.

Brain Injury Association of America (BIAA)
1608 Spring Hill Road, Suite 110
Vienna, VA 22182
1-703-761-0750; fax: 1-703-761-0755
www.biausa.org

BIAA is an advocacy organization whose mission is to improve the quality of life for persons with head injuries and their families, and to develop programs to prevent head injuries. To fulfill its mission, the BIAA focuses its efforts on education, support and information, public awareness, prevention, research, and training.

Huntington's Disease Society of America (HDSA)
505 Eighth Avenue, Suite 902
New York, NY 10018
1-800-345-4372 or 1-212-242-1968; fax: 1-212-239-3430
www.hdsa.org

HDSA is a national voluntary organization providing support and services to patients and families. HDSA also supports research and education, disseminates information, and has a network of local chapters across the United States.

Lewy Body Dementia Association (LBDA)
912 Killian Hill Road, SW
Lilburn, GA 30047
1-404-935-6444; fax: 1-480-422-5434
1-800-539-9767 (LBD Caregiver Link)
www.lbda.org

LBDA is a national voluntary organization providing support and services to patients with Lewy body dementia and their families.

National Academy of Elder Law Attorneys (NAELA)
www.naela.org

NAELA provides a searchable database to assist in finding an elder law attorney.

National Association of Professional Geriatric Care Managers (NAPGCM)
3275 West Ina Road, Suite 130
Tucson, AZ 85741-2198
1-520-881-8008; fax: 1-520-325-7925
www.caremanager.org

Private case managers are certified to provide an array of assessment and social services, ranging from obtaining in-home health help to linking with financial, legal, and other long-term-care services.

National Cell Repository for Alzheimer's Disease (NCRAD)
Division of Heriditary Genomics
Health Information and Translational Sciences Building
410 West 10th Street, HS 4000
Indianapolis, IN 46202-3002
1-800-526-2839
http://ncrad.iu.edu
E-mail: alzstudy@iupui.edu

NCRAD has been funded by the National Institute on Aging since 1990 to learn more about the genes that may increase the risk of developing Alzheimer disease. NCRAD is involved in various ongoing research studies, including studies focusing on families with a strong family history of Alzheimer disease.

National Council on Aging (NCOA)
1901 L Street NW, 4th Floor
Washington, DC 20036
1-202-479-1200
www.ncoa.org

NCOA is a private, nonprofit organization that serves as a resource for information, training, technical assistance, advocacy, and leadership in all aspects of aging.

National Health Information Center (NHIC)
P.O. Box 1133
Washington, DC 20013-1133
1-800-336-4797 or 1-301-565-4167; fax: 1-301-984-4256
www.health.gov/nhic
E-mail: info@nhic.org

NHIC has a link to Healthfinder.gov, which provides a starting point for consumers and health professionals seeking information on home health care. Currently available books and additional organizations that can provide further information are cited. Financial issues and how to find home health care providers are discussed.

National Organization for Rare Disorders (NORD)
55 Kenosia Avenue
P.O. Box 1968
Danbury, CT 06813-1968
1-800-999-6673 or 1-203-744-0100; fax: 1-203-798-2291
www.rarediseases.org

NORD is a federation of voluntary health organizations dedicated to helping people with rare "orphan" diseases. NORD serves as a clearinghouse for information and is committed to the identification, treatment, and cure of rare disorders through programs of education, advocacy, research, and service.

National Parkinson Foundation (NPF)
Bob Hope Parkinson Research Center
1501 NW 9th Avenue
Bob Hope Road
Miami, FL 33136-1494
1-800-327-4545 or 1-305-243-6666; fax: 1-305-243-6073
www.parkinson.org
E-mail: contact@parkinson.org

NPF provides educational services and information in the form of support groups, publications, and workshops. NPF also supports Parkinson disease research.

National Stroke Association (NSA)
9707 E. Easter Lane, Suite B
Centennial, CO 80112
1-800-787-6537; fax: 1-303-649-1328
www.stroke.org
E-mail: Info@stroke.org

NSA is a nonprofit organization whose mission is to reduce the incidence and impact of stroke on individuals and on society. It supports stroke research in all areas, develops and distributes educational materials, and is an information and referral clearinghouse.

State Agencies

State Department of Human Services
www.dhs.state.[2-letter state code].us

State offices provide linkage to state-administered and subsidized programs, including community care and adult day care, elder abuse and neglect programs, and nursing home and other residential care programs under Title XX.

State Department on Aging
(See state governmental listing in local telephone or Web directories.)

These agencies in each state funnel federal dollars to local area agencies on aging for disbursement to community agency services and programs for elders. Some programs may be dementia specific. This agency is a good entry point for information and referral for aging services.

State Alzheimer Programs

The following states have Alzheimer programs within their Department of Human Services that provide a variety of services, including information and referral: California, Connecticut, Delaware, Florida, Kansas, Massachusetts, Missouri, New Hampshire, New Jersey, New York, North Carolina, Pennsylvania, Texas, and Wisconsin.

Nursing Home Ombudsman Programs

These programs provide information regarding quality of care in nursing homes, lists of nursing homes, checklists, and so forth. Contact the nearest Area Agency on Aging for information on the ombudsman program in a specific area. Detailed information concerning the past performance of every Medicare- and Medicaid-certified nursing home in the United States is available at www.medicare.gov/nhcompare.

Other Sources of Information

Alzheimer's Disease Research Centers
www.nia.nih.gov/Alzheimers/ResearchInformation/ResearchCenters

The National Institute on Aging funds Alzheimer's Disease Centers (ADCs) throughout the United States. ADCs offer opportunities to participate in Alzheimer research, and some provide diagnosis and medical management as well as various support programs, such as caregiver support groups.

Alzheimer Research Forum
www.alzforum.org

A compendium of information for researchers, physicians, and the general public, the site includes news, articles, discussion forums, interviews, a diagnostic and treatment guide, a directory of drugs and clinical trials, and research advances. It also provides access to such unique tools as directories of genetic mutations, antibodies, patents, and conferences.

Area Agency on Aging of Pasco-Pinellas (Fla.)
Recommended Reading and Viewing for Alzheimer's Caregivers
www.agingcarefl.org/caregiver/alzheimers/reading

This listing is a source for readings and videos to support caregivers.

Hospice Care
www.nhpco.org

The National Hospice and Palliative Care Organization offers information on end-of-life issues and state-specific advance directives.

Planning for Long-Term Care

www.nia.nih.gov/Alzheimers/Resources/Lists/services.htm

This Web site from the National Institute on Aging explores the options for long-term care, with articles on planning ahead, making the right choice, and making a smooth transition.

Clinical Trials.gov

www.clinicaltrials.gov

Persons with Alzheimer disease, family members, and members of the public can find current trials and research. The searchable database provides the name and purpose of the study, eligibility details, and contact information. In addition, the site indicates whether the study is recruiting and includes citations from published works.

Index

*Page numbers printed in **boldface** type refer to tables or figures.*